Lecture Notes in Computer Science 10983

Commenced Publication in 1973
Founding and Former Series Editors:
Gerhard Goos, Juris Hartmanis, and Jan van Leeuwen

Hsinchun Chen · Qing Fang
Daniel Zeng · Jiang Wu (Eds.)

Smart Health

International Conference, ICSH 2018
Wuhan, China, July 1–3, 2018
Proceedings

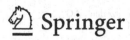 Springer

Editors
Hsinchun Chen
University of Arizona
Tucson, AZ, USA

Daniel Zeng
University of Arizona
Tucson, AZ, USA

Qing Fang
Wuhan University
Wuhan, China

Jiang Wu
Wuhan University
Wuhan, China

ISSN 0302-9743   ISSN 1611-3349 (electronic)
Lecture Notes in Computer Science
ISBN 978-3-030-03648-5   ISBN 978-3-030-03649-2 (eBook)
https://doi.org/10.1007/978-3-030-03649-2

Library of Congress Control Number: 2018960425

LNCS Sublibrary: SL3 – Information Systems and Applications, incl. Internet/Web, and HCI

This Springer imprint is published by the registered company Springer Nature Switzerland AG
The registered company address is: Gewerbestrasse 11, 6330 Cham, Switzerland

Preface

Advancing informatics for health care and health-care applications has become an international research priority. There is increased effort to leverage information systems and data analytics to transform reactive care to proactive and preventive care, clinic-centric to patient-centered practice, training-based interventions to globally aggregated evidence, and episodic response to continuous well-being monitoring and maintenance. The annual International Conference for Smart Health (ICSH), which originated in 2013, intends to provide a forum for the growing international smart health research community to discuss the technical, practical, economic, behavioral, and social issues associated with smart health.

ICSH 2018 was organized to mainly discuss the principles, frameworks, new applications, and effects of using big data and AI technology to address health-care problems and improve social welfare. It successfully attracted scholars working on smart hospital, online health community, mobile health, medical big data and health-care machine learning, chronic disease management, and health informetrics. We are pleased that many high-quality papers were submitted, accompanied by evaluations with real-world data or application contexts. The work presented at the conference encompassed a healthy mix of information system, computer science, health informetrics, and data science approaches.

ICSH 2018 was held in Wuhan, China. The two-day event encompassed presentations of 35 papers. The organizers of ICSH 2018 would like to thank the conference sponsors for their support and sponsorship, including the School of Information Management at Wuhan University and the China National Science Foundation Project No. 71573197. We further wish to express our sincere gratitude to all Program Committee members of ICSH 2018, who provided valuable and constructive reviews.

November 2018

Hsinchun Chen
Qing Fang
Daniel Zeng
Jiang Wu

Organization

Conference Co-chairs

Hsinchun Chen   University of Arizona, USA
      and Tsinghua University, China
Qing Fang   Wuhan University, China
Daniel Zeng   University of Arizona and Chinese Academy of Sciences, China

Program Co-chairs

Jiang Wu   Wuhan University, China
Chunxiao Xing   Tsinghua University, China
Xiangbin Yan   University of Science and Technology Beijing, China
Eric Zheng   University of Texas at Dallas, USA

Workshop Co-chairs

Xitong Guo   Harbin Institute of Technology, China
Wei Lu   Wuhan University, China
Jingdong Ma   Huazhong University of Science and Technology, China
Yong Zhang   Tsinghua University, China

Honorary Co-chairs

Feicheng Ma   Wuhan University, China
Zhanchun Feng   Huazhong University of Science and Technology, China
Gang Li   Wuhan University, China
Ting-Peng Liang   National Sun Yat-Sen University, China
Douglas R. Vogel   Harbin Institute of Technology, China

Publication Co-chairs

Zhaohua Deng   Huazhong University of Science and Technology, China
Ruhua Huang   Wuhan University, China
Xiaolong Zheng   Chinese Academy of Sciences, China

Publicity Co-chairs

Hao Li   Wuhan University, China
Hsin-Min Lu   National Taiwan University, Taiwan
Harry Wang   University of Delaware, USA
Kang Zhao   University of Iowa, USA

Local Arrangements Co-chairs

Yiwei Gong   Wuhan University, Chnia
Dan Ke   Wuhan University, China
Lihong Zhou   Wuhan University, China

Program Committee

Muhammad Amith   Texas Medical Center, USA
Lu An   Wuhan University, China
Mohd Anwar   North Carolina A&T State University, USA
Ian Brooks   University of Illinois at Urbana-Champaign, USA
Jingxuan Cai   Wuhan University, China
Lemen Chao   Renmin University of China, China
Michael Chau   University of Hong Kong, SAR China
Chien-Chin Chen   National Taiwan University, Taiwan
Qikai Cheng   Wuhan University, China
Chih-Lin Chi   University of Minnesota, USA
Shengli Deng   Wuhan University, China
Yimeng Deng   National University of Singapore, Singapore
Prasanna Desikan   Blueshield of California, USA
Shaokun Fan   Oregon State University, USA
Qianjing Feng   Southern Medical University
Chunmei Gan   Sun Yat-sen University, China
Mingxin Gan   University of Science and Technology Beijing, China
Gordon Gao   University of Maryland, USA
Liang Hong   Wuhan University, China
Jiming Hu   Wuhan University, China
Zhongyi Hu   Wuhan University, China
Jiahua Jin   University of Science and Technology Beijing, China
Hung-Yu Kao   National Cheng Kung University, China
Chunxiao Li   Arizona State University, USA
Jiao Li   Chinese Academy of Medical Sciences, China
Jiexun Li   Western Washington University, USA
Mingyang Li   University of South Florida, USA
Xin Li   City University of Hong Kong, SAR China
Yan Li   City University of Hong Kong, SAR China
Ye liang   Beijing Foreign Studies University, China
Yu-Kai Lin   Florida State University, USA
Hongyan Liu   Tsinghua University, China
Luning Liu   Harbin Institute of Technology, China
Xiao Liu   University of Utah, USA
Yidi Liu   City University of Hong Kong, SAR China
Long Lu   Wuhan University, China
Quan Lu   Wuhan University, China
James Ma   University of Colorado, Colorado Springs, USA

Jin Mao	Wuhan University, China
Abhay Mishra	Georgia State University, USA
Robert Moskovitch	Ben-Gurion University, Israel
Cath Oh	Georgia State University, USA
V. Panduranga Rao	Indian Institute of Technology Hyderabad, India
Raj Sharman	State University of New York, University at Buffalo, USA
Xiaolong Song	Dongbei University of Finance and Economics, China
Alan Wang	Virginia Polytechnic Institute and State University (Virginia Tech), USA
Xi Wang	Central University of Finance and Economics
Yu Wang	Virginia Polytechnic Institute and State University (Virginia Tech), USA
Zoie Wong	St. Luke's International University
Dan Wu	Wuhan University, China
Yi Wu	Tianjin University, China
Dong Xu	University of Arizona, USA
Jennifer Xu	Bentley College, USA
Kaiquan Xu	Nanjing University, China
Lucy Yan	Indiana University at Bloomington, USA
Weiwei Yan	Wuhan University, China
Siluo Yang	Wuhan University, China
Jonathan Ye	University of Auckland, New Zealand
Shuo Yu	University of Arizona, USA
Anna Zaitsev	University of Sydney, Australia
Qingpeng Zhang	City University of Hong Kong, SAR China
Tingting Zhang	University of Science and Technology Beijing, China
Xiaofei Zhang	Harbin Institute of Technology, China
Zhiqiang Zhang	Harbin Engineering University, China
Yang Zhao	Wuhan University, China
Yiming Zhao	Wuhan University, China
Lina Zhou	University of Maryland, Baltimore County, USA
Bin Zhu	Oregon State University, USA
Hongyi Zhu	University of Arizona, USA
Hou Zhu	Sun Yat-sen University, China
Zhiya Zuo	University of Iowa, USA

Contents

Smart Hospital

Drug-Drug Interactions Prediction Based on Similarity Calculation
and Pharmacokinetics Mechanism. 3
   Quan Lu, Liangtao Zhang, Jing Chen, and Zeyuan Xu

Augmented Reality: New Technologies for Building Visualized
Hospital Knowledge Management Systems. 15
   Long Lu and Wang Zhao

The Design of Personalized Artificial Intelligence Diagnosis
and the Treatment of Health Management Systems Simulating
the Role of General Practitioners. 26
   Shuqing Chen, Xitong Guo, and Xiaofeng Ju

Automatic Liver Segmentation in CT Images
Using Improvised Techniques. 41
   Prerna Kakkar, Sushama Nagpal, and Nalin Nanda

Bone Fracture Visualization and Analysis Using Map Projection
and Machine Learning Techniques 53
   Yucheng Fu, Rong Liu, Yang Liu, and Jiawei Lu

Online Health Community

Why Does Interactional Unfairness Matter for Patient-Doctor Relationship
Quality in Online Health Consultation? The Contingencies of Professional
Seniority and Disease Severity 61
   Xiaofei Zhang, Xitong Guo, Kee-hung Lai, and Yi Wu

Exploring the Factors Influencing Patient Usage Behavior
Based on Online Health Communities 70
   Yinghui Zhao, Shanshan Li, and Jiang Wu

Using Social Media to Estimate the Audience Sizes of Public Events
for Crisis Management and Emergency Care 77
   Patrick Felka, Artur Sterz, Oliver Hinz, and Bernd Freisleben

Exploring the Effects of Different Incentives on Doctors' Contribution
Behaviors in Online Health Communities. 90
   Fei Liu, Xitong Guo, Xiaofeng Ju, and Xiaocui Han

Cross-Cultural Comparison of User Engagement in Online
Health Communities   96
    Xi Wang and Yushan Zhu

Mobile Health

Development of Text Messages for Mobile Health Education
to Promote Diabetic Retinopathy Awareness and Eye Care Behavior
Among Indigenous Women   107
    Valerie Onyinyechi Umaefulam and Kalyani Premkumar

Why People Are Willing to Provide Social Support in Online Health
Communities: Evidence from Social Exchange Perspective.   119
    Tongyao Zhao and Rong Du

Strategic Behavior in Mobile Behavioral Intervention Platforms:
Evidence from a Field Quasi-experiment on a Health Management App.   130
    Chunxiao Li, Bin Gu, and Chenhui Guo

How Using of WeChat Impacts Individual Loneliness and Health?   142
    Meng Yin, Qi Li, and Xiaoyu Xu

Smart and Connected Health Projects: Characteristics
and Research Challenges   154
    Jiangping Chen, Minghong Chen, Jingye Qu, Haihua Chen,
    and Juncheng Ding

Medical Big Data and Healthcare Machine Learning

Designing a Novel Framework for Precision Medicine
Information Retrieval.   167
    Haihua Chen, Juncheng Ding, Jiangping Chen, and Gaohui Cao

Efficient Massive Medical Rules Parallel Processing Algorithms   179
    Xin Li, Guigang Zhang, Chunxiao Xing, and Zihan Qu

Intelligent Diagnosis and Treatment Research of Knee Osteoarthritis
Based on Big Data   185
    Xin Li, Guigang Zhang, Chunxiao Xing, and Yong Zhang

Use of Sentiment Mining and Online NMF for Topic Modeling Through
the Analysis of Patients Online Unstructured Comments   191
    Adnan Muhammad Shah, Xiangbin Yan, Syed Jamal Shah,
    and Salim Khan

What Affects Patients' Online Decisions: An Empirical Study of Online
Appointment Service Based on Text Mining.   204
  Guanjun Liu, Lusha Zhou, and Jiang Wu

Bayesian Network Retrieval Discrimination Criteria Model
Based on Unbalanced Information.   211
  Man Xu, Dan Gan, Jiang Shen, and Bang An

Readmission Prediction Using Trajectory-Based Deep
Learning Approach   224
  Jiaheng Xie, Bin Zhang, and Daniel Zeng

ICSH 2018: LSTM based Sentiment Analysis for Patient Experience
Narratives in E-survey Tools   231
  Chenxi Xia, Dong Zhao, Jing Wang, Jing Liu, and Jingdong Ma

A Deep Learning Based Pipeline for Image Grading
of Diabetic Retinopathy.   240
  Yu Wang, G. Alan Wang, Weiguo Fan, and Jiexun Li

A Deep Learning-Based Method for Sleep Stage Classification
Using Physiological Signal.   249
  Guanjie Huang, Chao-Hsien Chu, and Xiaodan Wu

Chronic Disease Management

Visualizing Knowledge Evolution of Emerging Information Technologies
in Chronic Diseases Research.   263
  Dongxiao Gu, Kang Li, Xiaoyu Wang, and Changyong Liang

Media Message Design via Health Communication Perspective:
A Study of Cervical Cancer Prevention   274
  Hua Ran, Shupei Geng, and Di Xiao

Information Systems and Institutional Entrepreneurship: How IT Carries
Institutional Changes in Chronic Disease Management.   286
  Kui Du, Yanli Huang, Liang Li, Xiaolu Luo, and Wei Zhang

The Development of a Smart Personalized Evidence Based Medicine
Diabetes Risk Factor Calculator   292
  *Lei Wang, Defu He, Xiaowei Ni, Ruyi Zou, Xinlu Yuan, Yujuan Shang,
  Xinping Hu, Xingyun Geng, Kui Jiang, Jiancheng Dong, and Huiqun Wu*

A Descriptive Tomographic Content Analysis Method in Chronic Disease
Knowledge Network: An Application to Hypertension.   301
  Liqin Zhou, Lu An, Zhichao Ba, and Zhiyuan Li

Health Informetrics

Visualizing the Intellectual Structure of Electronic Health Research:
A Bibliometric Analysis.................................... 315
  Tongtong Li, Dongxiao Gu, Xiaoyu Wang, and Changyong Liang

How Corporations Utilize Academic Social Networking Website?:
A Case Study of Health & Biomedicine Corporations 325
  Shengwei Yi, Qian Liu, and Weiwei Yan

Meta-analysis of the Immunomodulatory Effect of *Ganoderma Lucidum*
Spores Using an Automatic Pipeline 332
  Rui Liu, Yumeng Zhang, Ziwen Chen, Liqiang Wang, Shuaibing He,
  Guifeng Hua, and Chang Liu

Section Identification to Improve Information Extraction from Chinese
Medical Literature...................................... 342
  Sijia Zhou and Xin Li

Evolution of Research on Smart Health: A Bibliometrics Analysis 351
  Xiao Huang, Ke Dong, and Jiang Wu

Author Index 359

Smart Hospital

Drug-Drug Interactions Prediction Based on Similarity Calculation and Pharmacokinetics Mechanism

Quan Lu[1], Liangtao Zhang[2], Jing Chen[3(✉)], and Zeyuan Xu[4]

[1] Center for Studies of Information Resources, Wuhan University,
Wuhan, People's Republic of China
[2] School of Information Management, Wuhan University,
Wuhan, People's Republic of China
[3] School of Information Management, Central China Normal University,
Wuhan, People's Republic of China
jchen@mail.ccnu.edu.cn
[4] Henry Samueli School of Engineering and Applied Science,
University of California, Los Angeles, CA, USA

Abstract. Drug-drug interactions (DDIs) are one of the major causes of adverse drug events (ADEs), therefore, the prediction of DDIs for avoiding the ADEs is an important issue, which can help medical researchers economize research related resources in clinical trials. This study aims to predict DDIs based on drug similarity and ontology reasoning, and accordingly gives some possible explanations to why these drugs have DDIs. we develop a DDIs ontology integrated with similar drugs and pharmacokinetics(PK) mechanism, and formulate rules for inferring DDIs. Our method extends the existing research ideas, not only adds extrapolation of unknown data, but also reduces reliance on known data, and innovatively combines similar drugs with PK mechanism, which proved to be useful for inferring DDIs and can give some possible explanations for these DDIs. Besides our study is less demanding for data type, and the rules are more concise.

Keywords: Drug-drug interactions · Pharmacokinetic mechanism Ontology · Inference · Similarity

1 Introduction

1.1 Background and Significance

With the coexistence of a variety of chronic diseases and underlying diseases, the clinical multi-drug compatibility has become generalized and routine, and the problem of DDIs has also become a prominent problem of clinical concern [1, 2]. In clinical trials, researchers often employ some mathematical frameworks and models like PBPK model [3] to conduct a series of experiments to study interactions between drugs. With the development of information technology, computational methods can play a key role in the identification, explanation and prediction of DDIs [4]. Those methods for DDIs

© Springer Nature Switzerland AG 2018
H. Chen et al. (Eds.): ICSH 2018, LNCS 10983, pp. 3–14, 2018.
https://doi.org/10.1007/978-3-030-03649-2_1

studies depend on the integrity of the data, however drug data in the online database may not be complete, for instance, some medication data may not be updated in real time, and some mechanism of drug action may not yet be found and so on,which makes it more difficult to predict the all relevant DDIs. In present, researching interactions between all drugs through the clinical trials will consume a lot of resources and times and be unrealistic. But people want to predict DDIs in advance to reduce resource consumption. So in this study, we propose a new method, which combining reasoning and similarity calculation in the explanation and prediction of DDIs. This method can provide a reference for researchers to experiment drug interactions, besides it also can remind clinicians to prescribe.

1.2 Literature Review

Medical clinical often beget ADEs and even serious side effects because of DDIs, which will aggravate the patient's condition [5], therefore, the study of DDIs is very important. DDIs are usually divided into three categories according to the principle and action mode of interaction [6]: pharmaceutical DDIs [7], pharmacokinetic (PK) DDIs [8] and pharmacodynamics (PD) DDIs [9]. Recently, there are two main research directions for the prediction of DDIs, which are based on data mining and reasoning.

Data mining methods can effectively predict DDIs. Machine learning is a good method to predict DDIs. Hunta et al. [10] propose enzyme action crossing attribute creation for DDIs prediction through support vector machine (SVM) and others machine learning methods, while in 2017, these people take actions of both enzymes and transporter proteins into account to predict DDIs and gain better results [11]. Besides text mining is a common way of data mining, which not only discovers uncovering DDIs, but also extracts various facts of drug metabolism to help predict potential DDIs [12]. Although prediction based on data mining can get better results, this type of approach lacks interpretations of DDIs.

Meanwhile, prediction based on reasoning can offset this shortcoming, most of approaches are achieved by creating production rules or ontology and rules. Drug interaction ontology (DIO) is developed for formal representation of pharmacological knowledge to infer DDIs. Yoshikawa et al. [13] develop a knowledge base using DIO to support hypothesis generation of DDI. Herrero-Zazo et al. have summarized the conceptual model of DDIs, these models have been created using different formalisms and languages, such as first order logic (FOL), Web Ontology Language (OWL), Semantic Web Rule Language (SWRL) and so on [14]. For example, Imai et al. [15] build a framework of PD ontology using OWL to infer possible DDIs. In comparison, Herrero-Zazo et al. [16] construct a DIO and address the representation of different types of mechanisms leading to both PK and PD DDIs. Although this type of approach may provide a possible explanation for the predicted DDIs, their results are generally worse compared with prediction based on data mining. Thus, both types of methods have their own advantages and disadvantages.

In some of the previous literatures, there is a basic idea that if two molecules have similar chemical structures, then they are likely to target common proteins [17, 18], and they may have similar biological properties [19, 20]. A number of studies have been conducted to try to integrate the chemical structures of drugs and protein sequences

[21–23], and have used different methods to calculate the similarity between drugs. Kim [24] indicates that drugs causing similar side effects are likely to target similar proteins. In summary, we have a basic idea that similar drugs may target similar proteins. We hope to predict DDIs and get their possible explanations, so we use the predicting method based on reasoning. At the moment, with the development of medicine and the improvement of technology, drug-related data is continuously updated, new drugs are constantly being developed, and previous drugs are also found new mechanism. However, Existing data in the web can't be kept up-to-date, so DDIs related data coverage is not complete. The basic idea that similar drugs may target similar proteins can offset this flaw. Besides target is one of the considerations for finding DDIs. In the process of developing drugs, as long as the target for the drug is found, the drug can be developed and designed according to the target's characteristics [25]. Therefore, drugs with similar targets are more likely to have the same PK mechanism. Previous studies haven't consider factors of similar drugs when making DDI reasoning, our study proposes an innovative method that integrates drug similarity based on targets and PK mechanism to predict DDIs. Moreover, we also evaluate the usefulness of our method in this type of project that using reasoning to predict DDIs. Finally, we will discuss the interpretations at the end of the paper. Figure 1 is our flow chart.

2 Objectives

The goal of this study is using similarity calculation and ontology reasoning technology to predict DDIs and give possible explanations. According to drug similarity calculation, the unknown drug mechanism is deduced from the known mechanism of drug action, and then the reasoning is performed to predict and explain the DDIs.

3 Materials and Methods

3.1 Drug-Drug Similarity Calculation Based on Target

Drug target is the binding site between the drug and the body biological macro-molecule, including gene loci, receptors, enzymes, ion channels and so on [26]. Drugs affect and change the human body, resulting in pharmacological effects by acting on these biological macromolecules. Some drugs can only act on a single target, and some drugs can act on multiple targets. The dataset in this paper contains 882 drugs and 739 targets. Cosine similarity uses the cosine of the angle between two vectors in vector space as a measure of the difference between two individuals, which can effectively evaluate the similarity of the related variables between the two samples [27]. This paper uses the cosine similarity to calculate the drug-drug similarity based on target.

Firstly, we can get a 882 * 739 matrix in which line coordinate represents drugs and column coordinate represents targets. Therefore, the target of drug 'x' can be expressed as vector $V1(v1,1, v1,2, v1,3...., v1,m)$, and the target of drug 'y' can be expressed as vector $V2(v2,1, v2,2, v2,3...., v2,m)$. If the target Ti is the target of x, then let v1,i = 1, otherwise let v1,i = 0. Then, the similarity between 'x' and 'y' can be expressed as the following Formulae (1):

$$similarity(x, y) = \cos <v1, v2> = \frac{v1 \cdot v2}{||v1||v2||} = \frac{\sum\limits_{i=1}^{m} (v_{1,i})(v_{2,i})}{\sqrt{\sum\limits_{i=1}^{m} (v_{1,i})^2} \cdot \sqrt{\sum\limits_{i=1}^{m} (v_{2,i})}} \quad (1)$$

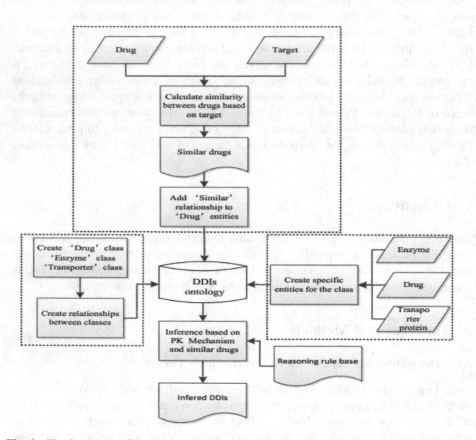

Fig. 1. The flow chart of our study. Firstly, we calculate the similarity between drugs based on targets, then we construct the DDIs ontology by creating related classes and adding instances for those classes. Finally, we establish reasoning rules of drug interactions to predict DDIs and give some possible explanations for DDIs.

The calculation results are nonnegative. DDIs are diverse, but because we only judged whether a group of drugs had any interaction, so long as the two drugs have an impact on the same target, we think they are similar to some extent.

3.2   DDIs Ontology

Ontology is a systematic explanation of objective existence, and it is concerned with the abstract essence of objective reality [28]. Ontology describes the connection between knowledge in a certain field through standard and accepted terms so as to reveal the abstract expression of knowledge in this field.

Pharmacokinetic DDI knowledge organizes PK DDI related knowledge including PK mechanism types like enzymes actions and transporter actions, besides it adds the object attribute of drug similarity relationship. This study constructs ontology of drug interactions, following steps are adopted: (1) identify basic concepts in PK DDI domain knowledge, (2) analyze and specify relationships between those concepts, (3) instantiate those concepts, (4) establish reasoning rules of drug interactions for those concepts. This study extracts PK mechanism related knowledge from DrugBank and introduces a mechanism of drug similarity. According to the existing literature [16], we have constructed a simple ontology. Basic concepts and relationships are shown by Fig. 2.

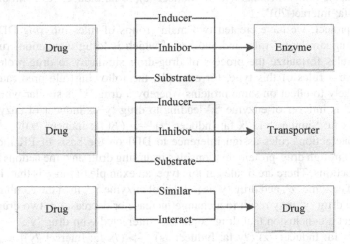

Fig. 2. The classes and their relationships in DDIs ontology.

In ontology, a class defines a group of individuals that have common properties, while properties can divide into data properties and object properties. Data properties describe the specific value or content of the attribute, and object properties clarify the relationship between individuals. This study uses the ontology building tool Protégé to build the basic ontology, and then in order to achieve the goal of reasoning DDI, 3 classes and 5 object properties are built. The relationships between 'Drug' class and 'Enzyme' class are 'Inducer', 'Inhibitor' and 'Substrate', yet similar to 'Drug' class and 'Transporter' class. Besides, this study defines two relations that 'Similar' and 'Interact' for 'Drug' class, which are respectively expressed as 'drug A may similar with drug B' and 'drug A may interact with drug B'.

According to the definition of a class, we can create specific entities for the class. This paper completes the filling of ontology instances by compiling owl ontology language. Owl is a network ontology language developed by the W3C for ontology semantic description [29]. Based on the compiling of owl ontology language, we have completed the filling of the entity and the relationship between the entities. Finally, there are 882 drugs, 106 enzymes and 63 transporter proteins in our ontology.

3.3 Rules for Inference of DDIs

To infer DDIs on the basis of pharmacokinetic mechanisms, it is necessary to model a set of rules expressing the effect of a precipitant drug on the absorption, distribution, and clearance of an object drug. Boyce et al. [30] use First Order Logic (FOL) to describe metabolic drug-drug interactions. Moitra et al. [31] demonstrate a set of rules to represent how one drug alters the metabolism of another drug based on the pharmacokinetics. In contrast, since the establishment of ontology, in our approach we build an ontology-based reasoning rule base. Each rule consists of the body and head, for example, [rule1:(?a fa: inducer ?c)(?b fa: inducer ?c) —> (?a fa: interact ?b)], among them, the body of rule is '(?a fa: inducer ?c)(?b fa: inducer ?c)', and the head of rule is '(?a fa: interact ?b)'.

In this project, we have created two main groups of rules inferring DDI, one of which is 'drug similarity' rule, and another of which is 'drug interaction' rule. 'Drug similarity' rules formalize the process of drug-drug similarity to drug-protein action and there are 3 rules of this type, for example, the following rule predicates similar drugs are likely to effect on same proteins whereby a drug 'x' is similar with drug 'y' and drug 'x' is inducer of enzyme 'z' leading to drug 'y' is inducer of enzyme 'z':

[rule: (?x fa: Similar ?y) (?x fa: Inducer ?z) —> (?y fa: Inducer ?z)]

'Drug interaction' rules assign inference to DDI on the basis of PK mechanism, represented through drug-protein relationships including drug-enzyme actions and drug-transporter actions. There are 6 rules of this type, an example of those is that, if drug 'x' is inducer of enzyme 'z', and drug 'y' is inducer of enzyme 'z', then the combined use of drug 'x' and drug 'y' may result to a change(increase or decrease) in two drug's effect, so we can get a conclusion that drug 'x' is may interacted with drug 'y':

[rule: (?x fa: Inducer ?z) (?y fa: Inducer ?z) —> (?x fa: Interact ?y)]

Finally, we have built 9 reasoning rules. There are many reasoning engines like JessCLIPS, Pellet for reasoning about rules, here we would use Jena ontology reasoning engine to actualize the inference of drug-drug interaction.

4   Results

In this section, we carry on the experiment that whether the combination of similarity and reasoning rules can be used to infer DDI and have a better effect. To do this, firstly, we calculate the drug-drug similarity based on target. As described in the paper above, we have 882 drug entities and 739 target entities, and each drug may act on multiple targets. After calculating cosine similarity, we get 12982 drug-drug similarity measurement data whose similarity value is greater than 0. We divide the similarity value into 20 intervals according to the range of 0–1, so as to use the incremental method to add those data to the ontology for reasoning. Table 1 describes the number of data contained in each interval.

Table 1. The number of data contained in each interval.

Interval	Num	Interval	Num
0–0.05	6	0.5–0.55	906
0.05–0.1	254	0.55–0.6	624
0.1–0.15	869	0.6–0.65	210
0.15–0.2	1252	0.65–0.7	139
0.2–0.25	1476	0.7–0.75	774
0.25–0.3	1467	0.75–0.8	88
0.3–0.35	1140	0.8–0.85	252
0.35–0.4	930	0.85–0.9	88
0.4–0.45	1329	0.9–0.95	57
0.45–0.5	374	0.95–1	747

Then, we create individuals for every class—'Drug', 'Enzyme' and 'Transporter', including 882 drugs, 106 enzymes and 63 transporter proteins. Besides we add the corresponding relationship to the ontology. There are 3 types of action that representing the role of drug in PK mechanism from DrugBank database, which are 'Inducer', 'Inhibitor' and 'Substrate'. From this we can learn that there are 3 relationships between drug and enzyme/transporter. Therefore, a drug with these actions will affect metabolite of other drugs. Here we use drug-enzyme actions to illustrate the impact mechanism [32]:

Substrate-Substrate: if drug 'x' is substrate of enzyme 'z', drug 'y' is substrate of enzyme 'z', then due to the competition of drugs, the metabolism of both 'x' and 'y' may be inhibited, resulting in the occurrence of drug interaction.

Inhibitor-Substrate: if drug 'x' is inhibitor of enzyme 'z', drug 'y' is substrate of enzyme 'z', then the metabolism of 'y' will be reduced, resulting in its existing time longer.

Inducer-Substrate: if drug 'x' is inducer of enzyme 'z', drug 'y' is substrate of enzyme 'z', then the metabolism of 'y' will be reduced and disappear earlier.

Inducer-Inducer: if drug 'x' is inducer of enzyme 'z', drug 'y' is inducer of enzyme 'z', then both drugs' metabolism will be accelerated, leading them to be earlier eliminated.

Inhibitor-Inhibitor: if drug 'x' is inhibitor of enzyme 'z', drug 'y' is inhibitor of enzyme 'z', then the metabolism of both drugs is reduced and the drugs remain longer in the body.

Inhibitor-Inducer: if drug 'x' is inhibitor of enzyme 'z', drug 'y' is inducer of enzyme 'z', then both drugs' effects will be weakened, affecting their own efficacy.

In addition, we have two other relationships that describe the connection between drugs, which are 'Similar' and 'Interact'. Finally, we have constructed 9 rules in the reasoning rule base and use Jena [33] to infer DDIs based on the ontology. We extracted from the DrugBank all the drug-drug interactions between 882 drugs and there are 65156 drug interactions. Next, we take the drug similarity into account to infer DDIs based on ontology. Then we use the incremental method to experiment. For example, we first add similar drugs in the 0.95–1 interval to the ontology, and then we use the 9 rules to predict DDIs and get results. We calculate the precision, recall and F1 values of the results next, and then repeat the above steps until all similar drugs are added to the ontology. Figure 3 depicts the evaluation results of inferred DDIs.

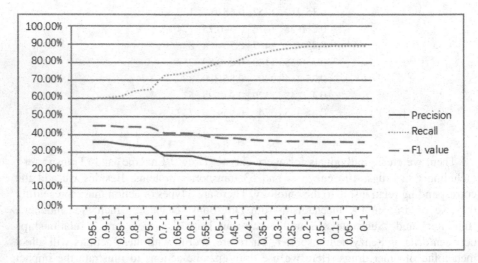

Fig. 3. The 'Precision', 'Recall' and 'F1 value' of our evaluation results. 'Precision' and 'F1 value' are basically on the decline, while 'Recall' is constantly increasing.

For the DDIs ontology with addition of drug similarity, as the number of similar drugs increases, the performance of reasoning is decreased in precision rate but increases in recall rate. For an analysis of such a large number of inferences, among the 65156 DDIs identified based on 882 drugs, at most 88.94% of the asserted DDIs have been correctly inferred. Compared with some previous studies, we used homologous data, and the amount of data is larger and the method is simpler, but a higher recall rate has been achieved, So to a certain extent, it can explain the superiority of our experiment.

5 Discussion

In this study, we construct a novel ontology integrated with drug similarity and PK mechanism for inferring DDIs. Our model collects drug targets, drug-enzyme actions, drug-transporter actions from DrugBank database. Then we infer potential interactions between drugs by integrating these resources into ontology. Finally we evaluate our results through the pairs of interacted drugs gathered from DrugBank and demonstrate that our approach have a more complete prediction rate of asserted DDIs compared with the previous research predicting DDIs based on PK mechanism and inference.

The aspect that this study differs from previous studies is we have combined two basic ideas which are 'similar drugs may target similar proteins' and PK mechanisms to expand the existing studies. We formulated 9 rules of reasoning and these rules have been also successfully applied to the inference of DDIs. Meanwhile, in our approach, the data type is relatively simple and the number of rules we set is small, but we get a relatively good result. This study demonstrated reasonable recall rates across the 65156 DDIs between 882 drugs, in terms of suggesting some possible explanation for these asserted interactions from the rule-making perspective by querying the relevant enzymes or transporter proteins actions between drugs. For example, if we have inferred that drug 'x' is interacted with drug 'y', we may be able to get some reasons why these two drugs have interaction through querying in the pharmacokinetic DDI ontology, probably because they both act on the same enzyme or transporter protein. Our results have the reference guidance for the conduct of clinical trials. Based on our results, clinicians can experiment with two specific drugs to see whether they interact in order to save resources. In addition, text mining of specific drug pairs can also be performed in periodical literature to identify uncovering DDIs.

One shortage of our approach is that there is a lower precision rate, and there are many reasons for this result. DDIs and their underlying mechanisms are complex pharmacological process [31]. This study only attempt to research PK DDIs and drug absorption and metabolism of PK mechanism in vivo. However, PK mechanism includes the absorption, distribution, metabolism and excretion of the drug in the organism, besides the remaining pharmaceutical interactions and PD interactions in DDIs study are not considered in our approach. Therefore, the DDIs related data is not comprehensive in this study.

Besides, there are some rule conflicts existing in rule making, for example, we can't determine drug y's effect on z if both [rule: (?x fa: Similar ?y) (?x fa: Inducer ?z) —> (?y fa: Inducer ?z)] and [rule: (?w fa: Similar ?y) (?w fa: Inhibitor ?z) —> (?y fa: inhibitor ?z)], but in this article, our predictions are generally divided into two drugs with interaction and two drugs without interaction, so as long as drug y has an impact on z, we can predict drug interactions. In future work, when studying what types of interactions exist between two drugs, we will make a detailed study of it.

In addition, the inferred DDIs which are not included in the asserted DDIs may not mean there are no interactions between them, probably because the DrugBank database may not contain all DDIs. After all, a database can't keep up-to-date updates because it will consume a lot of manpower and resource. Moreover, there is another reason that some DDIs are not yet clinically tested and therefore we don't know whether these drugs interacted or not. This is also a limitation of our study.

6 Conclusions

The DrugBank database offers comprehensive information about PK DDIs, however, there is a need for increased awareness of the update of the data and the comprehensiveness of knowledge. This paper is predictive and interpretive of DDIs, and has a more comprehensive recall rate of DDIs.

In our future work we will identify further information about DDI-related data from more biomedical databases such as DrugBank, STITCH, drugs.com, CHEMBL and so on and integrate the data to describe the DDIs' underlying mechanisms such as PK and PD, so that we can formulate the corresponding and more detailed rules to infer DDIs and further automate inference of explanations for DDIs for pharmacovigilance studies.

Acknowledgments. The authors gratefully acknowledge the financial support for this work provided by National Natural Science Foundation of China (No: 61772375 and 71420107026) and the MOE Project of Key Research Institute of Humanities and Social Sciences at Universities (No: 17JJD870002).Conflicts of InterestThe authors declare they have no conflicts of interest in this research.

Protection of Human and Animal Subjects Neither human nor animal subjects were included in this project.

Rule Appendix

[rule1:(?x   http://www.owl-ontologies.com/drug_action.owl#Similar   ?y)(?x   http://www.owl-ontologies.com/drug_action.owl#Inducer?   z)-> (?y   http://www.owl-ontologies.com/drug_action.owl#Inducer ?z)]

[rule2:(?x   http://www.owl-ontologies.com/drug_action.owl#Similar   ?y)(?x   http://www.owl-ontologies.com/drug_action.owl#Inhibitor   ?z)-> (?y   http://www.owl-ontologies.com/drug_action.owl#Inhibitor ?z)]

[rule3:(?x   http://www.owl-ontologies.com/drug_action.owl#Similar   ?y)(?x   http://www.owl-ontologies.com/drug_action.owl#Substrate   ?z)-> (?y   http://www.owl-ontologies.com/drug_action.owl#Substrate ?z)]

[rule4:(?x   http://www.owl-ontologies.com/drug_action.owl#Inducer ?z)(?y http://www.owl-ontologies.com/drug_action.owl#Inducer   ?z)-> (?x   http://www.owl-ontologies.com/drug_action.owl#Interact ?y)]

[rule5:(?x   http://www.owl-ontologies.com/drug_action.owl#Inducer ?z)(?y http://www.owl-ontologies.com/drug_action.owl#Inhibitor   ?z)-> (?x   http://www.owl-ontologies.com/drug_action.owl#Interact ?y)]

[rule6:(?x   http://www.owl-ontologies.com/drug_action.owl#Inducer ?z)(?y http://www.owl-ontologies.com/drug_action.owl#Substrate   ?z)-> (?x   http://www.owl-ontologies.com/drug_action.owl#Interact ?y)]

[rule7:(?x   http://www.owl-ontologies.com/drug_action.owl#Inhibitor ?z)(?y http://www.owl-ontologies.com/drug_action.owl#Inhibitor   ?z)-> (?x   http://www.owl-ontologies.com/drug_action.owl#Interact ?y)]

[rule8:(?x   http://www.owl-ontologies.com/drug_action.owl#Inhibitor ?z)(?y http://www.owl-ontologies.com/drug_action.owl#Substrate   ?z)-> (?x   http://www.owl-ontologies.com/drug_action.owl#Interact ?y)]

[rule9:(?x   http://www.owl-ontologies.com/drug_action.owl#Substrate ?z)(?y http://www.owl-ontologies.com/drug_action.owl#Substrate   ?z)-> (?x   http://www.owl-ontologies.com/drug_action.owl#Interact ?y)]

References

1. Matsuki, E., Tsukada, Y., Nakaya, A., et al.: Successful treatment of adult onset Langerhans cell histiocytosis with multi-drug combination therapy. Internal Med. **50**(8), 909–914 (2011)
2. Ito, K., Iwatsubo, T., Kanamitsu, S., et al.: Prediction of pharmacokinetic alterations caused by drug-drug interactions: metabolic interaction in the liver. Pharmacol. Rev. **50**(3), 387 (1998)
3. Nestorov, I.: Whole body pharmacokinetic models. Clin. Pharmacokinet. **42**(10), 883–908 (2003)
4. Percha, B., Altman, R.B.: Informatics confronts drug–drug interactions. Trends Pharmacol. Sci. **34**(3), 178 (2013)
5. Filippatos, T.D., Derdemezis, C.S., Gazi, I.F., et al.: Orlistat-associated adverse effects and drug interactions: a critical review. Drug Saf. **31**(1), 53 (2008)
6. Beijnen, J.H., Schellens, J.H.: Drug interactions in oncology. Lancet Oncol. **5**(8), 489 (2004)
7. Luo, H., Zhang, P., Huang, H., et al.: DDI-CPI, a server that predicts drug-drug interactions through implementing the chemical-protein interactome. Nucleic Acids Res. **42**(Web Server issue), W46 (2014)
8. Hisaka, A., Ohno, Y., Yamamoto, T., et al.: Prediction of pharmacokinetic drug-drug interaction caused by changes in cytochrome P450 activity using in vivo information. Pharmacol Therapeut. **125**(2), 230–248 (2010)
9. Huang, J., Niu, C., Green, C.D., Yang, L., Mei, H., Han, J.D.: Systematic prediction of pharmacodynamic drug-drug interactions through protein-protein-interaction network. PLoS Comput. Biol. **9**(3), e1002998 (2013)
10. Hunta, S., Aunsri, N., Yooyativong, T.: Drug-drug interactions prediction from enzyme action crossing through machine learning approaches. In: International Conference on Electrical Engineering/Electronics, Computer, Telecommunications and Information Technology, 24–27 June 2015, pp. 1–4. IEEE, Hua Hin (2015)
11. Hunta, S., Aunsri, N., Yooyativong, T.: Integrated action crossing method for drug-drug interactions prediction in noncommunicable diseases based on neural networks. In: International Conference on Digital Arts, Media and Technology, 1–4 March 2017, pp. 259–262. IEEE, Chiang Mai (2017)
12. Tari, L., Anwar, S., Liang, S., et al.: Discovering drug–drug interactions: a text-mining and reasoning approach based on properties of drug metabolism. Bioinformatics **26**(18), i547–i553 (2010)
13. Yoshikawa, S., Satou, K., Konagaya, A.: Drug interaction ontology (DIO) for inferences of possible drug-drug interactions. Stud. Health Technol. Inform. **107**(Pt 1), 454 (2004)
14. Herrerozazo, M., Segurabedmar, I., Martínez, P.: Conceptual models of drug-drug interactions: a summary of recent efforts. Knowl.-Based Syst. **114**, 99–107 (2016)
15. Imai, T., Hayakawa, M., Ohe, K.: Development of description framework of pharmacodynamics ontology and its application to possible drug-drug interaction reasoning. Stud. Health Technol. Inform. **192**(1), 567 (2013)
16. Herrerozazo, M., Segurabedmar, I., Hastings, J., et al.: DINTO: using OWL ontologies and SWRL rules to infer drug-drug interactions and their mechanisms. J. Chem. Inf. Model. **55**(8), 1698 (2015)
17. Keiser, M.J., Roth, B.L., Armbruster, B.N., et al.: Relating protein pharmacology by ligand chemistry. Nat. Biotechnol. **25**(2), 197 (2007)
18. Johnson, M.A., Maggiora, G.M.: Concepts and applications of molecular similarity. Am. Math. Mon. **12**, 96–97 (2005)

19. Martin, Y.C., Kofron, J.L., Traphagen, L.M.: Do structurally similar molecules have similar biological activity? J. Med. Chem. **45**(19), 4350 (2002)
20. Vilar, S., Cozza, G., Moro, S.: Medicinal chemistry and the molecular operating environment (MOE): application of QSAR and molecular docking to drug discovery. Curr. Top. Med. Chem. **8**(18), 1555–1572 (2008)
21. Faulon, J.L., Misra, M., Martin, S., et al.: Genome scale enzyme–metabolite and drug–target interaction predictions using the signature molecular descriptor. Bioinformatics **24**(2), 225–233 (2008)
22. Bleakley, K., Yamanishi, Y.: Supervised prediction of drug–target interactions using bipartite local models. Bioinformatics **25**(18), 2397–2403 (2009)
23. Fokoue, A., Sadoghi, M., Hassanzadeh, O., Zhang, P.: Predicting drug-drug interactions through large-scale similarity-based link prediction. In: Sack, H., Blomqvist, E., d'Aquin, M., Ghidini, C., Ponzetto, S.P., Lange, C. (eds.) ESWC 2016. LNCS, vol. 9678, pp. 774–789. Springer, Cham (2016). https://doi.org/10.1007/978-3-319-34129-3_47
24. Kim, S., Jin, D., Lee, H.: Predicting drug-target interactions using drug-drug interactions. PLoS One **8**(11), e80129 (2013)
25. Rask-Andersen, M., Almén, M.S., Schiöth, H.B.: Trends in the exploitation of novel drug targets. Nat. Rev. Drug. Discov. **10**(8), 579 (2011)
26. Overington, J.P., Al-Lazikani, B., Hopkins, A.L.: How many drug targets are there? Nat. Rev. Drug. Discov. **5**(12), 993 (2006)
27. Cosine similarity, 4 October 2017. https://en.wikipedia.org/wiki/Cosine_similarity
28. Maedche, A.: Ontology Learning for the Semantic Web. IEEE Intell. Syst. **16**(2), 72–79 (2002)
29. Mcguinness, D.L., Harmelen, F.: OWL web ontology language overview **63**(45), 990–996 (2004)
30. Boyce, R.D., Collins, C., Horn, J., et al.: Modeling drug mechanism knowledge using evidence and truth maintenance. IEEE Trans. Inf. Technol. Biomed. **11**(4), 386–397 (2007)
31. Moitra, A., Palla, R., Tari, L., Krishnamoorthy, M.: Semantic inference for pharmacokinetic drug-drug interactions. In: IEEE International Conference on Semantic Computing, 16–18 June 2014, pp. 92–95. IEEE, Newpoet Beach (2014)
32. Preissner, S., Kroll, K., Dunkel, M., Senger, C., Goldsobel, G., Kuzman, D., et al.: SuperCYP: a comprehensive database on Cytochrome P450 enzymes including a tool for analysis of CYP-drug interactions. Nucl. Acids Res. **38**, D237 (2010)
33. Li, H., Qiang, S.: Parallel mining of OWL 2 EL ontology from large linked datasets. Knowl.-Based Syst. **84**, 10–17 (2015)

Augmented Reality: New Technologies for Building Visualized Hospital Knowledge Management Systems

Long Lu[✉] and Wang Zhao

Wuhan University School of Information Management, Wuhan, China
bioinfo@gmail.com

Abstract. Augmented reality has developed rapidly in recent years and has been widely used. The knowledge management system of the hospital is a knowledge management system based on the theory and method of knowledge management and the latest information technology and visualization method. This paper introduces the technology architecture and recognition algorithm of augmented reality technology, and studies the application of augmented reality technology in the hospital knowledge management system.

Keywords: Augmented reality · Visualization
Knowledge management sytem

1 Introduction

With the development of science and technology and the arrival of a knowledge economy. Knowledge replaces traditional elements such as capital and labor and becomes an important strategic resource. Many organizations have strengthened the management of knowledge resources. In order to improve the sharing and use of knowledge, various knowledge management systems have been developed. Hospital is a highly intensive unit of knowledge, including the knowledge of medicine, pharmacy, management and so on. It has a wide connection with the humanities, ethics, law and information science. Therefore, the hospital needs to establish a knowledge management system to improve the overall knowledge application level of the hospital and promote the development of the hospital [1]. Because the hospital knowledge management involves a large number of human body structure, medical image and other aspects of knowledge, so the visualization method can be used to enhance the doctor and patient's rapid understanding of medical knowledge and improve the relationship between doctors and patients. Augmented reality is the latest research focus of visualization technology. It has a wide range of application prospects in the fields of education, medical treatment, transportation, book publishing and other industries. The hospital knowledge management system can make use of augmented reality technology to improve the application of medical knowledge and promote knowledge sharing.

© Springer Nature Switzerland AG 2018
H. Chen et al. (Eds.): ICSH 2018, LNCS 10983, pp. 15–25, 2018.
https://doi.org/10.1007/978-3-030-03649-2_2

2 Augmented Reality

Augmented reality technology is a new visualization technology based on virtual reality technology [2]. It superimposes the virtual world constructed by computer and the real world, strengthens user's cognition of reality, and increases all kinds of information of the real world.

Augmented reality technology has three important characteristics: authenticity, interactivity and practicality. Authenticity is that augmented reality is based on the real world. Interactivity mainly refers to human-computer interaction, which mainly embodies the interactive process between the user and the augmented reality system. Through interactivity, the user can obtain the best information he wants. Practicality refers to the combination of augmented reality system and practical application, which can promote the development of social economy, and has high practical value. Many devices now support augmented reality systems, such as smart phones or tablet computers. Head mounted displays (HMD) also support augmented reality systems. HMD installs display devices in helmets or glasses, and users wear them on their heads when they are used. The advantage is that the display is in front of the eye and is an immersive experience. Google Glass is a kind of HMD equipment, and many university medical centers are using it to explore the application of in medical care and medical education [3].

2.1 Augmented Reality Architecture

The architecture of augmented reality consists of seven main parts, which are interdependent and collaborated to complete the augmented reality, as shown in Fig. 1.

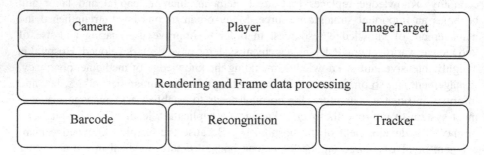

Fig. 1. Augmented reality technology architecture

- Camera module is responsible for collecting image binary stream data, and encapsulates PC, iOS and Android camera devices across platforms.
- Player module supports video playback programs, including multiple types of video files.
- ImageTarget module is mainly configured to identify target maps, mainly for target detection and recognition.

- Rendering and Frame data processing module is responsible for processing the binary frame data collected from the camera, and rendering it to the interface through the OpenGL graphics engine.
- Barcode module is a two-dimensional code recognition module, which is
- responsible for the recognition of two-dimensional code.
- Recongnition module is the image recognition module, and it is the core part of the system. It can support local image recognition and cloud recognition.
- Tracker module is the image tracking module, which tracks the location movement of images.

2.2 Augmented Reality Image Recognition Algorithm

Augmented reality image recognition algorithm is similar to image search algorithm, including two key words, image fingerprint and Hamming distance. The image fingerprint is the same as the human fingerprint, which is the symbol of identity, and the image fingerprint is simply a set of binary digits which are obtained by the arithmetic of hash.

Hamming distance is the number of steps passed from A to B. This value can measure the difference between the two pictures, and the smaller the Hamming distance, the higher the similarity. If Hamming distance is 0, that is to say, the two picture is exactly the same.

Image fingerprint algorithm uses the average hash value (aHash) algorithm, which is based on the comparison of each pixel and the average value of the grayscale map. The algorithm process is as follows:

- Reduce the picture: keep the structure, remove the details, remove the difference of size and aspect ratio, and zoom the picture to 8 * 8, a total of 64 pixels.
- Transform to grayscale map: transform the zoomed image to the 256 level grayscale map.

  Grayscale map correlation algorithm (R = red, G = green, B = blue).

  Floating-point algorithm: Gray = R * 0.3 + G * 0.59 + B * 0.11

  Integer method: Gray = (R * 30 + G * 59 + B * 11) / 100

  The shift method: Gray = (R * 76 + G * 151 + B * 28) $\gg$ 8

  Mean value method: Gray = (R + G+B) / 3

  Only take green: Gray = G
- Calculate the average value: calculate the average value of all pixels of the picture after grayscale processing.
- Compare the pixel gray level value: traversing each pixel of the grayscale picture, if it is greater than the average value, record 1, otherwise record 0.
- Get information fingerprint: combine 64 bits, and keep consistency in sequence.
- Contrast fingerprint: calculate the fingerprints of two pictures and calculate the Hamming distance, if the longer the Hamming distance, the more inconsistent the picture is, and conversely, if the Hamming distance is smaller, the more similar the picture is. When the distance is 0, the picture is exactly the same. Usually, the distance is more than 10, which means two different pictures.

3 Hospital Knowledge Management System

3.1 Knowledge Management

Knowledge management is developed from the accurate expression of knowledge connotation. Knowledge management is developed from the accurate expression of knowledge connotation. It Based on information technology and theoretical innovation. It aims to promote the development, dissemination and use of knowledge, and ultimately achieve knowledge sharing. The purpose is to improve the resilience and innovation ability of the organization.

Knowledge management in narrow sense refers to the management of knowledge itself, including knowledge creation, acquisition, processing, storage, dissemination and application management. On this basis, the broad knowledge management also includes the management of various resources and intangible assets related to knowledge, involving knowledge organization, knowledge facilities, knowledge assets, knowledge activities, and people involved in knowledge management.

The practical means of knowledge management include recognition, acquisition, development, decomposition, use and storage, which are characterized by accumulation, sharing and communication. Improving work efficiency is the ultimate goal [4].

With the challenge of knowledge economy to the hospital and the impetus of information technology to the development of knowledge management, the hospital knowledge management is becoming more and more important, and it has become a new research hotspot.

The hospital knowledge includes explicit knowledge and tacit knowledge. Explicit knowledge includes encoded text, images, symbols, sound and other forms. It exists in books, databases, disks, CD-ROM and other carriers, such as books, magazines, medical records, images, electronic databases and other documents. Tacit knowledge is mainly the intangible and non coding knowledge that exists in the human brain, such as the clinical experience, diagnosis and treatment methods and skills of the medical and nursing staff [5].

3.2 Hospital Knowledge Management System

The knowledge management system is the platform of knowledge management. It takes the human intelligence as the dominant, the information technology as the means. It is a man-machine combined management system. It integrates a variety of knowledge resources such as explicit knowledge and tacit knowledge in the enterprise to form a dynamic knowledge system,. It promotes knowledge innovation and promotes the improvement of labor productivity through the continuous innovation capability. Thus ultimately improve the core competitiveness of the hospital.

Knowledge management system is a comprehensive system composed of technology platform, information platform and management system [6]. The hospital knowledge management system is a platform to realize the efficient management of the hospital knowledge. Through the effective knowledge management mechanism, and relying on the computer network, data warehouse, data mining, statistical analysis and other information technology, the hospital knowledge management is highly integrated and flexible. Through the establishment of hospital knowledge management system, all kinds of knowledge and data in hospital can be accumulated and preserved for a long time. The wisdom and experience of hospital experts can be passed on to young doctors through knowledge sharing. The establishment of hospital knowledge management system can also promote academic exchange and innovation, increase knowledge wealth, and effectively protect the hospital knowledge assets [1].

The hospital knowledge management system mainly includes disease management system, medical imaging system, medical diagnosis and treatment system, online consultation system, medical literature system, medical knowledge system, medical teaching system, expert knowledge system, decision support system.

The disease management system includes knowledge and treatment methods for various diseases. Medical imaging system mainly manages image files and related knowledge of CT and MRI. Medical diagnosis and treatment system mainly includes knowledge of clinical diagnosis and treatment. Online consultation system is a system for doctors in hospitals to answer questions about medical knowledge. Medical literature system includes medical papers, medical monograph, electronic journals, medical books, etc. Medical knowledge system is mainly managed by doctors' tacit knowledge, especially medical treatment experience. Medical teaching system is a system for experts and doctors to impart medical knowledge to other doctors and patients. Expert knowledge system is based on the rich knowledge of medical experts, providing authoritative knowledge answers to doctors and patients. Decision support system relies on all kinds of knowledge resources to provide decision support for all kinds of business and development direction of hospitals.

3.3 Visual Hospital Knowledge Management System

A small part of the information obtained by human beings comes from the sense of touch, the other is from the hearing, and most of them come from the visual [7]. "One map wins thousands of words" is the truth. The information contained in a picture is more than one thousand sentences. People mainly get information through the vision. People know the world and the world of perception in an intuitive way. Human brain structure is more sensitive to image cognition, so people prefer to recognize things in graphic or image ways.

Knowledge visualization is developed on the basis of scientific computing visualization, data visualization and information visualization. The object of knowledge visualization is human knowledge. It refers to all the graphical means that can be used to construct and transmit complex views. It is a new stage of the development of visualization technology, and the purpose is to promote the dissemination of knowledge and the use of knowledge. Knowledge visualization tools include concept map, mind map, cognitive map, semantic network, thinking map, knowledge map, etc. [8].

The hospital knowledge management system stores and manages a large number of medical knowledge, including CT, MRI image knowledge, clinical diagnosis and treatment knowledge, drug knowledge, medical literature, and various business knowledge accumulated by medical and nursing staff. These knowledge is relatively suitable for visualization and dissemination through visualization technology. Visualization method can promote the understanding and use of medical knowledge, and finally improve the utilization of knowledge.

With the rapid development of computer graphics and visualization technology, from simple graphical user interface to visual display of various medical knowledge, such as 3D reconstruction of medical images, visualization techniques and methods have played a more and more important role in the hospital knowledge management system.

In the design of hospital knowledge management system, visualization tools and resources can be treated as resource repository. Visualization is planned as a basic module or visualization layer. Users can visualize and manage various resources of the hospital knowledge management system through this basic module or visual layer, including video, audio, interface buttons, icons and other resources. Various medical knowledge is transformed into a matching visual form through the basic module or visualization layer, which is used by the business layer. Its system frame is shown in Fig. 2.

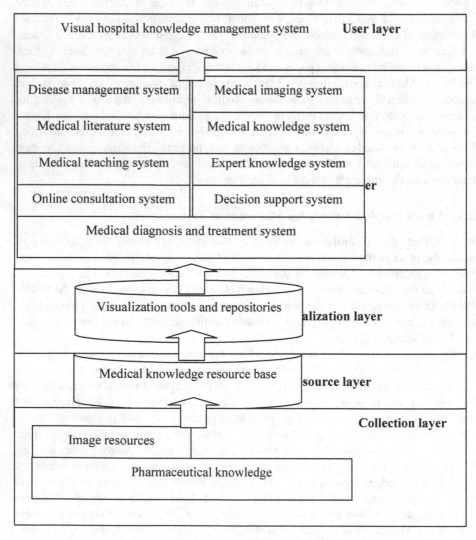

Fig. 2. Framework of visual hospital knowledge management system

The collection layer is mainly to collect all kinds of knowledge resources, including CT, MRI image knowledge, pharmaceutical knowledge, clinical diagnosis and treatment knowledge, medical literature and the knowledge accumulated by medical staff and so on.

The resource layer mainly stores and manages knowledge resources collected and processed by the collection layer. It uses big data technology and tools to efficiently store and utilize knowledge resources.

The visualization layer contains visual algorithms, tools, development packages, visual resources and so on. It provides a variety of visual display for the knowledge resources. Augmented reality is included in the visualization layer.

The business layer includes various business systems, including disease management system, medical imaging system, medical diagnosis and treatment system, online consultation system, medical literature system, medical knowledge system, medical teaching system, expert knowledge system, decision support system and so on.

The user layer is the main interface of the platform, that is, the user's user interface, mainly referring to the website and system interface.

The application of visualization technology and method in the hospital knowledge management system needs to make full use of various medical knowledge resources, provide various knowledge in the visual form, meet the various knowledge needs of the system users, and realize the efficient sharing of knowledge.

Augmented reality technology is the latest visualization technology. The application of augmented reality technology in the hospital knowledge management system promotes the use of knowledge and improves the effect of medical service.

4 Application of Augmented Reality Technology

4.1 Application Characteristics

- Openness
  Augmented reality technology should provide open support in the platform. It provides a comprehensive data read interface, and can also provide self media services for doctors and patients.
- Practicability
  Augmented reality technology is in accordance with the actual needs of doctors and patients. It aims at solving the practical problems of medical services.
- Mobility
  Through mobile terminals, such as mobile phones, doctors and patient users can use APP with augmented reality function, which is not limited by time and place.
- Interaction
  Doctors and patients can interact with each other through augmented reality programs, and programs will respond accordingly. This is an important application feature of augmented reality technology.
- Individualization

Doctors and patient users can customize the content and business functions of the augmented reality program according to their own needs. For example, the doctor can choose the parts of the 3D human model to be displayed.

4.2 Application Scene

- Medical knowledge display

Augmented reality can display all kinds of medical knowledge in the hospital knowledge management system in the real scene, and can display a variety of additional knowledge on the human body or medical image. This will improve the efficiency of doctors' acquisition of medical knowledge.In particular, various organ models reconstructed by image files can clearly display the comprehensive information and internal structure information of the organ.

For example, augmented reality technology is used to display complete three-dimensional liver tissue and structural information. It supports accurate quantification of liver tissue. It helps doctors to grasp the medical knowledge of liver, as shown in Fig. 3.

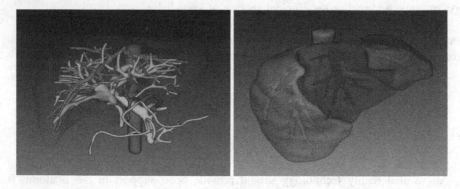

Fig. 3. Liver structural display

- Surgical simulation

Doctors can simulate and guide the various processes involved in medical operations through augmented reality technology, including operation planning, operation rehearsal drill, operation teaching, operation skills training, intraoperative guidance, postoperative rehabilitation, etc.

Using augmented reality technology and imaging equipment to display patient images and models, doctors immerse in three-dimensional scenes and learn the actual operation through visual, auditory and tactile operations. Doctors can practice repeatedly before performing complex operations on patients, improve the proficiency and accuracy of the operation, and reduce the cost and risk of surgical training and treatment. In this way, doctors can improve the skills and accuracy of clinical diagnosis and treatment, making the difficult operation easier. Now, some remote consultation systems using augmented reality technology have entered the application stage.

- Surgical navigation

Medical operation is highly risky and can not be repeated. Therefore, surgical navigation is of high practical value. By using augmented reality, doctors can obtain the internal structure of the organs that the naked eye can not see in the operation. It can obtain the three-dimensional information and accurate position of the surgical site, and the accuracy can reach the millimeter level, which can meet the needs of the actual operation. According to the experience and knowledge provided by the augmented reality technique, the doctor decides the size of the incision, avoids the important nerve and the vascular area, and chooses the safe operation path, thus reducing the surgical trauma, shortening the operation time and improving the quality of the operation. Surgical navigation based on augmented reality technology has been applied in neurosurgery, otolaryngology and radiology [9].

- Postoperative rehabilitation

In the field of postoperative rehabilitation, the application of augmented reality technology, on the one hand, can provide a vivid and realistic rehabilitation training environment for patients, and fully mobilize the enthusiasm of the patients training. On the other hand, the intelligent system, which combines the rehabilitation equipment and the augmented reality, provides all kinds of rehabilitation knowledge in the course of rehabilitation training to realize the therapeutic effect of combining the passive traction with the active training of the patients [10].

- Medical teaching and training

Medical education attaches great importance to practice, and has high requirements for teaching methods, students' learning effects and experimental conditions [11].

Medical teaching has many characteristics, such as many nouns, complex structures, and special subjects. Augmented reality technology can provide advanced teaching methods for medical teaching, reduce teaching cost and save experimental resources. To provide students with more intuitive, closer to the real clinical and experimental scenarios, such as touch, voice and image. And it is more suitable for heuristic teaching, improving teaching efficiency and medical education level [12]. For example, augmented reality technology is used to display human organs and structures in medical teaching and training, which can promote training staff's understanding of medical knowledge.

So as to enhance the enthusiasm of learners, improve their perception and imagination, and even enable students to regulate their learning rhythm and improve their teaching quality. The application of augmented reality can simulate some rare cases of rapid and correct treatment, training the relevant clinical skills repeatedly, mastering the key points of operation, and improving the proficiency. At the same time, the application of augmented reality system can carry out standardized training for some new technical operations, such as the training of clinical skills related to anesthesiology, emergency medicine, battlefield medicine and other related disciplines, which can avoid many risks [13].

Using augmented reality technology, we can overcome the limitation of space. Students can dynamically observe the internal conditions of objects, such as the molecular structure of drugs. It can also break through the time limit and can show the situation in a very short time that may be need take a long time to appear [13]. For example, to verify some of the results of biological genetics, it often takes a few months to experiment with animals, and the use of augmented reality can be achieved in a few hours.

- Medical equipment management

By augmented reality, doctors can visualized a variety of complex medical devices, especially expensive equipment, and doctors can simulate the use of these devices for various exercises and operations. It is beneficial to the maintenance and management of medical equipment.

- Expert online

Through the three-dimensional reconstruction of the patient's CT and MRI images, artificial intelligence algorithm and augmented reality can be used to display the disease area in real time. The expert can explain and communicate with the patient online, reduce the patient's medical cost and establish a good relationship between the doctor and the patient.

The use of expert online training for young doctors, especially in small hospitals and remote hospitals, can improve the efficiency and quality of medical knowledge dissemination and solve the problem of imbalance in the development of medical level [14].

- Multimedia entertainment

Augmented reality supports video and animation form [15], and also provides all kinds of games. Using the visual and multimedia functions of augmented reality technology, doctors and patients can view various medical videos and animations through the network, such as medical online class, famous medical teaching forum, and medical excellent courses, to obtain all kinds of medical and health care knowledge. To meet the needs of personalized medical information service.

5 Conclusion

Information technology is being deeply integrated into our work and life. We need to master the development trend of augmented reality technology and apply the augmented reality technology to the hospital knowledge management system. We should make full use of all kinds of knowledge resources to explore the combination of augmented reality and medical knowledge, so as to achieve efficient knowledge sharing. To provide diversified and rich medical knowledge to meet users' needs, we should improve the efficiency and quality of knowledge utilization, and give full play to the potential value of knowledge.

References

1. Guo, Z.: Construction of hospital knowledge management system. Chinese Journal of Hospital Management (11), 775–776 (2005)
2. Li, Q., Zhang, L.: An empirical study of mobile learning based on augmented reality. China Educ. Technol. **01**, 116–120 (2013)
3. Ma, L., Li, G.: Application of augmented reality in medical teaching. Beijing Med. **39**(10), 1073–1074 (2017)
4. Liu, S., Wei, J.: Construction of medical information service system based on knowledge management theory. J. Med. Inform. **30**(04), 32–35 (2009)
5. Li, S., Yu, W.: A summary of the research on Hospital Knowledge Management. Chin. J. Med. Books Inf. **19**(05), 36–39+48 (2010)
6. Du, F., Sun, Z.: Research on the framework of hospital knowledge management system. Inf. Mag. (05), 55–57 (2005)
7. Fang, L.: The application of information tree in information visualization. Books Inf. (02), 85–88+106 (2007)
8. Li, X., Qiu, J.: On intelligent library and knowledge visualization. Inf. Inf. Work. (01), 6–11 (2014)
9. Niu, Y., Wang, Y., Duan, H.: Surgical navigation technology based on Augmented Reality. Chin. Med. Device J. (01), 50–54 (2004)
10. Song, X., Cao, H., Zhang, Y., Liu, P.: The application of virtual reality technology in medicine. Shandong Sci. **22**(06), 79–82 (2009)
11. Yuan, Y., Weng, D., Wang, Y., Liu, Y.: Navigation system for minimally invasive endoscopic sinus surgery based on augmented reality. J. Syst. Simul. **20**(S1), 150–153 (2008)
12. Bai, X., Li, Z.: Application and discussion of virtual reality technology in medical education. Health Vocat. Educ. **35**(12), 32–34 (2017)
13. Zhang, D.: The wide application and significance of virtual reality technology (VR) in medical education and experiment. Sci. Technol. Innov. Her. (30), 211 (2008)
14. Tan, K., Guo, G., Wang, Y., Wu, P.: Application of virtual reality technology in medical surgery simulation training. Acad. J. PLA Postgrad. Med. Sch. (01), 77–79 (2002)
15. Zhang, B., Hui, R.: The exploration of augmented reality technology and its teaching application. Exp. Technol. Manag. (10), 135–138 (2010)

The Design of Personalized Artificial Intelligence Diagnosis and the Treatment of Health Management Systems Simulating the Role of General Practitioners

Shuqing Chen[✉], Xitong Guo, and Xiaofeng Ju

School of Management, eHealth Research Institute,
Harbin Institute of Technology, Harbin, China
chenshuqing_hit@qq.com

Abstract. Artificial Intelligence (AI) has continuously been used as a method in the fields of medical and clinical research to improve patients' health outcomes. However, the evidence of its effectiveness in self-health management through strengthening one's subconscious mind to change his/her health behavior is not well supported. This paper will use a design science method to describe The Design of Personalized Artificial Intelligence Diagnosis and the Treatment of Health Management Systems Simulating the Role of General Practitioners (AIHMS) that assists in providing tailored interventions to enhance health related behavioral changes. Findings from AI healthcare studies have shown promising insights, particularly in improving self-management and some health outcomes. In fact, AIHMS has not only promoted the happiness of patients, but eased the relationship between doctors and patients, improved patient's satisfaction and other benefits, with far-reaching theoretical and practical implications. Furthermore, AI technology service innovation will improve the wellbeing of patients.

Keywords: AI · Design science · Self-health management · Behavior change
Service innovation

1 Introduction

Chronic diseases, also known as Noncommunicable Diseases (NCDs), are often referred to as diseases that are long lasting and closely related to genetics, as well as physiological, environmental, and behavioral factors. The development of chronic diseases is milder than that of acute diseases, and hence the resulting serious harmful effects are easily overlooked. Regarding the harmful effects of chronic diseases, we perceive that according to the statistics of the World Health Organization (WHO), 70% of the world's annual deaths are caused by chronic diseases. The four main chronic diseases are cardiovascular diseases, cancer, chronic respiratory diseases, and diabetes. These four chronic diseases cause 80% of the premature deaths from chronic diseases. In China, the harmful effects of chronic diseases are more severe than those of developed countries. The mortality rates of the four major chronic diseases are as high

© Springer Nature Switzerland AG 2018
H. Chen et al. (Eds.): ICSH 2018, LNCS 10983, pp. 26–40, 2018.
https://doi.org/10.1007/978-3-030-03649-2_3

as 87% while their premature mortality is 19%. Moreover, the age-standardized death rates from cardiovascular diseases, cancer, and diabetes have been seen to increase in recent years. Chronic diseases are one of the major public health problems that threaten the health of China's residents. The high disease incidence and long-term medical expenditure have become the main causes of the impaired life expectancy of our residents, as well as resulting in poverty due to illness, and the return of poverty due to illness. China has a large population base as well as a large number of patients suffering from chronic diseases. However, medical resources are tight, with unevenly distributed medical resources, while the relationship between doctors and patients is strained. As a result, patients with chronic diseases lack effective chronic disease management.

To cope with the major public health threat posed by chronic diseases, to strengthen the prevention and treatment of chronic diseases, as well as to reduce the burdens of disease, and improve the life expectancy of residents, the General Office of the State Council issued the "Mid-term and Long-term Plan for Prevention and Treatment of Chronic Diseases in China (2017–2025)", in January 2017. With regard to the current shortage of medical resources, the plan encourages key breakthroughs in key technologies such as precision medicine, "Internet +" health care, and big data; and moreover supports the promotion and application of new technologies in the prevention and treatment of chronic diseases. The "New Generation Artificial Intelligence Plan" issued by the State Council in July 2017 clearly puts forward new methods to promote the use of artificial intelligence in the treatment of new modes. The plan also establishes a rapid and accurate smart medical system, while strengthening group intelligent health management, and generating breakthroughs in the analysis of healthy big data, as well as developing smart medical services and smart health management.

The serious harmful effects of chronic diseases have led to the huge demand for chronic disease management. The current situation of the restricted medical resources in China has promoted research as well as the application of key technologies such as big data and artificial intelligence in the management of chronic diseases. These studies and applications are still in the initial stage. Based on the characteristics of chronic diseases, our research will study the application of AI that integrates big data, artificial intelligence, and mobile health in chronic disease management, as well as comprehensively and systematically integrate health information, decision support, and service delivery. We focus on four aspects of self-management to explore the methods and mechanisms of chronic disease management based on AIs, thus providing a theoretical basis and practical guidance for exploring new chronic disease management models, and to alleviate the shortage of medical resources, as well as to improve the management effects of chronic diseases.

However, as we all know, the best intelligent medical platform in the world is IBM Watson. The vision of this platform is to focus on improving its interaction, discovery and decision-making capabilities so as to provide patients with more personalized and convenient services. But our AIHMS platform has several differences and advantages:

(1) Based on the characteristics of the disease: The platform is more targeted and focused, providing personalized diagnosis and treatment services for patients, and its diagnosis and treatment effect is better. For example, the e-commerce platform (Taobao, JD.com, Amazon, etc.) meets this requirement and make all customers

convenient to use. We also compared many large-scale medical health management platforms in China (such as haodaifu.com, xywy.com, guahao.com, etc.), its coverage is too rich and comprehensive, so that users can not be very precise to find what they want, and this also do not agree to be accepted by users. We believe that the future medical profession needs to be more focused.

(2) Based on the characteristics of the crowds: The platform has more usability and is more suitable for the needs and psychology of the elderly. In general, patients with chronic diseases tend to be ageing. Too complicated technology is a burden for them. They don't even know how to use it. This makes it harder to please customers even with intelligent high-end systems.

(3) Based on the characteristics of environment: Since the cold area is a high-risk area for vascular diseases, and economic conditions are backward, and the shortage of medical resources. Therefore, we would like to make this platform plays the role of a general practitioner and provide patients with a full-process medical service. A good service to the patient also supplements the current status of domestic general practitioner resources.

In addition, we acknowledge that the platform is inferior to Watson's high-end due to technical and team composition, but we believe it will also help Watson apply it in a wider range of medical applications.

The paper proceeds as follows. First, we review existing literature. This is followed by a review of the systematic development of the AI system. In the remaining sections we present the design and development, the hypotheses, experimental design, and results of the preliminary system evaluation. The paper ends with a discussion of the results and a conclusion.

2 Literature Review

The long-term and refractory nature of chronic diseases is an important factor leading to poor continuity in self-management and poor compliance with chronically ill patients (Horne et al. 1999). However, studies have shown that chronic diseases are preventable, detectable, and manageable. Moreover, a good management approach can improve the health status of chronically ill patients (Ghimire et al. 2017). Therefore, effective chronic disease management methods are crucial to the health management of patients with chronic diseases.

Bardram pointed out that the traditional medical care model is mainly based on face-to-face or telephone communication. Although this chronic disease management model solves certain problems, there are still many inadequacies such as inefficiency and inability to synchronize data (Bardram 2008). The introduction of Internet and mobile technologies into the public health and medical fields has resulted in a new service model for chronic disease management, which is known as telemedicine (Lee 2004), and can be used anywhere. For any user, with the help of mobile Internet technology, new carriers such as wearable devices, social media, and medical big data platforms can record and analyze personal health data at any time, providing patients with new medical services such as for the prevention, diagnosis, and treatment of healthcare, as well as for prognosis management. It also renders medical services more convenient (Kang et al. 2012) and promises to play an important role in the daily lives of people with chronic diseases (Lee et al. 2007). Through mobile healthcare, patients can better understand their own conditions and strengthen their contact with doctors, thus effectively improving the interaction between doctors and patients and the relationship between doctors and patients. Telemedicine also helps patients to better comply with treatment plans, and to eventually form a long-term and stable effect.

With advances in artificial intelligence technology, artificial intelligence applications that can freely 'talk' with people on the Internet are one of the key projects and a recent development of many technology companies. Artificial intelligence and healthcare have begun to deepen integration (Jianwei 2017). The earliest chat robot for medical treatment that was developed using artificial intelligence technology was ELIZA, which was known to mimic a psychologist (Weizenbaum 1966).

Studies have shown that chatbots based on artificial intelligence as an innovative health management method can provide patients with simpler, more convenient, and more effective health management services, as well as providing long-term health management for patients. Such interventions change the health behavior of patients resulting in a healthy lifestyle, and enabling them to overcome the limitations of current mobile health technology-based management practices (Fadhil et al. 2017). With the rise in mobile technologies and artificial intelligence technologies, medical service systems are able to directly collect patient-generated real-time health data and input them into electronic medical records (ECR), which play the role of family doctors and health advisors in patient health management. In the process of chronic disease management, the integration of mobile technologies and artificial intelligence technologies is crucial (Milani et al. 2016; Kim et al. 2015).

3 Theoretical Background

The AIHMS that we have developed focuses on the rehabilitation effects of patients experiencing heart bypass surgery. Heart bypass surgery is a chronic disease with a difficult recovery process (Mohr et al. 1999a,b), which requires lifelong therapy, and regular follow-up appointments, and other treatments. Some patients, however, tend to discontinue their rehabilitation plans and such poor premature compliance, causes unpredictable clinical outcomes. The factors influencing patients' discontinuation behavior may include slow recovery effects, depression, unrealistic expectations, and self-efficacy (Mohr et al. 1996; Mohr et al. 1997; Mohr et al. 1998; Mohr et al. 1999a, b; Mohr et al. 2000; Mohr et al. 2001). Moreover, each patient may be influenced by a different combination of the preceding factors. The objective of our AIHMS is to provide tailored interventions for patients to motivate them into continuing with their rehabilitation.

In this paper, we selected heart bypass surgery and rehabilitation to illustrate the research paradigm of integrating a behavioral model and Web technologies for health promotion. We attempt to explain how the (Knowledge-Attitude/Belief-Practice) KAP can be integrated into the AIHMS to support health promotion in a general sense. Therefore, the scope of this study is not restricted to specific diseases or rehabilitation.

After researching and comparing a variety of behavioral theories and models, the Knowledge-Attitude/Belief-Practice (KABP/KAP) was chosen as the theoretical foundation for our study. The KABP/KAP framework is one of the earliest comprehensive attempts to explain healthcare behavior based on expectancy value principles (Guinea et al. 2014). It has been widely applied to study all types of healthcare behaviors, such as contraceptive use, diet, and exercise (Bansal et al. 2010). It has also been applied in other diverse areas, and the model appears to have implications for work motivations as well as a broad range of human behaviors (Paul 2006).

The KABP/KAP framework is derived from the Health Belief Model (HBM) which integrates theoretical perspectives such as the Needs Motivation Theory, the Cognitive Theory and the Value Expectation Theory (Xu et al. 2008). There are three key elements in this framework: knowledge, attitude and belief, which are the basis of the KABP/KAP framework. It proposes that healthcare knowledge and information are the basis for establishing positive and correct beliefs and attitudes, and subsequently changing health-related behaviors; while beliefs and attitudes are the driving forces of behavioral change (Frank 2004; Johnston and Warkentin 2010). There exist many psychological activities that can lead to health related behavioral change. For example, Xu et al. (2008) found that perceived severity, perceived susceptibility, perceived benefits, perceived barriers, and self-efficacy are antecedents to behavioral change. Since the persistency of these habilitation plans of chronic diseases can be regarded as a form of long-term behavioral change, applying the KAP in this study is justified. The KAP holds promise for the development of effective interventions to enhance rehabilitation persistency.

4 Design and Development

Seven steps were involved in the AIHMS software development process (see Fig. 1). The V-Model demonstrates the relationships between each phase of the developmental life cycles and its associated phase of testing. The horizontal and vertical axes represent time or project completeness (left-to-right) and level of abstraction (coarsest-grain abstraction uppermost), respectively. The double-headed arrows between Design, Coding, and Testing reflect reciprocal relationships, indicating that several iterations of design, coding, and testing might be needed before completion of the system development.

4.1 Software Objectives

The AIHMS was designed to solve the problem of poor self-health management. It was expected to continuously interact with patients, followed by intelligent diagnosis and treatment of patients. Therefore, the objectives of the software development are as follows: The first objective is for AI to play the role of a general practitioner, and thus solve the problem of a shortage of general practitioners. This is because the combination of AI technology and medical specialists renders patient health management simple and effective. The second objective is to enable, AI to optimize medical approaches. In other words in using AI for patient management, patients are able to enjoy the best medical services without leaving home. It also simplifies the patient review process, effectively supervises patients' personal health management, as well as developing good habits that focus on patients' personal health. At the same time, AI can lighten the workload of doctors. After receiving a patient's health report, doctors do not need to spend too much time communicating with patients. They only need to provide feedback of the results of the diagnosis and treatment through AI. Third, at the social level, AI assists the Government and the National Health Planning Commission, and other government departments to formulate a sound medical system policy, to create benefits for doctors and patients, and to improve the overall level of medical health in China as a whole.

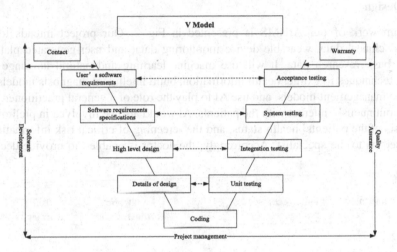

Fig. 1. Software development process

4.2 Requirement Study and Analysis

Before developing the AIHMS, we found it essential to conduct a thorough requirement study and analysis. Accordingly, our Phase I study was carried out following Berger et al. (2004). The objectives of the Phase I study were to accurately assess the motivations and influencing factors of the patients' ongoing self-diagnosis and to determine their most risky treatment programs. The findings from the Phase I study are briefly described below.

In order to identify the variables that might be related to discontinuation, we used a variety of methods to understand patients' specific needs, including: a survey, interviews, observation methods, market research, and other approaches. In addition, we factored the diversity in terms of respondents, patients, physicians, hospital managers, medical students, nurses, ordinary citizens and businessmen involved in the medical field. The final research and design framework was formed by the modification of multiple rounds of requirement documents.

The requirements of the AIHMS were determined by the objectives of the software and the needs of the project.

Below are some primary requirements:

(1) The AIHMS needs to incorporate a mobile terminal system.
(2) The AIHMS needs to be able to dynamically generate interventions on structures and contents for each individual patient based on the patient's Stage of Change, perceived importance of continuation, and balance of decisions.
(3) The AIHMS should incorporate adequate security.
(4) The AIHMS needs to include session control to ensure data integrity for each patient.
(5) The AIHMS should have a database to save intervention contents and patient data.

4.3 Design

The framework of our AIHMS is presented in Fig. 2. Our project intends to use patients' clinical data, wearable device monitoring data, and user-generated platform data as basic research data. It will use machine learning and natural language processing techniques to extract health information, build intelligent diagnosis models and dialogue management models, and use AI to play the role of a general practitioner, who would continuously interact with the patients. AI would also be involved in preliminary diagnosis of the patients' health status, and the screening of critical risk information to be passed on to the specialist. Accordingly, the doctor is enabled to provide decision

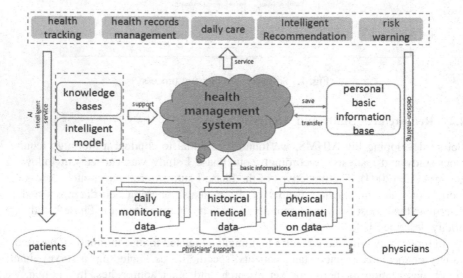

Fig. 2. The structure framework of AIHMS

support for the patients. In this way, AI health management mimicks the role of a general practitioner platform to build an AI smart health management ecosystem.

The execution of our AIHMS process is as follows:

(1) **Health data integration:** This section mainly uses the AI platform to synchronize the wearable device data, the automatic entry of clinical data, and the incentives to collect patients' diet and medication data without interference. In addition, desensitization or privacy operations are performed on health data to promote the effective use of health data.

(2) **Extraction of professional knowledge related to health management:** This section mainly focuses on information extraction of unstructured clinical medical data. The data involving diet, exercise, and medication are mainly structured data, and processing is relatively easy. In health management, key information entities such as diseases, symptoms (including sites, severity and duration), test results, and drugs (including frequency and dosage) require special attention. This information, also known as a medical entity, is the path taken from clinical data to the most reliable path. The clinical data is different from open field data. The conventional natural language processing tools based on the machine learning model will not be successful. Therefore, here, we mainly complete the construction of the model for the extraction of information on clinical data. Classical supervised learning tasks are used, and in the order of progression, they include: the extraction of information to be extracted, the construction of an annotated corpus, and the construction of an information extraction model based on machine learning methods.

(3) **AI intelligent diagnosis and treatment mode:** The interactions between patients and AI often involve multiple rounds of dialogues and interactions. The contents of the dialogues should be relevant and also consistent with the contexts. Accordingly, this section focuses on research on dialogue management methods. Our research content mainly comprises multiple rounds of dialogue. It is the user's intention to identify and track methods, as well as the automatic generation of dialogue content during multiple rounds of dialogue. Accurately identifying the user's intentions includes understanding the intent of the user's consultations, which could involve describing the symptoms, seeking consultations on the test results, selection of appropriate diet plans, exercise programs, or the seeking of consultations on prescribed drugs. The user also needs to select the classification methods according to his/her intentions. In addition, through the design of dialogue scenario rules and the dialogue content generation model based on the combination of statistical generation models and rules, a model study was constructed to provide patients with specific diagnoses and treatment services. Figure 3 shows the details functional design of AIHMS.

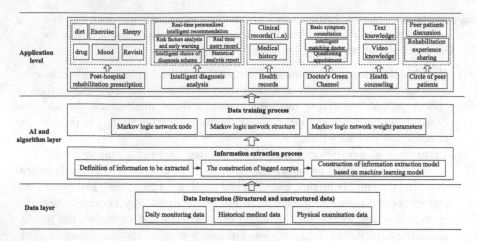

Fig. 3. The details functional design of AIHMS

4.4   Coding, Testing, and Deployment Plan

Coding Plan: Coding refers to the implementation of a software design. Active Server Pages, SQL, NLP, deep learning and ActiveX are used to implement the algorithms of our code. In addition, HTML, JavaScript, and CSS are used to create the user interface of the code, while Visual Basic, ActiveX Data Object, and SQL are used to access the relational database.

Testing Plan: Extensive testing was undertaken after the first version of the system was coded. Two Ph.D. students and a professor, a clinical specialist, a leader of a medical university and 15 medical students, the chairman of the health management center and several staff members and two IT professionals from an IT consulting company tested the software against the software requirements. A good representative sample of all possible scenarios was fed into the software to examine the software performance. The testing was a repetitive process. After 15 rounds of testing and revisions, the system performance was assessed by KAP experts and was considered to have met the system's requirements.

Deployment Plan: Before the system was deployed, several text changes were made according to suggestions generated by another review.

5   Preliminary Evaluation

5.1   Hypotheses

In the actual investigation of the hospital of our research, we learned that the diagnosis and treatment of chronic diseases is a lengthy process, requiring long-term rehabilitation training and return visits over time. Therefore, we undertook long-term monitoring and intervention for patients with chronic diseases, and made comparisons of the different visits at monthly, three-monthly, and six-monthly periods, etc., to monitor their health indicators. Studies have shown that doctors' interventions have a positive effect on the health of patients, and that our AI system simulates the role of general practitioners, by continuing to interact with patients, and involving long-term interventions in patients' rehabilitation behavior.

Hence, we propose that:

H1. Patients who receive AIHMS supported interventions have a longer and continuous rehabilitation training than those who do not receive AIHMS interventions.
H2. Patients who receive interventions supported by AIHMS have better health indicators than those who do not receive AIHMS interventions.

5.2 Experimental Designs and Anticipated Results

This section intends to use laboratory experiments to explore the impacts of patients' use of self-health management in the context of AI applications. The platform is mainly focused on the health management of patients with chronic diseases. The pilots and assessments in the early stage mainly consist of patients undergoing bypass surgery. There are several reasons for this:

(1) Cardiovascular disease is a serious chronic disease. The population of patients has a large base, long in duration and difficult to cure, which makes it difficult for patients to persist in long-term self-health management. Such as hypertension, hyperlipidemia and hyperglycemia are the inducement factors of cardiovascular disease, so we believe that if we can do well in the health management of cardiovascular disease, it will also play a good effect in other diseases. In patients with cardiovascular disease, postoperative health management is the most important. Therefore, we chose this group as the experimental group.
(2) The samples we choose have certain representativeness. The Department of Cardiology of the Second Affiliated Hospital of Harbin Medical University ranks in the top 10 in the country. Due to its location in cold areas, it has a high incidence rate and a serious degree of illness. Based on this sample, it has certain persuasiveness. In addition, in the recent progress of the work, we also expanded the platform to the Department of Cardiology and Endocrinology at the same time. The Department of Cardiology in the Second Hospital of Medicine is the top three in the country and also has a universality.

5.2.1 Laboratory Experiment

We randomly selected about 300 patients with the same disease, the same disease characteristics and similar personal characteristics. While they participated in the experiment, they did not participate in related experiments before this experiment. As perceived in Table 1, the subjects were randomly divided into eight groups. The number of men and women in each group was the same. There was one control group and eight test groups. The subjects of the experiment simulated the interaction process and strictly controlled for variables that were not related to the experiment. After the trial was completed, compliance was measured according to the users' diet records and the behavioral changes were measured according to whether the users' behavioral changes were recorded.

Table 1. Experimental design

	DC	Intelligent				Randomized			
		TR	IR	MR	RiW	RRa	RRc	RM	RaW
CG	√								
EG 1	√	√							
EG 2	√		√						
EG 3	√			√					
EG 4	√				√				
EG 5	√					√			
EG 6	√						√		
EG 7	√							√	
EG 8	√								√

Note*: EG represents Experimental group; CG represents Control groups; DC represents Daily Care; TR represents Timed Reply; IR represents Intelligent Recommendations; MR represents Message Reminders; RiW represents Risk Warnings; RRa represents Randomized Reply; RRc represents Randomized Recommendations; RM represents Randomized Message; RaW represents Randomized Warnings;

5.2.2 Analysis of Econometric Methods

In this section, we explore the causal relationship between the use of AI (system characteristics and human-computer interaction characteristics) and self health management (health behavioral changes) from the perspective of an empirical analysis. Moreover, the experiments of chronic disease health management were conducted. We collected the data of the patients' personal characteristics and the recorded data of AI usage before and after the AI applications, and followed this with the propensity score matching method to pair the intervention groups with the control groups in the experiment. After the matching, we did not expect, any significant differences between the intervention and the control groups. Following this, we used the double difference method, i.e., we first used the differences between the patients both before and after the application of AI, to eliminate the errors caused by the individual heterogeneity. Next, we collected the differences between the experimental group and the control group again to eliminate the errors caused by each individual's time trend, and finally arrived at the actual impacts of self-health management generated by the application of AI.

6 Discussion

The AIHMS is fundamentally transforming the healthcare system. Continuous interactions with patients through AI enables the delivery of health information to patients through its system. This paper describes the design and evaluation of the AIHMS that enhances chronic disease self-health management. The AI diagnosis and treatment strategy is built into the system after careful planning and research. The results of preliminary system evaluations indicate that the AIHMS can reduce the patients' compliance discontinuation rate and move more patients forward to the stage where discontinuation is less likely to happen. The findings suggest that the integration of behavioral theories and the AIHMS can make a significant contribution to healthcare delivery for the public. In addition, our research has implications for the development of AI diagnosis and the treatment of health management systems in general. Our research demonstrates that complicated theory-based knowledge can be embedded into AI diagnosis and treatment health management systems and also distributed through technology.

6.1 Theoretical Contributions

This paper presents two theoretical contributions. First, we designed a new diagnosis and treatment system of self-health management program for chronic diseases, based on AI, and this is an innovation service for mHealth and a breakthrough in the AI medical field. Thus this breakthrough offers great benefits for health management. Second, while the original health management methods have been mainly applied at the individual level, we have extended these methods at the organizational and social levels, Accordingly, there are far-reaching and significant implications for the health research field in future research.

6.2 Practical Contributions

Our study finds three practical contributions. First, we verify that to a certain extent, AI can ease the problem created by a shortage of general practitioners. At present, the number of general practitioners in China is too small and renders it impossible for them to establish effective contact with patients in order to meet their health needs. The combination of AI technology and specialists allows for simple and effective patient health management. Second, AI can optimize medical approaches. In fact, traditional methods of health management are time-consuming and laborious and do not yield positive results. The use of AI for patient management enables patients to enjoy the best medical services without leaving their homes. It also simplifies the patient review process, by effectively enabling patients' personal health management, and assists patients to develop good habits that focus on improving their health. At the same time, AI can lighten the work of doctors. In fact, after receiving their patients' health reports, doctors save time in communicating with their patients. This is because they only need to provide feedback and treatment options through AI. Third, at the social level, AI helps the Chinese Government and the National Health Planning Commission and other government departments to formulate a sound policy for a medical system, so as to create benefits for doctors and patients, and to improve the overall level of medical health in China generally.

6.3   Limitations and Suggestions for Future Research

There are some limitations in our study. First, the data collection may be limited, and we need to use multivariate data for an empirical test in future research. Second, the universality of the research findings needs further verification. Our study which focuses only on patients experiencing heart bypass surgery, indicates good compliance. In future research, we will need to verify the effects of multiple diseases.

In summary, mHealth has great potential for assisting patients with health management and for motivating healthy behaviors. However, further work is needed to: (1) prove the effectiveness of this AIHMS system; (2) integrate the use of the AIHMS used by health care providers into the health care delivery system; and (3) provide consumers with systematic and reliable information about the safety and medical utility of mobile health applications.

7   Conclusion

In this paper, we developed an AIHMS system to assist patients to management their health. And proved that patients who receive AIHMS supported interventions have a longer and continuous rehabilitation training, and have better health indicators. This paper mainly elaborated the design and development, the preliminary evaluation, and the discussions and conclusions. Further, we will extend the single-disease health management model to a general health management model, assisting the implementation and landing of national health reform policies.

References

Bansal, G., Zahedi, F.M., Gefen, D.: The impact of personal dispositions on information sensitivity, privacy concern and trust in disclosing health information online. Decis. Support Syst. **49**(2), 138–150 (2010)

Johnston, A.C., Warkentin, M.: Fear appeals and information security behaviors: an empirical study. MIS Q. **34**(3), 549–566 (2010)

Horne, R., Weinman, J.: Patients' beliefs about prescribed medicines and their role in adherence to treatment in chronic physical illness. J. Psychosom. Res. **47**(6), 555 (1999)

Ghimire, S., Castelino, R.L., Jose, M.D., Zaidi, S.T.R.: Medication adherence perspectives in haemodialysis patients: a qualitative study. BMC Nephrol. **18**(1), 167 (2017)

Bardram, J.E.: Pervasive healthcare as a scientific discipline. Methods Inf. Med. **47**(3), 178–185 (2008)

Lee, T.S.: Present state and prospects of mobile healthcare. In: Proceedings of KIEE, vol. 53, no. 9, pp. 36–42 (2004)

Kang, S.M., Kim, M.J., Ahn, H.Y., et al.: Ubiquitous healthcare service has the persistent benefit on glycemic control and body weight in older adults with diabetes. Diabetes Care **35**(3), e19 (2012)

Lee, T.S., Hong, J.H., Cho, M.C.: Biomedical digital assistant for ubiquitous healthcare. In: International Conference of the IEEE Engineering in Medicine and Biology Society, p. 1790 (2007)

Milani, R.V., Bober, R.M., Lavie, C.J.: The role of technology in chronic disease care. Prog. Cardiovasc. Dis. **58**(6), 579–583 (2016)

Kononenko, I.: Machine learning for medical diagnosis: history, state of the art and perspective. Artif. Intell. Med. **23**(1), 89–109 (2001)

Min, T.: Application research of wechat robot in real-time virtual reference service in the library: taking shanghai minhang district library as an example. New Century Libr. (2015)

Kwakkel, G., Kollen, B.J., Krebs, H.I.: Effects of robot-assisted therapy on upper limb recovery after stroke: a systematic review. Neurorehabilitation Neural Repair **22**(2), 111 (2008)

Lo, A.C., Guarino, P.D., Richards, L.G., et al.: Robot-assisted therapy for long-term upper-limb impairment after stroke. N. Engl. J. Med. **362**(19), 1772–1783 (2010)

Odusola, A.O., Hendriks, M., Schultsz, C., et al.: Perceptions of inhibitors and facilitators for adhering to hypertension treatment among insured patients in rural Nigeria: a qualitative study. BMC Health Serv. Res. **14**(1), 1–16 (2014)

Kim, H.S., Cho, J.H., Yoon, K.H.: New directions in chronic disease management. Endocrinol. Metab. **30**(2), 159–166 (2015)

Bellos, C., Papadopoulos, A., Rosso, R., et al.: Heterogeneous data fusion and intelligent techniques embedded in a mobile application for real-time chronic disease management. Conf. Proc. IEEE Eng. Med. Biol. Soc. **2011**(4), 8303–8306 (2011)

Sobrinho, Á.A.D.C.C., Silva, L.D.D., Medeiros, L.M.D.: MultCare a mobile assistant as a tool to aid early detection of chronic kidney disease. Procedia Technol. **5**, 830–838 (2012)

Fadhil, A., Gabrielli, S.: Addressing challenges in promoting healthy lifestyles: the al-chatbot approach. In: Proceedings of the 11th EAI International Conference on Pervasive Computing Technologies for Healthcare, pp. 261–265. ACM (2017)

Frank, E.: Physician health and patient care. JAMA **291**(5), 637 (2004)

Weizenbaum, J.: ELIZA—a computer program for the study of natural language communication between man and machine. Commun. ACM **9**(1), 36–45 (1966)

陈建伟: 人工智能与医疗深度融合. 中国卫生 (9), 102–103 (2017)

Mohr, D.C., Dick, L.P., Russo, D., et al.: The psychosocial impact of multiple sclerosis: exploring the patient's perspective. Health Psychol. Off. J. Div. Health Psychol. Am. Psychol. Assoc. **18**(4), 376–382 (1999a)

Mohr, D.C., Goodkin, D.E., Likosky, W., et al.: Therapeutic expectations of patients with multiple sclerosis upon initiating interferon beta-1b: relationship to adherence to treatment. Mult. Scler. **2**(5), 222 (1996)

Mohr, D.C., Goodkin, D.E., Likosky, W., et al.: Treatment of depression improves adherence to interferon beta-1b therapy for multiple sclerosis. Arch. Neurol. **54**(5), 531 (1997)

Mohr, D.C., Likosky, W., Boudewyn, A.C., et al.: Side effect profile and adherence to in the treatment of multiple sclerosis with interferon beta-1a. Mult. Scler. J. **4**(6), 487–489 (1998)

Mohr, D.C., Goodkin, D.E., Masuoka, L., et al.: Treatment adherence and patient retention in the first year of a Phase-III clinical trial for the treatment of multiple sclerosis. Mult. Scler. J. **5**(3), 192–197 (1999b)

Mohr, D.C., Likosky, W., Bertagnolli, A., et al.: Telephone-administered cognitive–behavioral therapy for the treatment of depressive symptoms in multiple sclerosis. J. Consult. Clin. Psychol. **68**(2), 356–361 (2000)

Mohr, D.C., Boudewyn, A.C., Likosky, W., et al.: Injectable medication for the treatment of multiple sclerosis: the influence of self-efficacy expectations and infection anxiety on adherence and ability to self-inject. Ann. Behav. Med. **23**(2), 125–132 (2001)

Fogg, B.J.: Persuasive technologies. Commun. ACM **42**(5), 26–29 (1999)

Kim, E., Kim, W., Lee, Y.: Combination of multiple classifiers for the customer's purchase behavior prediction. Decis. Support Syst. **34**(2), 167–175 (2003)

King, P., Tester, J.: The landscape of persuasive technologies. Commun. ACM **42**(5), 31–38 (1999)

Bental, D., Cawsey, A.: Personalized and adaptive systems for medical consumer applications. Commun. ACM **45**, 62–63 (2002)

Healthcare satisfaction study 2000: Harris Interactive/ARiA marketing, World Wide Web (2000), http://www.harrisinteractive.com/news/downloads/HarrisAriaHCSatRpt.pdf

Abrams, D.B., Mills, S., Bulger, D.: Challenges and future directions for tailored communication research. Ann. Behav. Med. Publ. Soc. Behav. Med. **21**(4), 299 (1999)

Rakowski, W., Andersen, M.R., Stoddard, A.M., et al.: Confirmatory analysis of opinions regarding the pros and cons of mammography. Health Psychol. Off. J. Div. Health Psychol. Am. Psychol. Assoc. **16**(5), 433 (1997)

Revere, D., Dunbar, P.J.: Review of computer-generated outpatient health behavior interventions: clinical encounters "in absentia". J. Am. Med. Inform. Assoc. **8**(1), 62–79 (2011)

Ryan, P., Lauver, D.R.: The efficacy of tailored interventions. J. Nurs. Scholarsh. **34**(4), 331–337 (2002)

De Vries, H., Brug, J.: Computer-tailored interventions motivating people to adopt health promoting behaviours: introduction to a new approach. Patient Educ. Couns. **36**(2), 99 (1999)

Kreuter, M.W., Skinner, C.S.: Tailoring: what's in a name? Health Educ. Res. **15**(1), 1 (2000)

Velicer, W.F., Diclemente, C.C.: Decisional balance measure for assessing and predicting smoking status. J. Pers. Soc. Psychol. **48**(5), 1279–1289 (1985)

Janis, I.L., Mann, L.: Decision making: a psychological analysis of conflict, choice, and commitment. Am. Polit. Sci. Assoc. **73**(1) (1977)

Bandura, A.: Self-efficacy: toward a unifying theory of behavioral change. Adv. Behav. Res. Ther. **1**(4), 139–161 (1977)

Bandura, A.: Self-Efficacy Mechanism in Human Agency. Am. Psychol. **37**(2), 122–147 (1982)

O'Keefe, R.M., Mceachern, T.: Web-based customer decision support systems. Commun. ACM **41**(3), 71–78 (1998)

Culnan, M.J.: Chauffeured versus end user access to commerical databases: the effects of task and individual differences. MIS Q. **7**(1), 55–67 (1983)

Wilson, E.V.: Asynchronous health care communication. Commun. ACM **46**(6), 79–84 (2003)

Friedman, R.H., Stollerman, J.E., Mahoney, D.M., et al.: The virtual visit: using telecommunications technology to take care of patients. J. Am. Med. Inform. Assoc. **4**(6), 413 (1997)

Guinea, A.O.D., Titah, R., Léger, P.-M.: Explicit and implicit antecedents of users' behavioral beliefs in information systems: a neuro psychological investigation. J. Manag. Inf. Syst. **30**(4), 179–210 (2014)

Paul, D.L.: Collaborative activities in virtual settings: a knowledge management perspective of telemedicine. J. Manag. Inf. Syst. **22**(4), 143–176 (2006)

Xu, D.J., Liao, S.S., Li, Q.: Combining empirical experimentation and modeling techniques: a design research approach for personalized mobile advertising applications. Decis. Support Syst. **44**(3), 710–724 (2008)

Automatic Liver Segmentation in CT Images Using Improvised Techniques

Prerna Kakkar[1(✉)], Sushama Nagpal[2], and Nalin Nanda[1]

[1] Electronics and Communication Department, NSIT, Dwarka, New Delhi, India
pkakkar95@gmail.com
[2] Computer Science Department, NSIT, Dwarka, New Delhi, India

Abstract. Computer aided automatic segmentation of liver can serve as an elementary step for radiologists to trace anomalies in the liver. In this paper, we have explored two techniques for liver segmentation - Region growing technique of Morphological Snake and a graph-based technique called Felzenszwalb. The aforementioned techniques have been modified by incorporating Artificial Neural Network (ANN) for automatic seed generation eliminating any user intervention. It has been tested on an open-source dataset of Liver CT Scans. Compared to the algorithms that have been used in past, the algorithms discussed in this paper are computationally much efficient in terms of time. Both algorithms were able to segment liver with high accuracy but Morphological Snake outperformed Felzenszwalb in terms of segmentation by achieving a dice index of 0.88 and a very high accuracy of 98.11%. However, Felzenszwalb computed results at a faster rate.

Keywords: Liver · Segmentation · Region-growing · Graph-based
Morphological Snake · Neural network

1 Introduction

Abdominal CT scans have been widely studied and researched by medical professionals in the recent years. CT scans have proved effective for the task of detection of liver abnormalities in patients [12] and can be inspected further to obtain a diagnosis. For the development of automatic system for liver lesion detection, segmentation of liver is usually the first and the most fundamental step in the model.

The prospect of segmentation of organ tissue from an image modality such as CT or MRI scans have always proved to be a formidable proposition. The high degree of variance in the medical images and low contrast level between organ tissue and neighbouring regions make it difficult for the task of segmentation. This is especially true in the case of liver segmentation from abdominal CT scans. Furthermore, the shape of liver fluctuates widely for each individual patient which makes the segmentation of liver particularly a non-trivial task. Additionally, the presence of organs other than liver such as lungs, spine, kidneys in the CT scan pose an additional challenge. This compounded with similar intensity levels of these organs as compared to liver makes it arduous to extract the liver alone.

© Springer Nature Switzerland AG 2018
H. Chen et al. (Eds.): ICSH 2018, LNCS 10983, pp. 41–52, 2018.
https://doi.org/10.1007/978-3-030-03649-2_4

The segmentation of organ tissue from medical imaging modality has been researched extensively over the years. Kong et al. [14] used region based fuzzy c-means technique for the segmentation of brain from MRI scans. Likewise, for segmentation of lung, Tong et al. [15] used region growing and morphological math algorithms to segment lung parenchyma. In the case of liver segmentation various techniques like adaptive threshold, fuzzy c-means with random walker algorithm and fully convolutional neural networks are exploited [3, 17, 19]. But not much work has been done on liver segmentation using relatively less used techniques like region growing and graph-based algorithms.

The goal of this paper is to explore techniques that can be used for liver segmentation in abdominal Computed Tomography (CT) images and make the process fully automated. A fully automated model is beneficial as it supplements radiologists' work and provides for more accurate diagnosis. We have employed two computationally fast algorithms - Morphological Snake [8] and Felzenszwalb algorithm [2] - for the purpose of segmentation and then compared the results of the two models. An artificial neural network that predicts the centroid of the liver contour is exploited to make the two methods fully automated.

The remaining paper is divided in following ways: Sect. 2 deals with the related work in the domain of biomedical segmentation. In Sect. 3, proposed model have been explained. In Sect. 4 our experimental setup has been elucidated while Sect. 5 discusses the analysis and comparison of our proposed methods. Finally the paper is concluded in Sect. 6.

2 Related Work

In recent years, use of computer vision for segmentation of various organ tissues such as lungs, breast, and brain has grown many folds. Fully convolutional neural network for segmentation of neuronal structures using U-Net architecture is used by Ronneberger et al. and is able to achieve a dice index of 0.94 [1]. Dheeba et al. [13] have used global thresholding technique for breast segmentation and have classified healthy and affected tissue using PSOWNN. In case of lung, techniques such as region-growing algorithms and thresholding followed by fuzzy clustering [15, 16] have been used.

In the past, segmentation of liver has drawn the attention of researchers. Selvathi et al. have used adaptive thresholding followed by morphological operations to achieve segmentation of liver on clinical dataset [17]. Moghbel et al. have used a hybrid of cuckoo optimization, Fuzzy c-mean algorithm, and random walker to carry out liver segmentation [19].

Felzenszwalb et al. [2] have come up with an efficient graph-cut technique which uses minimum spanning tree for creating mask. This technique is computationally efficient and has performed well on other image segmentation dataset and is yet to be explored in the field of biomedical imaging.

Abd-Elaziz et al. have used region growing technique to segment liver and is able to achieve a very high accuracy of 96.2% [3]. Jayanthi and Kanmani have also used region growing technique followed by morphological operation to extract image components using erosion and dilation and is able to achieve good segmentation results

[4]. Gambino et al. [18] used a similar region growing technique. They have used Gray Level Co-occurrence Matrices to extract texture features from the image and then applied seeded region growing techniques.

3 Methodology Used

The overall methodology used in this paper is discussed in the following section. The overall model pipeline used in this paper is illustrated in the Fig. 1.

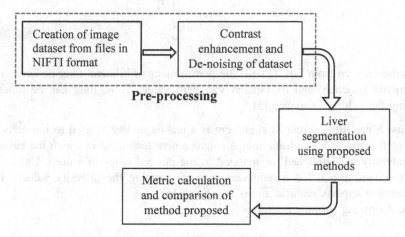

Fig. 1. Model pipeline overview

3.1 Preprocessing

CT scan images are affected by gaussian noises. Therefore, suitable preprocessing is required to smoothen the image and to preserve the edges. It makes segmentation an effortless process and improves results many folds. The granular noises are eliminated using 'Bilateral Filter' technique. To even out the intensity of the image we have used 'Contrast stretching' for equalization. Figure 2 shows the effect of preprocessing on the CT images.

Bilateral Filter. In order to remove noise Bilateral filter is used which is a non-linear method of denoising the image. It considers similarities between local neighborhood pixels such as gray level intensities and distance between the pair of pixels. The process is defined by the following equations:

$$w(i) = w_s(i).w_r(i) \tag{1}$$

$$w_s(i) = \exp\left(-\frac{|i_o - i_n|^2}{2\sigma_s^2}\right) \tag{2}$$

$$w_r(i) = \exp\left(-\frac{|y(i_o) - y(i_n)|}{2\sigma_r^2}\right) \tag{3}$$

Here, w(i) is the weighting signal used for smoothening while i is the pixel value of the image element under consideration.

w(i) consists of spatial function ws(i) and radiometric function wr(i). y(i) is a function that gives the pixel value at position i. The pixel intensity values are replaced by the new weights w(i). This is normalized by following equation:

$$\hat{x} = \sum_{n=i-N}^{i+N} w(i) \cdot \frac{y(i)}{\sum_{n=i-N}^{i+N} w(i)} \tag{4}$$

As can be seen from Eqs. (1)–(4) the performance of bilateral filter depends on σr (radiometric variance) and σs (spatial variance) value. Thus, filter can be tuned by changing the value of variance [5].

Contrast Stretching. Contrast stretching is a technique that is used to normalise the pixels of the image. It is a basic image enhancement technique in which the values of pixel intensity are 'stretched' or mapped to the desired range of values. Unlike Histogram equalisation it has a nonlinear way of mapping the intensity values. Thus, normalisation appears realistic and is less harsh [6].

The following formula is used:

$$P_{out} = \frac{(P_{in} - c)(b - a)}{d - c} + a \tag{5}$$

Where c and d are the minimum and maximum pixel intensity present in the input image. a and b are the minimum and maximum value of pixel intensity to which pixels of Pin are mapped to obtain Pout.

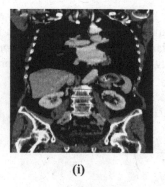 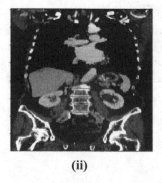

(i)   (ii)

Fig. 2. (i) CT scan of coronal view of liver before preprocessing (ii) after preprocessing

3.2   Liver Segmentation

The liver contour is extracted from the coronal views of the image dataset using two techniques - region growing algorithm and graph-based approach of segmentation. The segmentation method proposed is shown in Fig. 3. To make our models fully automated, we first employ an Artificial Neural Network (ANN) used for prediction of centroid of the liver.

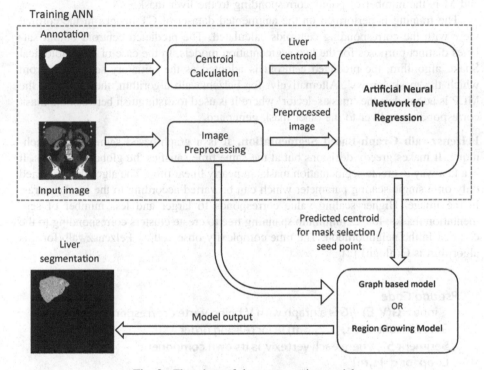

Fig. 3. Flowchart of the segmentation model

Artificial Neural Network for Centroid Prediction. Artificial Neural Network (ANN) are a computation model inspired by the building blocks that make up the brain i.e. neurons and the interconnections they form inside it. Neural network can be visualized as a weighted directed graph in which the hidden neurons are the nodes, while the directed neuron connections or edges - stipulated by the network weights - are the connections between the input and the output of the network [7]. ANN layers also consist of an activation function that maintains the output in the desired range.

In the proposed method, the neural network is utilized to predict the centroid of the liver tissue with the CT image given as the input to the network. The centroid was calculated for each image by employing the corresponding segmentation mask annotations by using the formula:

$$x_{centroid} = \frac{1}{M} \cdot \sum_i x_i \cdot \text{Image}(x_i, y) \tag{6}$$

$$y_{centroid} = \frac{1}{M} \cdot \sum_i y_i \cdot \text{Image}(x, y_i) \tag{7}$$

where Image(x, y) is the intensity of the image at the corresponding (x, y) coordinates and M is the number of points corresponding to the liver mask.

The training is performed on the augmented dataset of CT images in the coronal view with the corresponding centroids calculated. The predicted centroid output satisfies distinct purposes for the two segmentation models. In the case of Morphological Snake algorithm, the predicted centroid is adopted as the initiatory seed point from which the mask 'grows'. Alternatively, for Felzenswalb algorithm, the output of the MLP is adopted as the 'mask selector' where it is used to distinguish between the mask corresponding to liver to the other mask generated.

Felzenszwalb Graph-Based Segmentation. It is a graph-based segmentation technique. It makes greedy decisions but at the same time satisfies the global properties. It is a fast way to create segmentation masks in nearly linear time. The algorithm is varied only on a single scaling parameter which can be varied according to the local contrast in the image. Higher scaling value corresponds to larger and less number of segmentation masks. It uses minimum spanning tree to create clusters corresponding to the contrast in the neighborhood. The time complexity observed by Felzenszwalb for this algorithm is $O(n\log n)$ [2].

```
Pseudo Code
    input=G(V,E) //G is a graph with V being vertex corresponding to pixels
    Sort E into π = (o1, ..., om) in increasing order
    Segment S°, where each vertex vi is its own component
    Loop for q=[1,m]
        //q is an edge connecting vertex vi and vj
        oq=(vi,vj) //ordering of vertex
        //Let Cq-1i be the component of Sq-1 containing vi and Cq-1j the
        component //containing vj
        if Cq-1i ≠ Cq-1j && w(oq) ≤ Mint(Cq-1i,Cq-1j) then,
            Merge Cq-1i and Cq-1j
        else
            Sq = Sq-1
    return S=Sm
```

Fig. 4. Pseudo code for Felzenszwalb

For pseudo code given in Fig. 4 to work it should satisfy the given property:

For a finite graph G (V, E) the segmentation produced should not be too coarse or too fine, where G (V, E) is the graph corresponding to the image.

Morphological Snake. Active contours or more commonly known as Snakes, are widely utilized tools in computer vision problems like object edge detection, tracking and segmentation. They work on the basis of an energy functional provided by the image that is minimized over the surface to achieve the solution to the problem. The shortcomings of Snakes were addressed by new approaches such as Geodesic Active Contour (GAC) [11] and the Active Contours without Edges (ACWE) [10]. In these, the curve is derived over the surface represented by a zero-level set, using time-dependent partial differential equations (PDE). The solution of the PDE are computationally quite expensive and have stability issues.

The Morphological Snakes [8, 9] are a family of contour evolution algorithms which use a set of morphological operations defined on a binary level-set. Morphological Snakes employ these morphological operations that derive fast and stable approximations to the PDE. In our model we have used the Morphological Active Contours without Edges (MACWE).

The PDE for the ACWE is given as

$$\frac{\partial u}{\partial t} = |\nabla u|(\mu \operatorname{div}\left(\frac{\nabla u}{|\nabla u|}\right) - v - \lambda_1 (I - c_1)^2 + \lambda_2 (I - c_2)^2) \tag{8}$$

Morphological operations like dilation, erosion and the curvature flow operator are used to approximate the given PDE. One can say, we provide the solution to contour evolution problems by morphologically solving them. The approximations are used for implementation of the segmentation method since they are computationally inexpensive, stable and quite robust.

4   Experimental Setup

In this section, the experimental setup is discussed which includes the dataset used, parameters of the algorithms involved and performance measures employed.

4.1   Dataset

The proposed techniques were tested on Liver Tumor Segmentation Challenge dataset consisting of 131 CT scan images for training and 70 for testing. Expert annotations of liver and tumor masks are provided for the training dataset. From the dataset, we have extracted the coronal view to use in our model.

4.2 Parameter Setting

See Table 1.

Table 1. Parameter setting for various steps involved

S no.	Process	Technique	Parameters
1.	Denoising	Bilateral filter	$\sigma_s = 0.15$; $\sigma_r = 15$
2.	Equalisation	Contrast stretching	a = 2% of histogram; b = 98% of histogram
3.	Centroid prediction	Artificial neural network	Epochs = 1000; batch size = 25; hidden layer = 1; 10-fold cross validated; loss = MSE
4.	Segmentation	Morphological Snake	Smoothing = 3; initial radius = 20; iterations = 40
5.	Segmentation	Felzenszwalb	Scaling factor = 330; $\sigma = 0.98$; minimum component size = 220

4.3 Performance Measures

The efficacy of the pipeline proposed by us is evaluated on following metrics:

(a) Dice Index: It is widely used in biomedical image segmentation to judge the accuracy of segmentation achieved.

$$DI = 2\frac{|P \cap Q|}{(|P| + |Q|)} \tag{9}$$

Where P is generated segment and Q is the corresponding ground truth

(b) Specificity: Specificity is calculated using the following formula:

$$Specificity = \frac{TN}{(TN + FP)} \tag{10}$$

(c) F1 score: F1 score can be defined as the harmonic mean of precision and recall given by:

$$F1 - score = 2\frac{(Recall * Precision)}{(Recall + Precision)} \tag{11}$$

Where Recall and Precision can be calculated as:

$$Precision = \frac{TP}{TP + FP} \tag{12}$$

$$Recall = \frac{TP}{TP+FN} \tag{13}$$

(d) Accuracy: Accuracy is defined as the total number of true predictions made by the model over all of the predictions made

$$Accuracy = \frac{(TP+TN)}{(TP+TN+FP+FN)} \tag{14}$$

Where TP is True Positive, FP is false positive, TN is true negative and FN is False negative

(e) Volume Overlap error: It is evaluated using the following formula:

$$VOE = 1 - \frac{|P \cap Q|}{|P \cup Q|} \tag{15}$$

(f) Relative volume difference: This parameter is a size-based evaluation metric which is basically evaluates the difference in size of ground truth and segmented image

$$RVD = \frac{(P-Q)}{Q} \tag{16}$$

5 Results and Analysis

The detection presented is reviewed on coronal view of liver. The accuracy achieved by 10 fold cross validation of the Artificial Neural Network (ANN) is (85.38% (+/− 14.78%)). The evaluation metrics for both the segmentation techniques are mentioned in Table 2.

Table 2. Evaluation metrics.

Segmentation model	Dataset used	Average DICE	Specificity	F1 score	Accuracy	Volume overlap error	Relative volume difference
Morphological Snake	LiTS	0.8803	0.9899	0.8771	0.98116	0.2137	−0.0044
Felzenszwalb	LiTS	0.8602	0.9942	0.8556	0.9758	0.2452	−0.1506
FCN-4s 3 slices [20]	Own clinical CT	0.87					

The corresponding ROC Curves (Fig. 5) for Morphological Snake and Felzenszwalb are as shown. Since these methods provide a binary classification of the pixels without probabilities present in the output, a 'sharp elbow' is seen in the ROC curve.

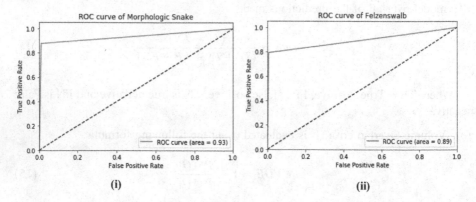

(i)   (ii)

Fig. 5. ROC curves of (i) Morphological Snake (ii) Felzenswalb

It can be seen that Morphological Snake achieved an average DICE index 0.88 with highest individual DICE index being as high as 0.97. Compared to that Felzenszwalb achieved a slightly lower average DICE index being 0.86 and the highest achieved is 0.96. Alternatively, Felzenswalb computed results at a faster rate than Morphological Snake. The segmentation masks created by Felzenszwalb is shown in Fig. 6 and that of Morphological Snake in Fig. 7.

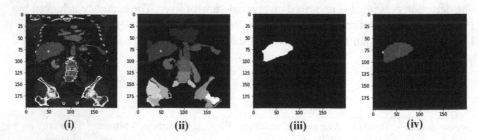

(i)   (ii)   (iii)   (iv)

Fig. 6. Stages of Felzenszwalb segmentation: (i) coronal view of liver with centroid predicted by ANN (ii) segmentation masks created (iii) extracted liver mask (iv) segmented liver from original image with DI = 0.95

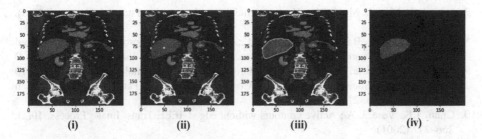

(i)   (ii)   (iii)   (iv)

Fig. 7. Stages of Morphological Snake segmentation: (i) coronal view of liver (ii) centroid as seed point (iii) liver contour obtained after region growing (iv) segmented liver from original image with DI = 0.96

6 Conclusion and Future Work

We have used two modified techniques for segmentation of liver-Felzenszwalb graph based segmentation and Morphological Snake method. These techniques have been automated to find out the seed points using neural network. Our proposed methods have achieved promising results on CT scan dataset and produce results in comparatively less time. The performance of algorithms are judged based on following evaluation metrics - Dice index, specificity, accuracy, F1 score, volume overlap error and relative volume difference. The two algorithms perform equally well but Morphological Snake out powers Felzenszwalb in terms of segmentation while latter outperforms in terms of computation achieving segmentation in linear time. The liver segmentation can be extended to find out lesion segmentations. Apart from CT scans it can be used in other domains on MRI and PET images.

References

1. Ronneberger, O., Fischer, P., Brox, T.: U-Net: convolutional networks for biomedical image segmentation. In: Navab, N., Hornegger, J., Wells, W.M., Frangi, A.F. (eds.) MICCAI 2015. LNCS, vol. 9351, pp. 234–241. Springer, Cham (2015). https://doi.org/10.1007/978-3-319-24574-4_28
2. Felzenszwalb, P.F., Huttenlocher, D.P.: Efficient graph-based image segmentation. Int. J. Comput. Vis. **59**(2), 167–181 (2004)
3. Abd-Elaziz, O.F., Sayed, M.S., Abdullah, M.: Liver tumors segmentation from abdominal CT images using region growing and morphological processing. In: 2014 International Conference on Engineering and Technology (ICET) (2014)
4. Jayanthi, M., Kanmani, B.: Extracting the liver and tumor from abdominal CT images. In: 2014 Fifth International Conference on Signal and Image Processing (2014)
5. Patanavijit, V.: The bilateral denoising performance influence of window, spatial and radiometric variance. In: 2015 2nd International Conference on Advanced Informatics: Concepts, Theory and Applications (ICAICTA) (2015)
6. Point Operations - Contrast Stretching. https://homepages.inf.ed.ac.uk/rbf/HIPR2/stretch.htm

7. Jain, A.K., Mao, J., Mohiuddin, K.M.: Artificial neural networks: a tutorial. Computer **29**(3), 31–44 (1996)
8. Márquez-Neila, P., Baumela, L., Alvarez, L.: A morphological approach to curvature-based evolution of curves and surfaces. IEEE Trans. Pattern Anal. Mach. Intell. **36**(1), 2–17 (2014)
9. Álvarez, L., Baumela, L., Henríquez, P., Márquez-Neila, P.: Morphological snakes. In: 2010 IEEE Computer Society Conference on Computer Vision and Pattern Recognition, San Francisco, CA, pp. 2197–2202 (2010)
10. Chan, T.F., Vese, L.A.: Active contours without edges. IEEE Trans. Image Process. **10**(2), 266–277 (2001)
11. Caselles, V., Kimmel, R., Sapiro, G.: Geodesic active contours. Int. J. Comput. Vis. **22**(1), 61–79 (1997)
12. Oliva, M.R., Saini, S.: Liver cancer imaging: role of CT, MRI, US and PET. Cancer Imaging **4**(Spec No A), S42–S46 (2004). PMC. Web. 4 Apr. (2018)
13. Dheeba, J., Singh, N.A., Selvi, S.T.: Computer-aided detection of breast cancer on mammograms: a swarm intelligence optimized wavelet neural network approach. J. Biomed. Inform. **49**, 45–52 (2014)
14. Kong, J., Wang, J., Lu, Y., Zhang, J., Li, Y., Zhang, B.: A novel approach for segmentation of MRI brain images. In: 2006 IEEE Mediterranean Electrotechnical Conference MELECON 2006, Malaga, pp. 525–528 (2006)
15. Tong, J., Da-Zhe, Z., Ying, W., Xin-Hua, Z., Xu, W.: Computer-aided lung nodule detection based on CT images. In: 2007 IEEE/ICME International Conference on Complex Medical Engineering, Beijing, pp. 816–819 (2007)
16. Amutha, A., Wahidabanu, R.S.D.: Lung tumor detection and diagnosis in CT scan images. In: 2013 International Conference on Communication and Signal Processing, pp. 1108–1112 (2013)
17. Selvathi, D., Malini, C., Shanmugavalli, P.: Automatic segmentation and classification of liver tumor in CT images using adaptive hybrid technique and contourlet based ELM classifier. In: 2013 International Conference on Recent Trends in Information Technology (ICRTIT), pp. 250–256 (2013)
18. Gambino, O., et al.: Automatic volumetric liver segmentation using texture based region growing. In: 2010 International Conference on Complex, Intelligent and Software Intensive Systems, Krakow, pp. 146–152 (2010)
19. Moghbel, M., Mashohor, S., Mahmud, R., Saripan, I.M.B.: Automatic liver tumor segmentation on computed tomography for patient treatment planning and monitoring. EXCLI J. **15**, 406–423 (2006)
20. Ben-Cohen, A., Diamant, I., Klang, E., Amitai, M., Greenspan, H.: Fully convolutional network for liver segmentation and lesions detection. In: Carneiro, G., et al. (eds.) LABELS/DLMIA-2016. LNCS, vol. 10008, pp. 77–85. Springer, Cham (2016). https://doi.org/10.1007/978-3-319-46976-8_9

Bone Fracture Visualization and Analysis Using Map Projection and Machine Learning Techniques

Yucheng Fu[1], Rong Liu[1,2], Yang Liu[1(✉)], and Jiawei Lu[3]

[1] Nuclear Engineering Program, Mechanical Engineering Department, Virginia Tech, 635 Prices Fork Road, Blacksburg, VA 24061, USA
liul30@vt.edu
[2] Department of Orthopaedics, PuRen Hospital Affiliated with Wuhan University of Science and Technology, No. 1 Benxi Road, Qingshan District 430080, Hubei, China
[3] Department of Orthopaedics, First Affiliated Hospital, Dalian Medical University, Dalian 116044, China

Abstract. Understanding intertrochanteric fracture distribution is an important topic in orthopaedics due to its high morbidity and mortality. The intertrochanteric fracture can contain high dimensional information including complicated 3D fracture lines, which often make it difficult to visualize or to obtain valuable statistics for clinical diagnosis and prognosis applications. This paper proposed a map projection technique to map the high dimensional information into a 2D parametric space. This method can preserve the 3D proximal femur surface and structure while visualizing the entire fracture line with a single plot. A total of 100 patients are studied based on the original radiographs acquired by CT scan. The comparison shows that the proposed map projection representation is more efficient and richer in information visualization than the conventional heat map technique. Using the proposed method, a fracture probability can be obtained at any location in the 2D parametric space, from which the most probable fracture region can be accurately identified. Based on the 2D parametric map, the principal component analysis is carried out to investigate the correlations of the fracture lines among different proximal femur regions.

Keywords: Intertrochanteric fracture · 2D map projection
Fracture line visualization · Principal component analysis

1 Introduction

Intertrochanteric fracture (IT) is a common severe injury among seniors that has received much attention due to its high morbidity and mortality. From 1999 to 2012, the IT fracture still yields a high mean one-year mortality rate of 23% [1]. The IT fracture requires great effort for orthopaedic surgeons to provide successful operation. Therefore, this study focuses on the visualization and analysis of IT fracture to obtain a better understanding of its distribution and mechanism. The IT fracture is referred to the fractures in the region lies below the proximal femur head and above the bottom transverse plane of the lesser trochanter.

© Springer Nature Switzerland AG 2018
H. Chen et al. (Eds.): ICSH 2018, LNCS 10983, pp. 53–58, 2018.
https://doi.org/10.1007/978-3-030-03649-2_5

In the past ten years, the fracture map technique has been developed to visualize fracture patterns and obtain statistical characteristics from large database [2]. One can map individual fracture lines to a standard bone template for visualization and analysis. With enough samples, the fracture line direction, pattern and frequency information can be visualized directly on the standard template. In the past decade, the fracture map technique has been applied to scapular fracture [3], tibia pilon fracture [2], and tibial plateau fracture [4], etc.

In fracture map technique, the selection of the view usually depends on the nature of the fracture patterns. If a fracture line is across several different views, two or more views are required to fully describe the fracture pattern [4]. With the consideration of different factors, such as age and gender, the visualization and analysis can become challenging with the existing fracture maps. Also, the scaling information is usually not kept by projecting the 3D model into a 2D representation. Further, it is difficult to obtain statistical information from a large amount of patients using these fracture maps. To address these issues, this paper proposes a new method to present the fracture map based on the map projection technique [5]. The proposed method unfolds a 3D bone mesh and maps it into a 2D parametric space, which retains all the geometrical and topological information of the fracture. The scaling factors are all kept in the mapping function for statistical analysis. Based on the acquired 2D parametric map, the principal component analysis is applied for investigating the correlation and distribution of different IT fracture lines.

2 Methods

2.1 Subjects

A total of 100 IT fracture cases are used in this study. The data are collected from PuRen Hospital (Wuhan, China) over an approximately three-year period from December 2013 to January 2017. The study is approved by the Institutional Ethics Committee of PuRen Hospital. The selected cases contain preoperative CT scan data, and the fracture region is confined to IT region which is the interest of this study. All the data are acquired by Siemens SOMATOM Sensation 16 CT. The CT scan images with a slice thickness of 1.5 mm or below are included to ensure the data quality.

A standard proximal femur template is used in this study for IT fracture visualization. The standard template is acquired from CT data of a normal right proximal femur. For each fracture case, the proximal femur is reconstructed from 2D CT images, and the fracture segments are reduced to the anatomical position. By referring to the patients' 3D reconstructed proximal femur mode, the fracture line is drawn on the standard template with a 4-mm-wide line. When all the fracture cases are superimposed onto the standard template, the heat map can be used for an intuitive representation of the fracture counts, fracture probability, etc.

2.2   2D Parametric Fracture Map

Conventional methods project the 3D bone mesh onto a 2D surface or a simplified 2D sketch template. The fracture lines are then superimposed onto the standard template. In this process, the fracture information could be lost while presenting the fracture lines with only one view. To improve the efficiency and accuracy of fracture line visualization, a map projection technique is developed aiming to visualize the complete fracture information of proximal femur in a 2D plane. The details of this mapping are shown in Fig. 1. In the figure, the proximal femur is first plotted in the Cartesian coordinate with axes of x, y, z. An unfold line is selected from the femoral head to the bottom, which is marked by a red dash line. This provides a reference line for the 2D parametric space. With the given standard proximal femur template, the cross-section shape at each specific height $z = z_i$ can be acquired. At each slice location $z = z_i$, the parameter z' in parametric space is set the same as z in the physical space. The second parameter s' is defined as:

$$s' = s/s_{max}(z'), \tag{1}$$

where s is the curve length along the boundary of the slice, starting from the unfolding point along a clockwise direction, and $s_{max}(z')$ is the perimeter of the slice at the height of $z' = z_i$. Using this mapping technique, every surface point in the physical space (x, y, z) is projected onto a unique point (z', s') in the 2D parametric space. The parameter z' shares the same range with z in the physical space, whereas the parameter s' has a range of $[0, 1]$.

Figure 1(b) shows the map of the standard 3D template in a 2D parametric space. The proximal femur is divided into six regions as shown in the image. For the convenience of discussion, the intertrochanteric region in this study excludes the greater and lesser trochanter as shown in the plot. As can be seen in the figure, the projected map includes both the anterior and posterior views of the 3D model. Different regions are completely visible in a single map. It should be noticed that the femoral head and the greater trochanter area are partially connected in the 2D parametric map. Since the surface is unfolded along the z direction, the slice may contain two separate regions: the femoral head and the other the greater trochanter. A dotted line is plotted in Fig. 1(b), which indicates that these two regions are separated by a finite distance in the physical space.

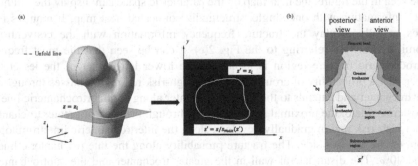

Fig. 1. (a) Pipeline of mapping surface in the physical coordinate to the parametric coordinate using 2D map projection, (b) the generated 2D parametric map. (Color figure online)

2.3   Principle Component Analysis

With the map projection technique, the principal component analysis (PCA) can be applied to the 2D parametric maps. The PCA method can transform a set of variables into linearly uncorrelated new combination of variables. For 2D parametric image, each image can be vectorized by concatenating the image matrix columns consecutively. Combined all the cases together, one can get a multi-dimensional data matrix $\mathbf{X}$ with the size of m by n. The m represents the number of pixels in a 2D parametric map and n represents the number of observation, which is 100 in this study. The steps of PCA is given below:

Step 1. Data normalization and bias remove:

$$z = \frac{x - \mu}{\sigma}, \tag{2}$$

where μ and σ are the mean and standard deviation of x.

Step 2. Calculate the covariance matrix of $\mathbf{X}$.

Step 3. Find the eigenvectors of the covariance matrix.

Step 4. Transfer the eigenvectors back to 2D parametric space as principal images for visualization.

By applying the PCA, one can better understand the correlation and distribution of fracture lines from the principal images. It can also benefit the classification of IT fracture since the principal images carry the information of the largest variance of change in different specific regions.

3   Results and Discussion

The fracture heat map is presented in Fig. 2 by combining all the 100 cases together. The color represents the probability of fracture, which is calculated by the number of fracture cases at each location divided by the total number of cases. The conventional four anatomical views: anterior, medial, posterior and lateral, are shown in Fig. 2(a) to (d). The heat map on the 2D parametric plane is shown in Fig. 2(e) for comparison. As can be seen in the figure, the heat map on the parametric space can display the full bone surface information with one single, structurally connected heat map. It requires four images to fully display the fracture frequency information with the conventional anatomical view. By referring to the Fig. 2(e), it can be seen that the most frequent intertrochanteric fracture region is located in the lower left corner of the lesser trochanter with a probability of around 70%. The high-risk red region passes through the lesser trochanter and extends to the greater trochanter along the intertrochanteric line on the posterior side of the proximal femur. Passing through the apex of greater trochanter, another high-risk region gradually develops along the intertrochanteric line from top to bottom on the anterior side. The fracture probability along the intertrochanteric line is around 40%. The distal lateral wall in the greater trochanter and the subtrochanteric region show a less frequent and more scattered fracture probability distribution in the map.

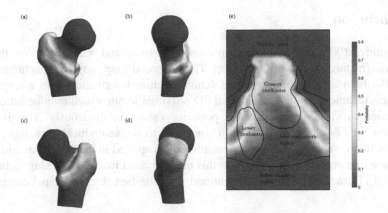

Fig. 2. Proximal femur fracture probability visualization with all 100 cases using four anatomical views: (a) anterior view, (b) medial view, (c) posterior view, (d) lateral view, and (e) the 2D parametric fracture heat map. (Color figure online)

The PCA analysis results based on the 100 cases are shown in Fig. 3. The first three major principal component images in 2D parametric space are presented. The principal component represents the largest possible variance of the observations. The regions with the same color in these images can represent the most frequent IT fracture patterns. In Fig. 3(a), the image shows that if IT fracture happens, it will either affect the intertrochanteric crest and intertrochanteric line, or the greater trochanter region at a time. Figure 3(b) indicates that the IT fracture happens along intertrochanteric crest and intertrochanteric line in near femoral neck or femur shaft side. It usually will not cross the ridge of the intertrochanteric crest and intertrochanteric line. The red region Fig. 3 (c) demonstrates the probability of injury on the greater trochanter. This can be caused by falling onto the greater trochanter due to aging and the loss of agility [6]. The blue region under the greater trochanter shows a mode of reverse obliquity fracture among IT fractures which run through the distal lateral wall in the intertrochanteric region.

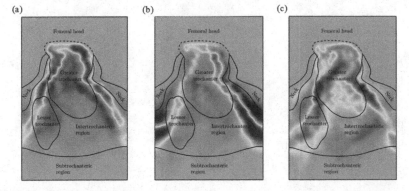

Fig. 3. The first three principal component images using 2D parametric space representation acquired from the principal component analysis. (Color figure online)

4 Conclusion

In this study, 100 cases of IT fractures are visualized and analyzed using the 2D parametric fracture probability heat map. The proposed map projection technique can project the high dimensional proximal femur fracture information onto a single 2D plane. This technique retains the original 3D proximal femur structure information and can be used to visualize anterior and posterior views simultaneously. This is more convenient for IT fracture visualization compared to the anatomical view representation. In addition, the principal component analysis is applied in the 2D parametric space for fracture line property analysis. With this unsupervised machine learning technique, the typical IT fracture patterns are identified with the first three principal component images.

References

1. Mundi, S., Pindiprolu, B., Simunovic, N., Bhandari, M.: Similar mortality rates in hip fracture patients over the past 31 years. Acta Orthop. **85**(1), 54–59 (2014)
2. Cole, P.A., Mehrle, R.K., Bhandari, M., Zlowodzki, M.: The pilon map: fracture lines and comminution zones in OTA/AO type 43C3 pilon fractures. J. Orthop. Trauma **27**(7), e152–e156 (2013)
3. Armitage, B.M., et al.: Mapping of scapular fractures with three-dimensional computed tomography. J. Bone Jt. Surg. - Ser. Am. **91**(9), 2222–2228 (2009)
4. Molenaars, R.J., Mellema, J.J., Doornberg, J.N., Kloen, P.: Tibial plateau fracture characteristics: computed tomography mapping of lateral, medial, and bicondylar fractures. J. Bone Jt. Surg. - Am. **97**(18), 1512–1520 (2015)
5. Sendra, G.H., Hoerth, C.H., Wunder, C., Lorenz, H.: 2D map projections for visualization and quantitative analysis of 3D fluorescence micrographs. Sci. Rep. **5**(July), 1–6 (2015)
6. Nevitt, M.C., Curnmings, S.R.: Type of fall and risk of hip and wrist fractures: the study of osteoporotic fractures. J. Am. Geriatr. Soc. **41**, 1226–1234 (1993)

Online Health Community

Why Does Interactional Unfairness Matter for Patient-Doctor Relationship Quality in Online Health Consultation? The Contingencies of Professional Seniority and Disease Severity

Xiaofei Zhang[1] , Xitong Guo[2] , Kee-hung Lai[3] , and Yi Wu[4]([⊠])

[1] Nankai University, Tianjin 30071, China
[2] Harbin Institute of Technology, Harbin 150001, China
[3] The Hong Kong Polytechnic University, Hung Hom, Hong Kong SAR
[4] Tianjin University, Tianjin 300072, China
yiwu@tju.edu.cn

Abstract. The development of online health platforms in recent years has drawn significant research attention to understanding patient participation. However, the unfairness in patient–doctor relationship development has been largely overlooked in the online health context. This study proposes and tests a model that examines how interactional unfairness (encompassing interpersonal unfairness and informational unfairness) influences online patient–doctor relationship quality and the contingent conditions of a doctor's professional seniority and disease severity on the unfairness–relationship quality link. Using objective data with 31,521 observations from a leading online health platform, this study employed rare-event logistic regression to test the model. The results show that interpersonal unfairness and informational unfairness have negative and positive effects on relationship quality, respectively, and a doctor's professional seniority and disease severity moderate the strength of the unfairness-relationship quality link. This study advances the knowledge of interactional unfairness in online health, and provides practical insights for online healthcare stakeholders into how to manage unfairness and consider the contingent factors to improve patient–doctor relationship in online health consultations.

Keywords: Online health consultation · Relationship quality
Interactional unfairness · Professional seniority · Disease severity

1 Introduction

The patient–doctor relationship is an important part of healthcare practices, and is essential for developing high-quality healthcare services [1, 2]. Given its practical significance, research efforts have been made to examine the antecedents and outcomes of patient–doctor relationships [3–6]. In recent years, the use of information and communication technologies (ICTs), e.g., online communities and online consultation, for healthcare has grown in popularity. The introduction of ICTs changes the previous

H. Chen et al. (Eds.): ICSH 2018, LNCS 10983, pp. 61–69, 2018.
https://doi.org/10.1007/978-3-030-03649-2_6

power structure in the traditional patient–doctor relationship in which doctors play a dominant role [7, 8]. Therefore, patients and doctors are encouraged to interact through a more equal status of "mutual participation" with shared power and responsibility [9]. Yet, little research has addressed the unique patient–doctor relationship in ICT-based contexts, and how a quality relationship between the two parties can be nurtured. Investigating this unique relationship, which determines the quality of healthcare services [10] and the quality of the existing patient–doctor relationship [11], is of significant practical relevance.

Among the different forms of ICTs implemented in healthcare, online health consultation (OHC) is an emerging service, and offers an alternative source of health information for patients and their relatives [41]. Through Web 2.0-based platforms, this service allows patients to inquiry into their health condition and obtain medical advice (e.g., recommendations and suggestions). Unlike patient–patient online communities, the health information in an OHC is mainly provided by health professionals [42], as if patients are consulting an Internet-doctor [43]. Examining the new patient–doctor relationship in an OHC is important because it differs from existing patient–doctor relationships in health literature: the online relationship is primarily formed through interactions between patients and doctors through an OHC and is influenced little by health institutions, treatments, and medicines (e.g., the waiting time in the hospital and the quality of the medicine).

The online context allows doctors and patients access to adequate resources, and they then develop a "roughly equal status" [12]. However, the interactions between doctors and patients are largely unfair because the former possess knowledge and power that the latter lack [13]. Therefore, the unfairness in the interaction between patients and doctors could be a common challenge in an OHC. Yet, little research has been conducted to examine the impact of the interactional unfairness on patient–doctor relationship development, particularly in the ICT-based contexts.

Although the significance of interactional (un)fairness has been widely studied [14, 15], its non-significant outcomes also show inconsistent results [16–22]. Thus, delineating the plausible explanations for the mixed findings is desirable. This study takes two steps to unravel these mixed findings. First, this study examines the subdimensions of interactional unfairness rather than treating it as a general concept, thereby providing a more finely tuned understanding of its impact on relationship development. In particular, interactional unfairness consists of two subdimensions: informational fairness (fairness perceptions on information) and interpersonal fairness (fairness perceptions on treatment) [23, 24]. Previous studies have shown that these two subdimensions have distinct relationships with organizational outcomes [25]. Second, we explore the boundary conditions under which interactional unfairness exerts different effects on relationship development.

To plug the research gaps previously mentioned, this study develops a theoretical model to investigate how interactional unfairness influences online patient–doctor relationship development and the moderating roles of two boundary factors on the unfairness influence for patient–doctor relationship quality. Specifically, this study aims to address the following research questions.

What are the impacts of interpersonal unfairness and informational unfairness on the quality of the online patient–doctor relationship?

How are these impacts contingent on a doctor's professional seniority and disease severity?

2   Research Model

Figure 1 shows the research model in this study.

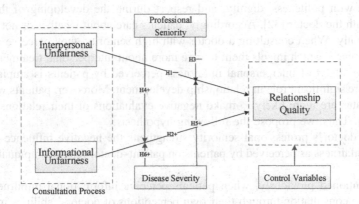

Fig. 1. Theoretical model

Individuals who have been treated unfairly by other people are motivated to terminate the relationship and reestablish a new fairness relationship with others [26]. When patients perceive low interpersonal fairness in an OHC, they will react to these perceptions, and negatively evaluate the interaction process [27]. Then, they generate negative evaluations toward their relationships with doctors and are less likely to enhance these relationships in the future. Otherwise, when patients are treated with politeness, dignity, and respect, and personally perceive that they are treated with fairly, they generate experience satisfaction with the relationship and will be motivated to enhance the it [28]. We thus propose the following hypothesis.

H1: Interpersonal unfairness as perceived by patients with doctors worsens their relationship quality with the latter in an OHC.

As mentioned previously, unfair personal treatment motivates patients to reestablish a fairer relationship [26]. Unlike the effect of interpersonal unfairness, informational unfairness in healthcare leads to "the setting up of a relationship of trust and confidence" [29] because the main purpose of an OHC is to obtain health information. Considering that patients do not have the same health knowledge as doctors (i.e., information asymmetry) [30], they evaluate the interaction process through their own perceptions of a doctor's abilities instead of directly observing of the consultation [29]. Then, they will believe that the doctor is doing his or her best in helping them [31]. When patients obtain inadequate information from the consultation, they trust that the doctor has the ability and is doing his or her best, and they attribute the reasons for the inadequate information to other factors, such as their failure to provide enough information to the doctor and the efficiency of the online consultation mechanism. Then, patients find new ways to obtain further information by enhancing their relationship with the doctor. Thus, we propose the following hypothesis.

H2: Informational unfairness as perceived by patients with doctors enhances their relationship quality with the latter in an OHC.

A doctor's professional seniority is represented the clinical title of doctor, and reflects a doctor's professional ability and experience. In an online consultation meeting with a doctor of professional seniority, patients are of a different status from the doctor. They perceive themselves as having a lower status relative to the doctor during the interaction. A lower status makes them pay more attention to whether they are treated with politeness, dignity, and respect during the developing of their relationship with the doctor [32]. Accordingly, patients care about whether or not they are treated equally. When consulting a doctor with high seniority, they perceive a greater status difference, which impels them to care more about interpersonal treatment. Then, the negative effect of interpersonal unfairness perceived by patients is amplified and plays a more significant role in relationship development. Moreover, patients who have a lower status are more likely to make negative evaluations of their relationship with others [33]. Thus, we propose the following hypothesis.

H3: A doctor's professional seniority strengthens the negative influence of interpersonal unfairness as perceived by patients on patient–doctor relationship quality in an OHC.

As mentioned previously, when patients perceive informational unfairness, they evaluate the consultation through their own perceptions of doctors' abilities instead of through direct observations [29]. In a consultation with a high-seniority doctor who is believed to have higher professional ability and richer clinical experience, patients perceive that the doctor is better able to address their diseases than doctors with lower seniority. Thus, when patients perceive a lack of information about their diseases because of inadequate information from the consultation, they are more likely to be motivated to obtain further information by enhancing their relationship with a high-seniority doctor compared with other doctors, given their stronger capability. Therefore, the effect of informational unfairness perceived by patients is amplified in the consultation with a high-seniority doctor. Thus, we propose the following hypothesis.

H4: A doctor's professional seniority strengthens the positive influence of informational unfairness as perceived by patients on patient–doctor relationship quality in an OHC.

Disease severity refers to the extent to which patients perceive the seriousness of their diseases [34]. Disease severity implies patients' perceived potential loss resulting from the diseases and serves as a contingent boundary of patients' evaluation of the consultation process [35]. Patients with high disease severity have a strong desire to deal with their diseases, and generally, have high expectations for online consultations [36]. When evaluating the interaction process, they rely more on the outcomes of the consultation than whether they were treated with politeness, dignity, and respect. Thus, when patients have high disease severity, the negative influence of interpersonal unfairness decreases. Therefore, we propose the following hypothesis.

H5: Disease severity lessens the negative influence of interpersonal unfairness as perceived by patients on patient–doctor relationship quality in an OHC.

Patients with high disease severity have high expectations of the online consultation with regard to obtaining adequate health information [36]. Given that inadequate information might be obtained from a doctor during an online consultation, patients with high disease severity have more information demands than patients with lower disease severity. Because they do not have the same health knowledge as the doctor (information asymmetry) [30], such patients tend to believe in the professional competency of the doctor. Accordingly, these patients are more proactive in enhancing their relationship with the doctor to obtain adequate information, such as by engaging in a phone consultation. Therefore, patients characterized by high disease severity are more prone to enhance the relationship by engaging in a phone consultation in view of the unfair information obtained through the online consultation. Therefore, we propose the following hypothesis.

H6: Disease severity strengthens the positive influence of informational unfairness as perceived by patients on patient–doctor relationship quality in an OHC.

3 Research Methodology

A JAVA based web crawler was developed to collect data from the website. To ensure validity, the respondents were confined to patients suffering from two diseases, lung cancer (a common cancer with high severity) and diabetes (a common chronic disease with low severity). The dataset includes two parts: the doctor's home page and the online consultation page. We collected online consultation data on these the two diseases that occurred from January 2014 to March 2015. To calculate the unfairness factors, we excluded topics with no more than one round (a question and an answer). In total, 31,521 topics with 93 doctors were collected.

Compared with an online consultation, a phone consultation with doctors is a more expensive and efficient approach. The transition from an online consultation to a phone consultation indicates that the patient holds the firm belief that the doctor can be relied on and an efficient and further interaction was worthy of the high expense, which implies a high-quality relationship [37]. Thus, we used whether or not the patient engaged in a phone consultation as a proxy of relationship quality. In the online service context, response time is an important predictor of service performance [38]. A rapid response implies that the doctor paid more attention to the patient's question, and the patient perceived politeness, dignity, and respect from the consultation [39]. Thus, we adopted the key factor of online service, the ratio of response time as a proxy for interpersonal unfairness. Informational unfairness refers to the unfairness perceptions of the information richness provided in an online consultation [23, 24]. Thus, we drew on the ratio of questions and replies in an online consultation to evaluate informational unfairness. The offline attributes and online experience of doctors were used as control variables. Table 1 summarizes the results of the rare-event logit regressions.

We find that interpersonal unfairness and informational unfairness have different effects on relationship quality. The effect of interpersonal unfairness is negative and significant ($\beta = -.226$, $p < 0.001$) (see Model 2), indicating that high interpersonal unfairness hinders the development of quality relationship. The effect of informational unfairness is positive and significant ($\beta = .270$, $p < 0.001$) (see Model 2), meaning that high informational unfairness contributes to the development of a quality relationship. Therefore, H1 and H2 are supported. The moderating effects of doctor seniority on the impacts of interpersonal unfairness ($\beta = -.010$, $p < 0.001$) and of informational

Table 1. Rare-event logit regressions results

Variables	Model estimating				Robustness check			
	Model 1	Model 2	Model 3-1	Model 3-2	Model 2R1	Model 2R2	Model 3-1R	Model 3-2R
Control variables								
Hospital level	.002 (.007)	−.003 (.010)	−.001 (.009)	−.005 (.009)		.002 (.008)	.008 (.019)	.003 (.013)
No. of Thank-you letter	−.163*** (.020)	−.287*** (.272)	−.325*** (.030)	−.289*** (.269)		.095* (.045)	−.355*** (.041)	−.390*** (.013)
No. of gift	.047*** (.005)	.052*** (.006)	.057*** (.007)	.051*** (006)		.040** (.012)	.039** (.014)	.070*** (.007)
Total patients	−.062 (.025)	.003*** (.032)	.017 (.033)	.034 (.032)		−.141** (.043)	.096 (.068)	.013 (.037)
Total visiting	.022 (.022)	−.022 (.027)	−.034 (.029)	.296*** (.026)		.054 (.042)	−.112 (.060)	−.040 (.032)
Professional seniority	.074*** (.008)	.258*** (.019)	.079*** (.016)	.259*** (.017)	.262*** (.018)	−.011 (.008)	.151*** (.025)	
Disease severity	.001* (.006)	.067*** (.009)	.080*** (.009)	−.006** (.013)	.069*** (.008)	.020* (.008)		−.043* (.018)
Independent variables								
Interpersonal unfairness		−.266*** (.040)	−.385*** (.026)	−.335*** (.034)	−.258*** (.034)	−.056* (.013)	.341*** (.018)	−.538*** (.035)
Informational unfairness		.270*** (.011)	.275*** (.009)	.276*** (.011)	.255*** (.010)	.028** (.007)	−.513*** (.050)	.361*** (.013)
Professional seniority* interpersonal unfairness			−.010*** (.002)				.003 (.010)	
Professional seniority* informational unfairness			.007*** (.001)				.009*** (.001)	
Disease severity * interpersonal unfairness				.011*** (.003)				.014*** (.004)
Disease severity * informational unfairness				.004** (.001)				.010*** (.001)
Number of observations	31521	31521	31521	31521	31521	31521	18665	16525
Log pseudo-likelihood	−2009	−1113	−1039	−1088	−1191	−1132	−565.5	−733.7
Pseudo R-square	.082	.491	.525	.503	.455	.102	.585	.554

Note: *p < .05 **p < .0l; ***p < .001 All testes are tailed.

Robust standard errors are in parentheses.

The Pseudo R-square we used in the paper is the R-square from logit regressions.

unfairness ($\beta = .007$, $p < 0.001$) (see Model 3-1) on quality relationship development are both significant, thus supporting H3 and H4. The moderating effects of disease severity on the impacts of interpersonal unfairness ($\beta = .011$, $p < 0.001$) and informational unfairness ($\beta = .004$, $p < 0.01$) (see Model 3-2) on quality relationship development are both significant, thus supporting H5 and H6.

We checked the robustness of the results in three different ways. First, we tested the robustness of Model 2 by dropping all of the control variables [40]. Model 2R1 in Table 1 shows consistent results with Model 2. Second, instead of measuring relationship quality by switching from an online consultation to a phone consultation, we used patients' giving of an online gift to the doctor as a dependent variable. Model 2R2 in Table 1 shows that the results are consistent with those of Model 2. Finally, the subsample of high disease severity (i.e., lung cancer) was used to test the robustness of Model 3-1, and the subsample of high-seniority doctors (i.e., senior doctor) was used to test the robustness of Model 3-2. Model 3-1R and Model 3-2R in Table 1 show the results. We find that most of our findings still hold, except for H3 in Model 3-1R.

4   Conclusion

This study presents four insightful key findings. First, as two components of interactional unfairness, interpersonal unfairness and informational unfairness have different effects on the development patient–doctor relationship. Second, both a doctor's professional seniority and the severity of the disease moderate the effects of interpersonal unfairness on relationship quality. Third, both the seniority of the doctor and the severity of the disease enhance the positive effects of informational unfairness on the development of relationship quality.

This paper makes several theoretical contributions. First, this study proposed and tested the patient–doctor relationship for unfairness and its online development, thus enriching our understanding of this newly shaped relationship. Second, as previously mentioned, some literature concluded mixed findings on the effects of interactional fairness, highlighting the need to specify the effect of interactional (un)fairness. By examining the effect of interactional unfairness from its subdimensions and boundary conditions, this study provided explanations for the mixed findings. Third, this study found the positive effect of informational unfairness on online patient–doctor relationship quality. Finally, this study also contributes to the fairness literature by using an objective method to measure unfairness.

The growing popularity of OHCs has changed the previous power equation between patient and doctor in healthcare. Even though patients have more authority in an OHC, their relationships with doctors are still unfair given the knowledge that doctors possess. However, few previous studies have explored this phenomenon in online healthcare. In addition, for the effects of interactional (un)fairness, previous literature has included many mixed findings that are left unexplained. Therefore, this study explored the interactional unfairness in an OHC and explained the mixed findings in the previous literature. This study contributes to online consultation, fairness theory, and patient–doctor interaction.

References

1. Onotai, L.O., Ibekwe, U.: The perception of patients of doctor-patient relationship in otorhinolaryngology clinics of the University of Port Harcourt Teaching Hospital (UPTH) Nigeria. Port. H. Med. J. **6**, 65–73 (2012)
2. Venkatesh, V., Zhang, X., Sykes, T.A.: "Doctors do too little technology": a longitudinal field study of an electronic healthcare system implementation. Inf. Syst. Res. **22**(3), 523–546 (2011)
3. Duan, G., Qiu, L., Yu, W., Hu, H.: Outpatient service quality and doctor-patient relationship: a study in Chinese public hospital. Int. J. Serv., Econ. Manag. **6**(1), 97–111 (2014)
4. Vick, S., Scott, A.: Agency in health care. Examining patients' preferences for attributes of the doctor–patient relationship. J. Health Econ. **17**(5), 587–605 (1998)
5. Pilnick, A., Dingwall, R.: On the remarkable persistence of asymmetry in doctor/patient interaction: a critical review. Soc. Sci. Med. **72**(8), 1374–1382 (2011)
6. Beckman, H.B., Markakis, K.M., Suchman, A.L., Frankel, R.M.: The doctor-patient relationship and malpractice: lessons from plaintiff depositions. Arch. Intern. Med. **154**(12), 1365–1370 (1994)
7. Burkhardt, M.E., Brass, D.J.: Changing patterns or patterns of change: the effects of a change in technology on social network structure and power. Adm. Sci. Q. **35**(1), 104–127 (1990)
8. Klecun, E.: Transforming healthcare: policy discourses of IT and patient-centred care. Eur. J. Inf. Syst. **25**(1), 64–76 (2016)
9. Rider, T., Malik, M., Chevassut, T.: Haematology patients and the internet – the use of on-line health information and the impact on the patient–doctor relationship. Patient Educ. Couns. **97**(2), 223–238 (2014)
10. Broom, A.: Virtually he@lthy: the impact of internet use on disease experience and the doctor-patient relationship. Qual. Health Res. **15**(3), 325–345 (2005)
11. Sreejesh, S., Mohapatra, S.: Theoretical development and hypotheses. Mixed Method Research Design, pp. 27–46. Springer, Cham (2014). https://doi.org/10.1007/978-3-319-02687-9_3
12. Ou, C.X., Pavlou, P.A., Davison, R.: Swift guanxi in online marketplaces: the role of computer-mediated communication technologies. MIS Q. **38**(1), 209–230 (2014)
13. Toombs, S.K.: The meaning of illness: a phenomenological approach to the patient-physician relationship. J. Med. Philos. **12**(3), 219–240 (1987)
14. Turel, O., Connelly, C.E.: Too busy to help: antecedents and outcomes of interactional justice in web-based service encounters. Int. J. Inf. Manag. **33**(4), 674–683 (2013)
15. Cropanzano, R., Ambrose, M.L., Greenberg, J., Cropanzano, R.: Procedural and distributive justice are more similar than you think: a monistic perspective and a research agenda. In: Advances in Organizational Justice, pp. 119–151. Stanford University Press, Stanford (2001)
16. Orth, U.: Secondary victimization of crime victims by criminal proceedings. Soc. Justice Res. **15**(4), 313–325 (2002)
17. Frenkel, S.J., Li, M., Restubog, S.L.D.: Management, organizational justice and emotional exhaustion among Chinese migrant workers: evidence from two manufacturing firms. Br. J. Ind. Relat. **50**(1), 121–147 (2012)
18. Leung, K., Smith, P.B., Wang, Z., Sun, H.: Job satisfaction in joint venture hotels in China: an organizational justice analysis. J. Int. Bus. Stud. **27**(5), 947–962 (1996)
19. Kuo, Y.-F., Wu, C.-M.: Satisfaction and post-purchase intentions with service recovery of online shopping websites: perspectives on perceived justice and emotions. Int. J. Inf. Manag. **32**(2), 127–138 (2012)
20. Mase, J.A., Ucho, A.: Job related tension, interactional justice and job involvement among workers of dangote cement company Gboko. Food Sci. Technol. **35**(ahead), 2105–2112 (2014)

21. Kwortnik, R.J., Han, X.: The influence of guest perceptions of service fairness on lodging loyalty in China. Cornell Hosp. Q. **52**(3), 321–332 (2011)
22. Zahra, S.A., Newey, L.R.: Maximizing the impact of organization science: theory building at the intersection of disciplines and/or fields. J. Manag. Stud. **46**(6), 1059–1075 (2009)
23. Colquitt, J.A.: On the dimensionality of organizational justice: a construct validation of a measure. J. Appl. Psychol. **86**(3), 386–400 (2001)
24. Greenberg, J.: Stealing in the name of justice: informational and interpersonal moderators of theft reactions to underpayment inequity. Organ. Behav. Hum. Decis. Process. **54**(1), 81–103 (1993)
25. Roch, S.G., Shanock, L.R.: Organizational justice in an exchange framework: clarifying organizational justice distinctions. J. Manag. **32**(2), 299–322 (2006)
26. Blau, P.M.: Exchange and Power in Social Life. Transaction Publishers, New Brunswick (1964)
27. Gouldner, A.W.: The norm of reciprocity: a preliminary statement. Am. Sociol. Rev. **25**(2), 161–178 (1960)
28. Oliver, R.L., Swan, J.E.: Consumer perceptions of interpersonal equity and satisfaction in transactions: a field survey approach. J. Mark. **53**(2), 21–35 (1989)
29. Arrow, K.J.: Uncertainty and the welfare economics of medical care. Am. Sociol. Rev. **53**(5), 941–973 (1963)
30. Rochaix, L.: Information asymmetry and search in the market for physicians' services. J. Health Econ. **8**(1), 53–84 (1989)
31. Kolstad, J.T., Chernew, M.E.: Quality and consumer decision making in the market for health insurance and health care services. Med. Care Res. Rev. **66**(1), 28–52 (2009)
32. Chen, Y.-R., Brockner, J., Greenberg, J.: When is it "a pleasure to do business with you?" The effects of relative status, outcome favorability, and procedural fairness. Organ. Behav. Hum. Decis. Process. **92**(1), 1–21 (2003)
33. Keltner, D., Gruenfeld, D.H., Anderson, C.: Power, approach, and inhibition. Psychol. Rev. **110**(2), 265–284 (2003)
34. Weissfeld, J.L., Brock, B.M., Kirscht, J.P., Hawthorne, V.M.: Reliability of health belief indexes: confirmatory factor analysis in sex, race, and age subgroups. Health Serv. Res. **21**(6), 777–793 (1987)
35. Jha, S., Balaji, M.: Perceived justice and recovery satisfaction: the moderating role of customer-perceived quality. Manag. Mark. **10**(2), 132–147 (2015)
36. Weinfurt, K.P., et al.: The correlation between patient characteristics and expectations of benefit from phase I clinical trials. Cancer **98**(1), 166–175 (2003)
37. Crosby, L.A., Evans, K.R., Cowles, D.: Relationship quality in services selling: an interpersonal influence perspective. J. Mark. **54**(3), 68–81 (1990)
38. Cooper, M.D.: Response time variations in an online search system. J. Am. Soc. Inf. Sci. **34**(6), 374–380 (1983)
39. Bies, R.J., Moag, J.S.: Interactional justice: communication criteria of fairness. Res. Negot. Organ. **1**(1), 43–55 (1986)
40. Shane, S.: Selling university technology: patterns from MIT. Manag. Sci. **48**(1), 122–137 (2002)
41. Lu, H.-Y., Shaw, B.R., Gustafson, D.H.: Online health consultation: examining uses of an interactive cancer communication tool by low-income women with breast cancer. Int. J. Med. Inform. **80**(7), 518–528 (2011)
42. Yan, L., Tan, Y.: Feeling blue? Go online: an empirical study of social support among patients. Inf. Syst. Res. **25**(4), 690–709 (2014)
43. Umefjord, G., et al.: Medical text-based consultations on the internet: a 4-year study. Int. J. Med. Inform. **77**(2), 114–121 (2008)

Exploring the Factors Influencing Patient Usage Behavior Based on Online Health Communities

Yinghui Zhao, Shanshan Li, and Jiang Wu[✉]

School of Information Management, Center for E-commerce Research and
Development, Wuhan University, Wuhan 430072, Hubei, China
jiangw@whu.edu.cn

Abstract. Online health community, as a new medical pattern, provides
patients with a platform for searching health-related information and seeking
medical help. Considering there is a causality loop between patients' doctor
choice behavior and patient review behavior, this study uses a simultaneous
equation system to explore the factors influencing patient usage behavior and the
reverse causality between patient choice and patient review. The results show
that online word-of-mouth of doctors is a principal factor that patients care about
when making online booking and consultation. In addition, our findings substantiate that there is a positive peer influence in the health field. This article
innovatively extends the online feedback mechanism from e-commerce to online
health field, and studies the patient usage behavior as an economic system,
which has a high significance for the theoretical study of online health
community.

Keywords: Online health community · Patient choice · Word-of-mouth
Information adoption theory · Simultaneous equations

1 Introduction

With the development of information technology, online health has changed the way
people obtain medical services, providing patients with a platform for seeking medical
help and getting informational and emotional support [1, 2]. Nevertheless, since online
health services contain high degrees of uncertainty and risk, it can be difficult for
patients to evaluate doctors' services and make decisions [3, 4]. Before making online
booking and consultation, patients regularly seek doctors' service quality information.
And after receiving medical services, patients will evaluate doctors' service quality
through the online review systems of online health communities, which thereby
affecting the doctors' online word-of-mouth.

Considering the relationship between patients' doctor choice behavior and patient
review behavior works in both directions, this paper uses a simultaneous equation
system [5] to fully capture the factors influencing patient choice and patient review, as
well as the reverse causality between the two behaviors.

H. Chen et al. (Eds.): ICSH 2018, LNCS 10983, pp. 70–76, 2018.
https://doi.org/10.1007/978-3-030-03649-2_7

2 Research Design

2.1 Research Model

In the online health community, patient usage behavior consists of patients' doctor choice behavior and patient review behavior. This article uses the number of appointments and votes as the measurement of patients' doctor choice behavior and patient review behavior, respectively. In order to better explain patient usage behavior, we introduce the information adoption model proposed by Sussman and Siegal [6]. Specifically, Fig. 1 presents the research model with the appointment quantity as dependent variable, and Fig. 2 shows the model taking the number of votes as dependent variable.

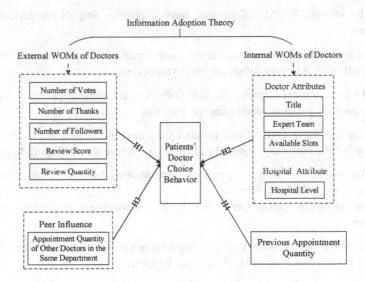

Fig. 1. The research model of patients' doctor choice behavior.

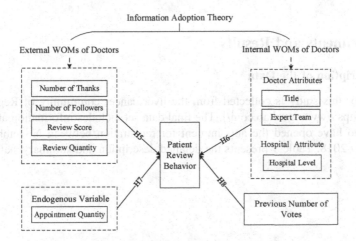

Fig. 2. The research model of patient review behavior.

2.2   Hypotheses

Online word-of-mouth (WOM) has been acknowledged as an important factor affecting consumer choice and sellers' reputation [7, 8]. Specifically, online WOMs can be divided into external WOMs hosted by consumers and internal WOMs hosted by sellers [9]. Based on this, the following hypotheses are made:

H1. The external WOMs of doctors have a positive impact on patients' doctor choice behavior.

H2. The internal WOMs of doctors have a positive impact on patients' doctor choice behavior.

H5. The external WOMs of doctors have a positive impact on patient review behavior.

H6. The internal WOMs of doctors have a positive impact on patient review behavior.

The medical level among doctors in the same department promotes each other [10]. In consideration of this peer influence, we hypothesize:

H3. The appointment quantity of other doctors in the same department has a positive impact on patients' doctor choice behavior.

Extant studies have verified that product sales are autocorrelated [5, 11]. In addition, online WOM also has transitivity [12]. So we derive the following hypotheses:

H4. The number of doctors' previous appointments have a positive impact on patients' doctor choice behavior.

H8. The number of doctors' previous votes have a positive impact on patient review behavior.

Besides, there is a causality loop existing between patients' doctor choice behavior and patient review behavior [13]. Hence, we hypothesize:

H7. The number of doctors' appointments have a positive impact on patient review behavior.

3   Experiments and Results

3.1   Description of the Data

The data for this study is collected from the liver cancer community of Registration Website (https://www.guahao.com/). The final data set includes information about 608 doctors who have opened the appointment for registration between November 2017 and January 2018. Table 1 presents the detailed description and summary statistics for our sample.

Table 1. Variables description and summary statistics.

Variable	Description	Mean	Std. dev.	Min	Max
BookNum	Cumulative appointment quantity in moment t-1	1964.93	4315.682	1	57000
Book_Num	Appointment increment from moment t-1 to t	32.93	44.31	0	367
Title	The title of the doctor (coded as 1 if the doctor is a chief physician or professor, 0 otherwise)	0.599	0.490	0	1
Expert	The expert team the doctor belongs to (coded as 1 if the doctor belongs to the expert team, 0 otherwise)	0.383	0.486	0	1
ArrangeNum	The available slots of the doctor in moment t-1	2.059	3.490	0	14
HosRank	The hospital ranking (tertiary hospital = 3, secondary hospital = 2, primary hospital = 1, general hospital = 0)	2.988	0.1328	1	3
VoteNum	The cumulative number of votes in moment t-1	13.217	31.775	0	388
Vote_Num	The increment of votes from moment t-1 to t	0.957	1.654	0	31
Followers	The followers number of the doctor in moment t-1	390.652	477.551	1	2821
Thanks	The thanks number of the doctor in moment t-1	0.226	0.887	0	9
RevScore	The review score of the doctor in moment t-1	9.290	0.483	7.1	10
RevNum	The review quantity of the doctor in moment t-1	152.283	327.960	5	4342
DepBnum	The appointment quantity of other doctors in the same department in moment t-1	2510.491	4293.351	0	28000

3.2   Empirical Model Specification

This article constructs the following two-equation system with the increment of appointments and votes as dependent variables, corresponding to the model 1 and model 2. In this study, we use panel data analysis method to explore the factors influencing patient usage behavior. Given that the ranges of some variables are much larger, we take logarithm of them.

$$Book\_Num_t = \beta_0 + \beta_1 * \text{Ln}(BookNum_{t-1}) + \beta_2 * Vote\_Num_t + \beta_3 *$$
$$\text{Ln}(Followers_{t-1}) + \beta_4 * Thanks_{t-1} + \beta_5 * RevScore_{t-1} + \beta_6 *$$
$$\text{Ln}(RevNum_{t-1}) + \beta_7 * \text{Ln}(DepBNum_{t-1}) + \beta_8 * Title_{t-1} + \beta_9 * \tag{1}$$
$$Expert_{t-1} + \beta_{10} * ArrangeNum_{t-1} + \beta_{11} * HosRank_{t-1} + \varepsilon_1$$

$$Vote\_Num_t = \alpha_0 + \alpha_1 * \text{Ln}(VoteNum_{t-1}) + \alpha_2 * Book\_Num_t + \alpha_3 *$$
$$\text{Ln}(Followers_{t-1}) + \alpha_4 * Thanks_{t-1} + \alpha_5 * RevScore_{t-1} + \alpha_6 *$$
$$\text{Ln}(RevNum_{t-1}) + \alpha_7 * Title_{t-1} + \alpha_8 * Expert_{t-1} + \alpha_9 * \tag{2}$$
$$HosRank_{t-1} + \varepsilon_2$$

3.3   Results and Discussions

This paper uses three stage least square (3SLS) to analyze the data, and the estimated results are shown in Table 2.

Table 2. Model results.

Independent variables	Book_Num$_t$	Vote_Num$_t$
Book_Num$_t$		0.011***
Vote_Num$_t$	1.575***	
Ln(BookNum$_{t-1}$)	0.812***	
Ln(VoteNum$_{t-1}$)		0.049***
Ln(Followers$_{t-1}$)	0.678***	0.076***
Thanks$_{t-1}$	0.036	0.003
RevScore$_{t-1}$	0.484	0.042
Ln(RevNum$_{t-1}$)	0.021**	0.052**
Ln(DepBnum$_{t-1}$)	0.761***	
Title $_{t-1}$	1.181**	0.028***
Expert $_{t-1}$	3.522*	0.05**
ArrangeNum $_{t-1}$	1.528***	
HosRank $_{t-1}$	1.652***	0.069***
_cons	−8.31	−0.428

Note: p < 0.1, *p < 0.05, **p < 0.01, ***p < 0.001

Analysis of the Influencing Factors on Patients' Doctor Choice Behavior. In terms of external WOMs of doctors, the number of doctors' votes, followers, and reviews all have a significant positive impact on patient choice. Contrastingly, there is no significant impact of the number of thanks and review scores on patient choice. This is because the variances of thanks and review scores are so small that it is difficult for patients to differentiate doctors' service qualities from them. Besides, the results indicate that internal WOMs of doctors have a significant positive effect on patient choice. As for the peer influence, the appointment quantity of other doctors in the same department has a significant positive impact on patient decision, which suggests that the appointment quantity among doctors in the same department promotes each other. In addition, our findings confirm that the number of appointments have a positive autocorrelation: the more historical appointments the doctor has, the more patients choose the doctor for registration.

Analysis of the Influencing Factors on Patient Review Behavior. As for the impact of doctors' external WOMs on patient review behavior, the results indicate that the number of doctors' followers and reviews have a significant positive effect on the number of patients votes for doctors. In contrast, the number of thanks and review scores have no significant influence on patient voting behavior, because the thanks and review scores gap among doctors is so small that there is no distinction. We also found there is a significant and positive impact of doctors' internal WOMs on patient review behavior. Besides, doctors' previous vote quantity has a significant positive effect on patient voting behavior. Moreover, doctors' appointment quantity has a significant positive impact on patient voting behavior. The results substantiate the existence of a reverse causality between patients' doctor choice behavior and patient review behavior.

4 Conclusions

This paper uses panel data analysis and simultaneous equation model to study the factors influencing patient usage behavior and the reverse causality between patient choice and patient review. The results provide us with valuable insight into the role of online word-of-mouth and peer influence in the online health community. Future studies may consider the regional development level as a moderating variable to explore the differences in the influences on patient usage behavior in different regions.

References

1. Xiao, N., et al.: Factors influencing online health information search: an empirical analysis of a national cancer-related survey. Decis. Support Syst. **57**(1), 417–427 (2014)
2. Ziebland, S., et al.: How the internet affects patients' experience of cancer: a qualitative study. BMJ **328**(7439), 564 (2004)
3. Cohen, R., Elhadad, M., Birk, O.: Analysis of free online physician advice services. PLoS ONE **8**(3), e59963 (2013)
4. Lederman, R., et al.: Who can you trust? Credibility assessment in online health forums. Health Policy Technol. **3**(1), 13–25 (2014)
5. Duan, W., Gu, B., Whinston, A.B.: Do online reviews matter? – An empirical investigation of panel data. Decis. Support Syst. **45**(4), 1007–1016 (2008)
6. Sussman, S.W., Siegal, W.S.: Informational influence in organizations: an integrated approach to knowledge adoption. Inf. Syst. Res. **14**(1), 47–65 (2003)
7. Chen, Y.F.: Herd behavior in purchasing books online. Comput. Hum. Behav. **24**(5), 1977–1992 (2008)

8. Dhanasobhon, S., Chen, P.Y., Smith, M.D.: An analysis of the differential impact of reviews and reviewers at Amazon.com. In: International Conference on Information Systems, ICIS, Montreal, Quebec, Canada, December 2007

9. Gu, B., Park, J., Konana, P.: Research note—the impact of external word-of-mouth sources on retailer sales of high-involvement products. Inform. Syst. Res. **23**, 182–196 (2012)

10. Bhatia, T., Wang, L.: Identifying physician peer-to-peer effects using patient movement data. Int. J. Res. Mark. **28**(1), 51–61 (2011)

11. Elberse, A., Eliashberg, J.: Demand and supply dynamics for sequentially released products in international markets: the case of motion pictures. Market. Sci. **22**(4), 544 (2003)

12. Bowman, D., Narayandas, D.: Managing customer-initiated contacts with manufacturers: the impact on share of category requirements and word-of-mouth behavior. J. Mark. Res. **38**(3), 281–297 (2001)

13. Soares, A.A.C., Costa, F.J.D.: The influence of perceived value and customer satisfaction on the word of mouth behavior: an analysis in academies of gymnastics. Energy Fuels **22**(3), 2033–2042 (2008)

Using Social Media to Estimate the Audience Sizes of Public Events for Crisis Management and Emergency Care

Patrick Felka[1(✉)], Artur Sterz[2], Oliver Hinz[1], and Bernd Freisleben[2]

[1] Goethe University Frankfurt, Frankfurt am Main, Germany
felka@wiwi.uni-frankfurt.de
[2] Technische Universität Darmstadt, Darmstadt, Germany

Abstract. Public events such as soccer games, concerts, or street festivals attract large crowds of visitors. In an emergency situation, estimations about current events and their numbers of visitors are important to be able to react early and effectively by performing adequate countermeasures. Previous research has proposed approaches to detect events like accidents and catastrophes by relying on user-generated content and reporting event-related information. To be proactive in case of an emergency, it is important to know what is happening in direct proximity, even if it is not yet affected by the catastrophe. Therefore, information about ongoing events and numbers of visitors in the surrounding environment is indispensable. We develop a system design that allows collecting and merging event-related information from social media to provide estimations of the audience sizes. We illustrate the potential of our approach by estimating the number of visitors of soccer games, fairs, street festivals, music festivals, and concerts, and by comparing it to the real numbers of visitors. Our results indicate that matching event-related user-generated content leads to improvements of the estimations. Finally, we demonstrate the usefulness of the system in a recent crisis scenario.

Keywords: Emergency and crisis management · Crisis coordination
Event estimation · Social media analysis

1 Introduction

Public events such as concerts, fairs, soccer games, or festivals attract large crowds of people and occur frequently. Information about ongoing events and their numbers of visitors is important for various reasons. Especially in case of an emergency, knowledge about ongoing and upcoming events and their corresponding numbers of visitors may play a crucial role in the planning of evacuation measures.

During the last years, social media have become major platforms for everyday communication. The most popular online social network (OSN) is Facebook (with 1.13 billion active users per day) [1]. Users often communicate their participation in events such as concerts, music festivals, exhibitions, or create their own events in social networks. The potential that lies in the utilization of these data sources for prediction purposes is tremendous.

© Springer Nature Switzerland AG 2018
H. Chen et al. (Eds.): ICSH 2018, LNCS 10983, pp. 77–89, 2018.
https://doi.org/10.1007/978-3-030-03649-2_8

Indeed, previous research analyzes the value of user-generated content (UGC) for emergency and crisis management. The vast number of approaches consider event detection as well as reporting of unplanned events to provide real-time information about the current situation. Using such approaches, researchers are able to detect, assess, summarize, or report messages of interest for emergency and crisis coordination [2–4]. Another stream of studies investigates the detection of catastrophes like earthquakes [5–7] or epidemics [8]. The large majority of existing approaches in the context of emergency management analyses UGC to provide information about detected events like accidents or catastrophes and the current situation. Therefore, these approaches are reactive and often support specific types of events (e.g., catastrophes and epidemics).

To be proactive in case of emergencies, such as terrorist attacks, tsunami warnings, or chemical accidents, it is also important to know what is happening in the direct proximity, even if it is not yet affected by the catastrophe. Therefore, planned events – such as street festivals, fairs, soccer matches, and concerts – also play an important role in emergency management. Such events attract large crowds of visitors and appear regularly. The audience size plays a decisive role in carrying out appropriate evacuation measures or for preventing further harm.

Therefore, our work investigates the ability to estimate the audience sizes of events based on Facebook events and presents a system design to collect and process the data effectively. Based on the collected data, our system is able to present information about ongoing and upcoming events on a web interface. The presented information helps to get an initial overview of the location of local events and their number of visitors. The estimates will be continuously updated and available at all times, even if no disaster occurs. If a disaster or a catastrophe occurs, this information serves as a starting point for countermeasures, such as an evacuation. The research question addressed in our work is highly relevant for emergency care and crisis management by enabling professional responders to react early and more precisely with countermeasures to save lives.

2   Related Work

The use of social media to support emergency and crisis management gained increased attention during the last few years. Much of the previous research in the area of social media and emergency management focuses on the detection of events or reports information about the detected event based on UGC for emergency or crisis management.

Cameron, Power, Robinson, and Yin [2], for instance, propose a system to detect, assess, summarize, and report messages of interest for crisis coordination on Twitter. The authors present a system, to extract and report relevant Twitter messages to the crisis management about an emergency incident as it unfolds. Another approach by Schulz, Ristoski, and Paulheim [3] makes use of semantic enrichment for real-time identification of small-scale incidents. Pohl, Bouchachia, and Hellwagner [4] study the detection of different sub-events based on metadata from Flickr and YouTube in critical situations using clustering methods. Earle, Bowden, and Guy [7] study the detection of earthquakes based on Twitter by monitoring tweets about earthquakes. Other studies also investigate the recognition of earthquakes or epidemics based on Twitter data [5, 6, 8].

Another stream of literature investigates the value and use of social media during emergency and crisis situations [9–11] or consider the value of social media by the government during emergencies and disasters [12–14].

Overall, these approaches are able to support the emergency care and crisis management teams at different levels. Some studies consider the benefits of social media by processing UGC, while others consider the benefits of social media to communicate with the public and other stakeholders in the event of an emergency or crisis. However, these approaches do not come without limitations. In particular, approaches to detect or report events are reactive and support only specific types of events, such as catastrophes or epidemics. Yet, planned events – such as street festivals, soccer matches, and concerts – represent the majority of events. These events may also have a major impact on the local environment and occur more frequently. Therefore, the goal of our approach is not to detect an unplanned event, but rather to provide information about planned events and their estimated audience size.

To the best of our knowledge, there is no system that can estimate or predict the number of visitors based on event-related UGC. Such a system is not only important for crisis management and emergency care but also for authorities which can benefit from our system to prevent other problems. For example, large cities like Munich [15] or Berlin [16] allocate their emergency personnel for events, such as doctors and paramedics based on the number of visitors, which is typically an estimation based on values of previous years or the number of sold tickets. These estimations are relatively precise for ticket events, where the number of visitors depends on the number of tickets sold. However, it can also deviate strongly in the case of no-ticket events, such as street festivals where the event takes place without any access restrictions.

3 System Design

Our approach aims to estimate the number of event visitors based on UGC. To provide a theoretical foundation for the estimation of the visitor numbers, we synthesize the findings of previous research on electronic Word-of-Mouth (eWOM) communication as one part of UGC. eWOM is the electronic form of Word-of-Mouth (WOM) and is defined as the informal, interpersonal communication between consumers about content such as products, brands, or services [17, 18]. Past studies already show a significant influence of WOM on users' information search and decision-making (e.g., Engel, Blackwell, and Kegerreis [19]; Lynn [20]). The concept of eWOM describes the exchange of interpersonal communication using electronic media such as social networks.

To estimate the visitor numbers of events, we rely on two major effects of eWOM in social media: (1) social media is often used for self-enhancement and self-representation purposes [21], (2) sharing content may be positively reflected to the sender of the message. By sharing the participation in an event, the user draws attention to an event but also shows the participation in the event. The latter is also an expression of self-representation in social media, which may seem favorable to the sender. Further, drawing attention to an upcoming event can influence other peoples' decision-making. We suggest that the volume of eWOM or rather UGC related to an event will be a suitable estimator for the number of visitors because it reflects the attention and participation in an event. We rely on these findings and use them as a starting point for our system design.

3.1 Methodology – Design-Science Approach

The research objective of this paper is to design, implement, and evaluate a system to structure and collect event-based data for estimation purposes. We will follow the principles of design science research using the methodology suggested by Hevner et al. [22]. The authors provide guidelines for effective and high-quality design science research. Our research is compliant with these guidelines which are described in more detail in [22].

3.2 An Event Visitor Estimation System

We aim to design a system that is able to collect event information and estimate their number of visitors. To achieve this and derive accurate estimations, our system needs to collect, update and match data about ongoing and upcoming events from UGC. In the following, we present a system design to process UGC from social media, describe the core idea, and explain each component in detail. Figure 1 gives a brief overview of the individual components of our system.

A fundamental component of the system is the data collection component. This element collects event-related UGC about upcoming or ongoing events from social media platforms like Facebook. Social media platforms offer the opportunity to create events, invite friends, and to send messages related to an event or location. Our system can capture this information and store it in the form of metadata. This includes data such as the number of messages related to an event, number of Likes, Shares, and Comments on Facebook events or the number of users who plan to attend events. However, this data is subject to constant change and must be updated continuously in order to provide accurate estimations. A core element of the system is the event repository with the matching engine. The event repository stores collected events as event objects. These objects are characterized by mainly three dimensions: time span, location, and category. We separate events into these three dimensions to match duplicate events by using similarity metrics or clustering methods. The matching of events takes place when an event occurs in the same location as another, the time of the two events overlap, and the events belong to the same category. This procedure intends to improve accuracy by avoiding event duplicates to be viewed as single events.

The estimation engine allows us to select a tailored training set of events and to apply estimation methods to the training set. The basic idea behind the selection is that events at the same place or in the same category behave similarly in terms of UGC and numbers of visitors. We make this assumption and estimate the audience size of events at the same location or within the same category. Furthermore, this is also useful to apply complex and time-consuming machine learning approaches with an increasing volume of event data. Therefore, an efficient selection of events for the training set is important. For example, if the number of visitors during a soccer game constitutes the prediction target, one possible selection would be to add previous events of the same

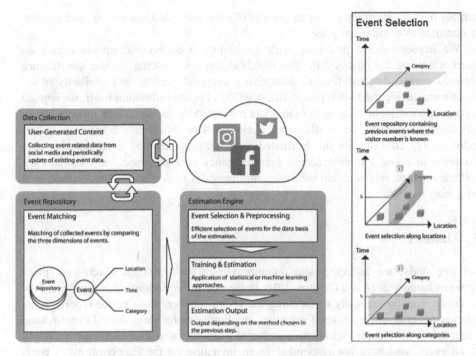

Fig. 1. Overview of our system design

Fig. 2. Efficient selection of events (Color figure online)

category or at the same location into the training set. Figure 2 demonstrates the selection of events among the event dimensions. The blue cubes illustrate past events for which activity in social networks and the number of visitors is known. The yellow cubes illustrate ongoing or upcoming events with unknown audience size. The diagram in the middle illustrates the selection of previous events at the same location; the lower diagram shows the selection of similar events at different locations. This training set is the basis for the subsequent estimation phase. The methods and approaches depend on the particular target, e.g., estimating the audience size by using statistical methods or data mining methods.

4 Proof of Concept

In essence, our prototype consists of three connected components: backend, frontend, and a database as a connecting element in between. Further, our prototype processes Facebook events as one possible source for event-related UGC. Social networks such as Facebook offer their users the opportunity to organize events, invite other users, inform participants about news, and promote an event. Other users on Facebook can announce their interest or intention to attend an event. Furthermore, users can post comments on the event page and interact with the event organizer or with other users. Thus, Facebook events have different indicators, such as the number of comments, number of users attending an event, number of users interested in an event, and number of comments on the event page.

We implemented a prototype with the ability to collect and update events on Facebook using the official API. For matching duplicate events, we use the distance between events, date and time to determine a temporal overlap, and similarity of the event name (using the Jaro Winkler distance [23]). For the estimation itself, we applied regression models. In contrast to many data mining methods, regression models can be estimated and interpreted to illustrate relationships or differences between variables more easily. To visualize the estimated data, we implemented a responsive web-frontend, to allow a mobile access for emergency care personnel. It visualizes the collected events, related event estimates, and provides basic event-related information on a map.

5 Dataset

For our study, we collected data on approximately 400 events which took place between January 2014 and October 2016, in Germany. For each event, we collected the audience sizes by manually researching the visitor numbers from police reports, news articles, ticket agencies, football statistics, etc. Furthermore, we collected event-related Facebook events. These include the number of users who attend an event, are interested in an event, and have not responded to an invitation on the Facebook event page. Table 1 provides a brief description of all the variables and data sources.

Table 1. Description of variables and sources

Variables	Source	Description
Attending	Collected using Facebook API	Number of Facebook users attending an event
home_attending *away_attending*		Number of Facebook users attending an event of home\away soccer team (available only for soccer events)
stadium Dummies		e.g., 1 = stadium1; 0 = otherwise
category Dummies	Classified manually	e.g., 1 = soccer_game; 0 = otherwise
Visitors	Collected manually	Number of visitors to an event

6 Evaluation

Our evaluation consists of three parts. The first part examines whether estimates based on UGC yield better results than estimates based on historical data. The second part evaluates our estimation model within the system design. In the last part of the evaluation, we demonstrate the potential of our system based on a case study.

6.1   Baseline

In the first part of the evaluation, we examine estimations based historical data at the same location as well as estimations based on UGC. Further, we examine estimation improvements by matching duplicate events with the matching engine.

For this part of the evaluation, we choose soccer matches for our base model. Soccer games have the advantage that they occur frequently. Furthermore, in contrast to other events like street festivals, where the number is often approximated, the visitor number of soccer games are publically available and very precise. Soccer games are also suitable for our investigation to evaluate the utility of the matching engine. This is due to the fact that soccer events on Facebook are usually created and disseminated by the soccer club. To promote the next game of the soccer club each club creates and share their own event on Facebook. Since two teams are involved in a soccer match and each club promotes one event on Facebook. As a result, there are often several events on Facebook which actually refer to the same event.

We estimate three different regression models, which we introduce in the following: Our first model illustrates a simple estimation based on the number of visitors in the past. Therefore, this model includes only dummy variables for each stadium. The second model additionally describes the relation between the number of visitors and the number of *home_attending* users on the Facebook events created by the home team. The final regression model considers the gain by an additional matching of redundant events on Facebook. Here, we add the variable *away_attending* to the model, which includes the number of attending users in the event of the opposing team.

We estimate our models using ordinary least square regression to explain the audience size represented by the number of visitors. We use cluster-robust standard errors to mitigate problems with heteroscedasticity. Table 2 presents the estimation results for all three models.

The results of the F-test ($p < .000$) show for all models that at least one of the variables can explain some variation in the dependent variable in a statistically significant way. The adjusted R^2 (96.8%–97.3%) indicates a very good fit. Our first model captures large parts of the variance explaining the visitor numbers by using dummy variables only. This is not surprising because a stadium has a maximum capacity of visitors and most teams have devoted fans like season ticket holders who lead to rather high minimum capacity utilization. Therefore, the visitor numbers in a stadium are quite stable and can be estimated accurately with a dummy variable for the single stadiums. The second model improves the results only to a very small extent by including the number of Facebook users attending an event of the home team.

Our third model illustrates the power of the matching engine by matching duplicate events on Facebook. Here, the results show that the already quite accurate estimate of previous models can be improved even further. The variable *away_attending* ($p < .01$) is highly significant and positively related to the number of visitors while *home_attending* is not statistically significant. This indicates that the dummy variable of the stadium can capture the variance related to visitor numbers of the home team, but variance related to the visitor numbers of the away team can be estimated using UGC. Therefore, for further improvement of the estimates, a combination of event data is indispensable.

Table 2. Estimation results

Variable	Model 1 Coef. (Std. Dev.)	Model 2 Coef. (Std. Dev.)	Model 3 Coef. (Std. Dev.)
home_attending	–	0.40 (0.23)	0.04 (0.18)
away_attending	–	–	1.33*** (0.26)
stadium = Stadium 1 (omitted)	–	–	–
Stadium 2	−17632.57*** (890.40)	−16322.71*** (1229.69)	−17069.44*** (1033.50)
Stadium 3	2773.308** (1277.52)	3268.10** (1299.83)	3143.37** (1256.57)
Stadium 4	32553.67*** (497.03)	31797.61*** (652.34)	32788.77*** (633.02)
Stadium 5	−2278.571 (1461.78)	−1624.188 (1492.94)	−1873.15 (1415.97)
Stadium 6	−19598.67*** (595.57)	−18197.72*** (1065.06)	−18273.01*** (862.76)
Stadium 7	−33877.08*** (506.42)	−32370.78*** (1071.26)	−32745.08*** (891.17)
Stadium 8	12662.93*** (528.74)	13068.18*** (647.26)	13100.74*** (622.41)
Stadium 9	5314.714*** (942.02)	5463.47*** (967.99)	5578.88*** (941.04)
Stadium 10	−7679.429*** (1733.31)	−6514.93*** (1886.58)	−7693.48*** (1489.14)
Stadium 11	7776.00*** (485.20)	8823.24*** (841.06)	6889.83*** (775.14)
Stadium 12	−31876.92*** (507.19)	−30689.28*** (913.44)	−31036.41*** (760.76)
Stadium 13	−20926.64*** (921.93)	−19384.50*** (1317.20)	−19986.50*** (1084.47)
Stadium 14	3486.77** (1621.70)	4058.90** (1647.50)	3801.67** (1580.54)
Stadium 15	−19792.79*** (592.14)	−18395.39*** (1049.04)	−18764.21*** (837.33)
Stadium 16	−7625.00*** (594.28)	−7167.91*** (683.61)	−7320.42*** (637.49)
Constant	48600*** (485.20)	46838.84*** (1229.69)	46486.27*** (1033.50)
N	207	207	207
Root MSE	3138.1	3116.2	2874.2
Adj. R^2	0.9678	0.9682	0.9730

Note: Standard errors in parentheses; * $p < .10$, ** $p < 0.05$, *** $p < 0.01$

To summarize, our analysis of soccer data indicates a strong positive relationship between Facebook users attending an event on Facebook and the real number of visitors attending the event. Furthermore, the analysis shows that matching duplicate events on Facebook can improve the estimation significantly.

6.2 Estimation Model

In our second analysis, we examine the visitor numbers for five different categories of events. The intention is to show a more general and complex use case compared to the previous analysis. For this part of the evaluation, we use the complete dataset described in Sect. 5 to estimate the audience size. Our regression model for this part of the evaluation is as follows:

$$visitors = \beta_0 + \beta_1 attending + \sum_{s=1}^{S} y_s attending * category_s + \sum_{s=1}^{S} z_s category_s + \varepsilon$$

Table 3. Estimation results

Variable	Coef.	Std. Dev.
Attending	6.68***	0.68
attending * category = soccer_game (omitted)	–	–
concert	−4.92***	0.80
fair	0.13	1.91
music_festival	−7.28***	1.06
street_ festival	216.51**	102.65
category = soccer_game (omitted)	–	–
concert	−10876.56***	5899.38
fair	194636.1***	23474.99
music_festival	69646.32**	35912.84
street_ festival	474078.1**	243099.2
Constant	26049.75***	1675.06
N	391	
Adj. R^2	0.5009	

Note: Standard errors in parentheses; * p < .10, ** p < 0.05, *** p < 0.01

As described in Sect. 5, the viewers counting method differs between the categories. To take this into account, we add the variable *attending* as well as *attending* depending on the *category*, i.e., as interaction effect. This allows us to quantify the individual effect of attending Facebook users on the visitor numbers in each category. The last part of the equation describes the constant depending on *category*.

Table 3 presents the estimation results for the presented model. The adjusted R^2 of the model is 50.09% and shows that our model captures large parts of the variance that explains the number of visitors. Furthermore, our results show a general positive effect of the number of attending people in UGC ($p < .01$) on the actual number of visitors. We also find an interesting difference for attending depending on the category music festivals ($p < .01$) and street festivals ($p < .05$). The coefficient for street festivals is much higher than for the other ones while the coefficient for music festivals is negative. One possible explanation lies in the different counting methods of the categories. People on multi-day street festivals are counted several times and usually, there are no access restrictions. In contrast, for music festivals, there are access restrictions and the ratio between users attending an event on Facebook and the actual number of visitors is much higher compared to soccer games. The category constants reveal significant differences between all categories. Fairs, music festivals, and street festivals are significantly larger compared to soccer games, while concerts are significantly smaller events.

Overall, our model can explain large parts of the variance and indicates a strong, significant relationship between visitor numbers and UGC. This confirms our assumption that events on Facebook reflect the public interest fairly, but also that events of the same category behave similarly in terms of UGC and visitor numbers.

6.3   Case Study

For our case study, we selected an amok run that took place in July 2016 in the city of Munich (Germany) to demonstrate the capabilities of our system. During this amok run, an 18-year-old student killed nine people at the Olympic Shopping Center (OEZ) in the district of Moosach. At 05:50 pm, the first shots were fired at a restaurant next to the shopping mall [24]. Two minutes after the first shots, the police received the first emergency calls [25]. The gunman disappeared and the police tried to locate him. At 06:35 pm, the police in Munich issued warnings to the population because the gunman was untraceable. The police were able to locate the gunman more than 2 h later at 08:30 pm. During this 2 h the gunman committed suicide [24]. The police were on the lookout for possible other perpetrators and continued the evacuation. During the evacuation, 64 shootings and 2 kidnappings were reported to the police and distributed to social media [26, 27]. At 01:31 am, the police gave the all-clear signal: the person who had killed himself was the only offender, and it turned out that all other reported shootings and kidnappings were false alarms.

After the first emergency calls, our system would have been able to provide information about nearby events immediately. Due to the fact that the whereabouts of the gunman was unknown, potential targets such as large events could be evacuated or protected. Figure 3 shows a screenshot with events (red circles) that took place during the shooting (yellow star). Our system identified two large events in the immediate vicinity and estimated their audience size. Based on this information, the police can evacuate or protect the events at an early stage. This is especially useful if not all the emergency care forces are on site, and evacuation is not possible for the entire area.

Fortunately, the gunman did not visit any other places to continue his amok run. But this case shows that previous approaches to detect unplanned events based on social media would be less useful in this scenario. The first emergency calls reached the police only 2 min after the first shots and thus the identification of the event is without difficulty. Second, due to the high volume of false reports about shootings and kidnappings in social media, such approaches would probably detect false events. Our system cannot be affected by this type of false alarms and could have given the operational forces important information to carry out countermeasures.

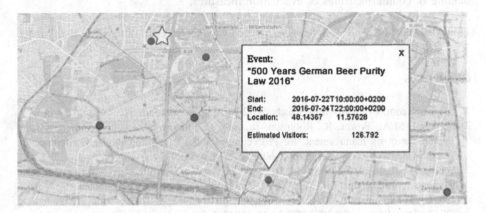

Fig. 3. Screenshot case study (Color figure online)

7 Conclusion

There are several approaches to make use of social media for emergency management. However, there is no general system with the ability to collect event information from social media and use this data for the estimation of audience sizes. We addressed this problem and presented a system design for processing and analyzing event-related data. By building a prototype and estimating the visitor numbers for different event categories, we highlighted the capabilities of our system. Further, we illustrated estimation improvements and demonstrated the benefits of our approach using a realistic scenario.

Our study does not come without limitations. We did not control for exogenous effects that might have an impact on the estimation results. For example, when the event takes place outdoors, the weather can have a strong impact on the audience size. Furthermore, we only investigated five event categories, while there are further event categories that are also relevant for emergency and crisis management. For example, demonstrations are often organized and promoted through social media to find fellow campaigners. Such events are also important for local authorities, emergency and crisis management.

Regarding future research, our system offers the possibility to quantify further influencing factors on the audience size. With a larger training set, it is probably possible to measure effects such as weekday effects, weather effects, or even cannibalization effects between competitive events.

Regarding practical implications, our system enables authorities to execute preventive actions. Events usually require a registration at local authorities with the expected number of visitors. This allows the detection of deviations between the expected and the estimated numbers of visitors. Since the number of local forces depends on the expected number of visitors, the local authority can preventively reduce or increase local forces. Furthermore, our system continuously updates the data repository for the estimations and allows instantaneous access. During a time-critical emergency, our system is able to provide near real-time estimations and support the planning of countermeasures or evacuation measures.

Acknowledgements. This work has been funded by the DFG as part of the CRC 1053 MAKI.

References

1. Facebook.com: Company Info. Facebook (2016) http://newsroom.fb.com/company-info/
2. Cameron, M.A., Power, R., Robinson, B., Yin, J.: Emergency situation awareness from Twitter for crisis management. In: Proceedings of the 21st International Conference on World Wide Web (WWW), pp. 695–698. ACM, Lyon (2012)
3. Schulz, A., Ristoski, P., Paulheim, H.: I see a car crash: real-time detection of small scale incidents in microblogs. In: Cimiano, P., Fernández, M., Lopez, V., Schlobach, S., Völker, J. (eds.) The Semantic Web: ESWC 2013 Satellite Events, pp. 22–33. Springer, Heidelberg (2013). https://doi.org/10.1007/978-3-642-41242-4_3
4. Pohl, D., Bouchachia, A., Hellwagner, H.: Automatic sub-event detection in emergency management using social media. In: Proceedings of the 21st International Conference on World Wide Web (WWW), pp. 683–686. ACM, Lyon (2012)
5. Sakaki, T., Okazaki, M., Matsuo, Y.: Earthquake shakes Twitter users: real-time event detection by social sensors. In: Proceedings of the 19th International Conference on World Wide Web (WWW), pp. 851–860. ACM (2010)
6. Sakaki, T., Okazaki, M., Matsuo, Y.: Tweet analysis for real-time event detection and earthquake reporting system development. IEEE Trans. Knowl. Data Eng. **25**, 919–931 (2013)
7. Earle, P.S., Bowden, D.C., Guy, M.: Twitter earthquake detection: earthquake monitoring in a social world. Ann. Geophys. **54**, 708–715 (2011)
8. Aramaki, E., Maskawa, S., Morita, M.: Twitter catches the flu: detecting influenza epidemics using Twitter. In: Proceedings of Empirical Methods in Natural Language Processing (EMNLP), pp. 1568–1576. Association for Computational Linguistics (2011)
9. Bird, D., Ling, M., Haynes, K.: Flooding Facebook-the use of social media during the Queensland and Victorian floods. Aust. J. Emerg. Manag. **27**, 27 (2012)
10. Yates, D., Paquette, S.: Emergency knowledge management and social media technologies: a case study of the 2010 Haitian earthquake. Int. J. Inf. Manag. **31**, 6–13 (2011)
11. Prentice, S., Huffman, E.: Social medias new role in emergency management. Idaho National Laboratory, pp. 1–5 (2008)
12. Kavanaugh, A., et al.: Social media use by government: from the routine to the critical. In: Proceedings of the 12th Annual International Digital Government Research Conference, pp. 121–130. ACM, Maryland (2011)
13. Lindsay, B.R.: Social Media and Disasters: Current Uses, Future Options, and Policy Considerations. Congressional Research Service, Washington, DC (2011)
14. Dalrymple, K.E., Young, R., Tully, M.: "Facts, not fear" negotiating uncertainty on social media during the 2014 Ebola crisis. Sci. Commun. **38**, 442–467 (2016)
15. Muenchen.de: Veranstaltungssicherheit - Muenchen.de (2016). https://www.muenchen.de/rathaus/dam/jcr:7ad4293a-5d02-4088-a35f-3f83aac74c61/Veranstaltungssicherheit_10MB.pdf

16. Berlin.de: Veranstaltung Erlaubnis (2016). https://service.berlin.de/dienstleistung/324911/
17. Arndt, J.: Word of mouth advertising: a review of the literature. Advertising Research Foundation (1967)
18. Bone, P.F.: Word-of-mouth effects on short-term and long-term product judgments. J. Bus. Res. **32**, 213–223 (1995)
19. Engel, J.F., Blackwell, R.D., Kegerreis, R.J.: How information is used to adopt an innovation. J. Advert. Res. **9**, 3–8 (1969)
20. Lynn, S.A.: Identifying buying influences for a professional service: implications for marketing efforts. Ind. Mark. Manag. **16**, 119–130 (1987)
21. Wojnicki, A., Godes, D.: Word-of-mouth as self-enhancement (2008)
22. Hevner, A.R., March, S.T., Park, J., Ram, S.: Design science in information systems research. MISQ **28**, 75–105 (2004)
23. Cohen, W., Ravikumar, P., Fienberg, S.: A comparison of string metrics for matching names and records. In: KDD Workshop on Data Cleaning, Record Linkage and Object Consolidation, pp. 73–78 (2003)
24. Polizei.Bayern.de: Übersicht der veröffentlichten Pressemeldungen zur Schießerei in München (2016). https://www.polizei.bayern.de/muenchen/news/presse/faelle/index.html/245254
25. Zeit.de: Polizei identifiziert 18-Jährigen als mutmaßlichen Täter (2016). http://www.zeit.de/gesellschaft/zeitgeschehen/2016-07/muenchen-schuesse-live
26. n-tv.de: Münchner Amoklauf und Fehlalarme - Polizei geht gegen Trittbrettfahrer vor (2016). http://www.n-tv.de/panorama/Polizei-geht-gegen-Trittbrettfahrer-vor-article18613041.html
27. BR.de: Ermittlungen wegen "Störung des öffentlichen Friedens" (2016). http://www.br.de/nachrichten/oberbayern/inhalt/amoklauf-hetze-internet-100.html

Exploring the Effects of Different Incentives on Doctors' Contribution Behaviors in Online Health Communities

Fei Liu[1,2]([✉]), Xitong Guo[1], Xiaofeng Ju[1], and Xiaocui Han[1]

[1] School of Management, Harbin Institute of Technology, Harbin, China
[2] Department of Management and Marketing,
The Hong Kong Polytechnic University, Hong Kong, Hong Kong
f.liu@connect.polyu.hk

Abstract. With the dramatic development of Web 2.0, the occurrence of online health communities (OHCs) appeal to increasing number of patients and physicians to involve in this new healthcare platform. Extant literature has primarily discussed the motivation of knowledge sharing from participants in OHCs. However, scant studies have been conducted to explore the motivations of doctors' contribution behaviors in OHCs. Drawing on motivation theory, knowledge sharing theory and social capital theory, we mainly examine the effects of monetary and reputational incentives on doctors' continuous participation in OHCs. In addition, we also investigate how online incentive factors and offline status of doctors can interact hereby motivating doctors to better serve in the OHCs. We will collect data from an OHCs in China. The findings will not only enrich the relevant theory, but also help us to understand physicians' motivation mechanisms in OHCs.

Keywords: Online health communities · OHCs · Offline status
Online rewards · Online contribution behaviors

1 Introduction

Online health community (OHCs) is likened as a new healthcare platform that participants share healthcare information, treatment experience, and healthy behaviors [1]. Additionally, patients can also provide online treatment to patients without temporal and locational constrains [2]. Increasing number of global organizations and individuals use OHCs to communicate and exchange health information and obtain online treatment [3]. According to Oh and Lee [4], patients prone to actively communicate with doctor in the OHCs, in turn leading to better doctor-patient relationships. OHCs provide a good platform for participants to exchange healthcare knowledge [5], share their own experiences related to disease treatment, health promotion and disease prevention [6, 7]. However, extant research primarily focuses on exploring the motivations of patients and ordinary users for sharing behaviors [8, 9], and rare studies have explored the motivational factors for doctors' participation in the online community [10]. Therefore, the purpose of this study is to investigate the motivators that encourage doctors to participate in the OHCs.

© Springer Nature Switzerland AG 2018
H. Chen et al. (Eds.): ICSH 2018, LNCS 10983, pp. 90–95, 2018.
https://doi.org/10.1007/978-3-030-03649-2_9

In OHCs, the treatment of doctors on patients is always embodied by knowledge sharing [11], which is regarded as one type of exchange behavior [12]. Participants in the OHCs perform knowledge sharing behaviors are triggered by intrinsic and extrinsic rewards [21]. Intrinsic rewards refer to internal fulfillment such as achievement, success and pleasure, etc. By contrast, extrinsic rewards refer to external stimuli such as money, reputation and promotion, etc. [11]. In many OHCs, physicians normally provide two types of services to patients: payable services and voluntarily sharing. Drawing upon knowledge sharing theory and motivation theory, extrinsic motivations exert a positive role in influencing people's participation behavior [12]. Additionally, physicians' participation in the OHCs is primarily influenced by personal factors (economical and reputational rewards) and social influence. Therefore, this research is designed to primarily investigate the effect of online incentives (reputational and monetary rewards) and offline status on doctors' contribution behavior in the OHCs. We also examine the interaction effect between online incentives and offline status on doctors' participation behavior.

2 Research Context and Hypothesis

In OHCs, doctors can obtain both online and offline rewards. Online incentives include reputational and monetary rewards and offline status include doctor title, hospital tiers, and location on doctors' contribution level. Additionally, evaluations and votes provided by users promote doctors to obtain reputational rewards, in turn enhancing the status in OHCs. By contrast, economic rewards are also very important factor that motivate doctors to participate in the OHCs. Specifically, patients can purchase online virtual presents (reputational rewards) to doctors. Besides, physicians can also attain economic rewards by providing patients with telephone consultation. As knowledge in this regard, we understand the motivations for doctors to participate in the OHCs include personal incentives (reputational and economic rewards) and social influence (physicians' social capital). For doctors who have different titles and social status, the effects of reputational and economic rewards on their contribution behavior tend to be different as well.

In OHCs, physicians expect to achieve anticipated objectives through performing contribution behaviors. It means physicians fully involve in the participation in the OHCs in order to attain personal values. The services provided by physicians in "Good Doctor Online" include: online consultation service, telephone consultation services, treatment transference appointment, share healthcare popular science knowledge, etc. physicians provide these services to patients in order to improve their contribution level and enhance their personal value. Additionally, patients choose applicable doctors in the "Good Doctor Online" OHCs based on the factors include doctors' online reputation, specialized knowledge, and status. Drawing on motivation theory, it indicates that extrinsic motivation significantly influences individuals' participation behaviors [13], which explains why doctors would like to participate in the OHCs. Prior literature related to exploring the motivations of individuals' participation in the online communities has demonstrated that reputational and economical rewards are the primary drivers for people's devotion online [14]. In the OHCs, the services doctors deliver to patients are mainly embodied by knowledge sharing [11]. Doctors normally provide two types of services, payable services and voluntary sharing, in "Good Doctor Online" OHCs. Patients can post their evaluations related to the quality of doctors' services after they receive online consultation services. Positive evaluations and feedback could provide references for other patients regarding to doctors' service quality, in turn increasing the online reputational rewards of doctors [15]. Therefore, online reputation is also likened as one of the significant motivators for doctors to participate in the OHCs. Apart from reputational rewards, economic rewards can also encourage doctors to perform participation behavior in the OHCs. Patients always buy virtual gifts for doctors to express their gratitude. These virtual gifts can be transferred monetary rewards for doctors. Additionally, doctors can also obtain economic rewards through telephone consultations. Based on the above reasoning, we propose:

H1a: Reputational rewards positively influence doctors' online contribution level.
H1b: Monetary rewards positively influence doctors' online contribution level.

In addition, social influence is also a principal element trigger individuals' participation behaviors [16]. Social influence factors include: social status, identity, social recognition, etc. Social influence factors facilitate people to attain social and affective supports through social ties. The different titles of physicians signify their different social identity. Social identity is often deemed as doctors' social capital, which motivates doctors to participate in the OHCs. Therefore, we purport:

H2: Offline identity positively influence doctors' online contribution level.

Further, psychology research has demonstrated that people have different regulatory foci that tend to have different levels of sensitivity to the same stimuli [17]. Based on the regulatory focus theory, individuals with promotion focus tend to focus on positive outcomes, such as success, achievement and happiness [18, 19]. Accordingly, doctors with different social status might perform different behaviors even to the same incentives. The social status of doctors might influence their contribution behaviors online. For doctors with high social status, they might pay more attention on achievement and self-fulfillment (internal motivation) rather than economical and reputational rewards (external motivation) [20]. Therefore, we hypothesize:

H3: As the increasing of social status of doctors, the effect of reputational rewards on doctors' contribution behaviors will decrease accordingly.
H4: As the increasing of social status of doctors, the effect of monetary rewards on doctors' contribution behaviors will decrease accordingly.

The participation of doctors in the OHCs help doctors achieve both reputational and monetary rewards, which are the main drivers that motivate doctors' contribution behaviors. Therefore, we propose:

H5: Reputational rewards and monetary rewards have complementary effect on doctors' contribution behaviors.

To summary, this research is designed to primarily investigate the effect of online incentives (reputational and monetary rewards) and offline status (doctor title, hospital tiers, and location) on doctors' contribution level. We also examine the interaction effect between online and offline status on doctors' contribution level. Figure 1 depicts our research model.

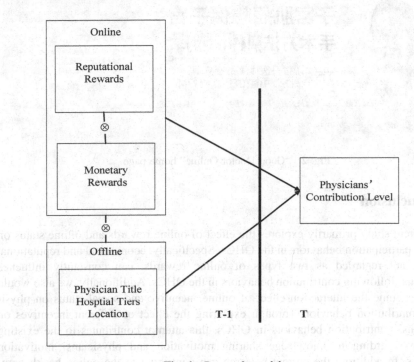

Fig. 1. Research model

3 Data Collection

We will collect data from "Good Doctor Online" OHCs (Fig. 2 displays the home page of "Good Doctor Online") using Locoyspider software, which is one of specialized web crawler tools. This software can help us fetch on data from structural text, picture and documents on webpages. We anticipate to collect data based on each doctor's identity document. The specific procedure will be: First, we will obtain each doctor's homepage address to attain all the relevant information about each doctor; Second, we will obtain the information about each doctor's location, affiliated hospital and hospital tiers; Finally, doctors' information and hospital tier will be integrated according to the same fields of two data table.

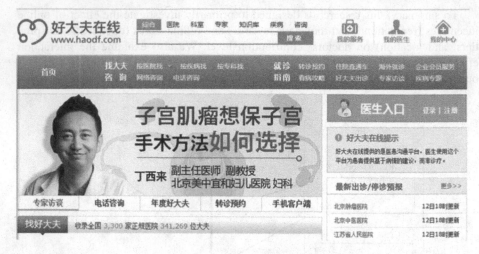

Fig. 2. "Good Doctor Online" home page

4   Conclusion

This current study primarily explores the effect of online rewards and offline status on doctors' participation behaviors in the OHCs. Specifically, economical and reputational rewards, are regarded as two types of online rewards, can constantly influence physicians' following contribution behaviors in the OHCs. Additionally, we also would like to examine the interaction effect of online incentive and social status on physicians' contribution behavior. Through exploring the effect of different incentives on physicians' contribution behaviors in OHCs, this attempt contributes to the existing literature regarding to knowledge sharing motivation and physicians' motivation behaviors. In addition, the current research can contribute to the online health communities research by improving the development of network platform and establishment of patient-doctor interaction mechanism, thereby stimulating doctors to actively contribute to the OHCs.

This study is still in progress. Future research will conduct to data collection and data analysis. Discussion, findings, theoretical implications & practical implications, limitations and conclusion also need to be addressed comprehensively.

References

1. Valaitis, R.K., Akhtar-Danesh, N., Brooks, F., Binks, S., Semogas, D.: Online communities of practice as a communication resource for community health nurses working with homeless persons. J. Adv. Nurs. **67**(6), 1273–1284 (2011)
2. Cao, X., Liu, Y., Zhu, Z., Hu, J., Chen, X.: Online selection of a physician by patients: empirical study from elaboration likelihood perspective. Comput. Hum. Behav. **73**, 403–412 (2017)

3. Ba, S., Wang, L.: Digital health communities: the effect of their motivation mechanisms. Decis. Support Syst. **55**(4), 941–947 (2013)
4. Oh, H.J., Lee, B.: The effect of computer-mediated social support in online communities on patient empowerment and doctor-patient communication. Health Commun. **27**(1), 30–41 (2012)
5. Ba, S., Pavlou, P.A.: Evidence of the effect of trust building technology in electronic markets: price premiums and buyer behavior. MIS Q. **26**(3), 243–268 (2002)
6. Armstrong, N., Powell, J.: Patient perspectives on health advice posted on internet discussion boards: a qualitative study. Health Expect. **12**(3), 313–320 (2009)
7. Yan, L., Tan, Y.: Feeling blue? go online: an empirical study of social support among patients. Inf. Syst. Res. **25**(4), 690–709 (2014)
8. Oh, S.: The characteristics and motivations of health answerers for sharing information, knowledge, and experiences in online environments. J. Assoc. Inf. Sci. Technol. **63**(3), 543–557 (2012)
9. Wicks, P., et al.: Perceived benefits of sharing health data between people with epilepsy on an online platform. Epilepsy Behav. **23**(1), 16–23 (2012)
10. He, W., Wei, K.-K.: What drives continued knowledge sharing? an investigation of knowledge-contribution and-seeking beliefs. Decis. Support Syst. **46**(4), 826–838 (2009)
11. Yan, Z., Wang, T., Chen, Y., Zhang, H.: Knowledge sharing in online health communities: a social exchange theory perspective. Inf. Manag. **53**(5), 643–653 (2016)
12. Bock, G.-W., Zmud, R.W., Kim, Y.-G., Lee, J.-N.: Behavioral intention formation in knowledge sharing: examining the roles of extrinsic motivators, social-psychological forces, and organizational climate. MIS Q. **29**(1), 87–111 (2005)
13. Ryan, R.M., Deci, E.L.: Intrinsic and extrinsic motivations: classic definitions and new directions. Contemp. Educ. Psychol. **25**(1), 54–67 (2000)
14. Sun, Y., Fang, Y., Lim, K.H.: Understanding sustained participation in transactional virtual communities. Decis. Support Syst. **53**(1), 12–22 (2012)
15. Gao, G., Greenwood, B., McCullough, J., Agarwal, R.: The information value of online physician ratings. (2011). Working paper
16. Centola, D., van de Rijt, A.: Choosing your network: social preferences in an online health community. Soc. Sci. Med. **125**, 19–31 (2015)
17. Higgins, E.T.: Promotion and prevention: regulatory focus as a motivational principle. Adv. Exp. Soc. Psychol. **30**, 1–46 (1998)
18. Higgins, E.T.: Beyond pleasure and pain. Am. Psychol. **52**(12), 1280 (1997)
19. Liang, H., Xue, Y., Wu, L.: Ensuring employees' it compliance: carrot or stick? Inf. Syst. Res. **24**(2), 279–294 (2013)
20. Sun, S.-Y., Ju, T.L., Chumg, H.-F., Wu, C.-Y., Chao, P.-J.: Influence on willingness of virtual community's knowledge sharing: based on social capital theory and habitual domain. World Acad. Sci. Eng. Technol. **53**, 142–149 (2009)
21. Kankanhalli, A., Tan, B.C., Wei, K.-K.: Contributing knowledge to electronic knowledge repositories: an empirical investigation. MIS Q. **29**(1), 113–143 (2005)

Cross-Cultural Comparison of User Engagement in Online Health Communities

Xi Wang[✉] and Yushan Zhu

School of Information, Central University of Finance and Economics,
Beijing, China
xiwang@cufe.edu.cn

Abstract. Online health communities have become major source for people having health related concerns to exchange social support. Different websites are designed for serving people around the world. However, the OHCs across different countries might have similarities and variances. This study analyzes user engagement in two OHCs of USA and China from a cross cultural perspective. The goal of the study is to explore pros and cons of OHCs in different cultural background. The outcome of the paper has implications for the website design.

Keywords: Online health communities · User behavior
Cross-cultural comparison

1 Introduction

Healthcare is a major challenge for modern society and has attracted the attention of stakeholders well beyond the healthcare industry. The ubiquitousness of the Internet has made it easier for individuals to obtain, process, and understand information related to health. According to a report from the Pew Research Center [1], 72% of United States adults have used the Internet for information about medical conditions. In addition to only seeking information through web portals, such as Wikipedia and WebMD, Internet users also interact with others online to obtain knowledge and support. People communicate through the Internet for common concerns forming online communities, such as discussion forums and bulletin boards. The online communities designed specifically for people with a health interest are referred to as Online Health Communities (OHCs).

The most widely accepted definition of an OHC is "a group of individuals with a common interest or a shared purpose, whose interactions are governed by policies in the form of rules, rituals, or protocols; who have ongoing and persistent interactions; and who use computer-mediated communication as the primary form of interaction to support and mediate social interaction and facilitate a sense of togetherness" [2]. Besides the broad reach and 24-h availability, OHCs have many advantages compared with offline support groups. First, all the previous posts are warehoused on the website,

---

Supported by Beijing Natural Science Foundation (9184032).

H. Chen et al. (Eds.): ICSH 2018, LNCS 10983, pp. 96–104, 2018.
https://doi.org/10.1007/978-3-030-03649-2_10

which means new users can retrieve past related information any time. Although medical knowledge may update rapidly over time, the stored data are still a good resource to provide possible solutions or support to newcomers of the community. Meanwhile, compared with Face-to-Face support group, labor and time costs are efficiently saved. In addition, Wright [3] points out that OHCs are beneficial in reducing users' embarrassment. Compared to face to face setting, online users may be more likely to express themselves in a straightforward and honest way about their concerns. In other words, OHCs can successfully mask physical appearance or disabilities that are a result of the health condition, which may be valuable for some users.

As a resource sharing platform of Big Data era, the OHCs have been welcomed around world. Multiple websites are designed in different languages for serving people in various countries. Although the format and content may be different across countries, the ultimate goal of these OHCs is to support people who have medical concerns. Due to different cultural or religion background, individuals from various countries may behave differently. For example, the American people emphasize more about independence of being adults – most of them move out from their parents after college, while the Chinese families prefer to live together, and the parents are used to pay all the living expenses for their children even after they get married. Then for the usage of OHCs, an interesting question would be, do people across countries behave differently?

This study aims to compare user engagements of OHCs between USA and China. With identifying the disparity of their behaviors, we will uncover the cultural impact on Internet users. The outcome of the paper will benefit for identifying the pros and cons of OHCs in different cultural backgrounds. Learning from each other's advantages and implementing them to improve design of domestic websites provides managerial implications for the community operators.

2 Background

As a special type of online community, OHCs share similarities with other online communities. The users can share knowledge and exchange feelings about the medical or treatment-related questions with the help of the Internet. But at the same time, OHCs feature some unique characteristics. First, in a peer to peer OHC, where users are mainly patients and caregivers, there is few monetary values for users to contribute. The altruism becomes the motivation of users to publish content [4]. Second, different from other knowledge sharing online communities, OHCs emphasize more about social support. Social support can help them adjusting to the stress of living with and fighting against their diseases [5–7], and it is a consistent factor for users' continued participation in OHCs [8]. Compared to western people, Chinese people usually have a higher level of family cohesion, where they can receive more support. Therefore, individuals from various cultural environment may have different levels of requirement or ways of exchanging social support in OHCs.

2.1 Social Support

Social support refers to the "exchange of resources between at least two individuals perceived by the provider or the recipient to be intended to enhance the well-being of the recipient" [9]. Based on the nature of exchanged "resources," community psychology researchers have identified different types of social support. For example, House [10] defined four types of social support: emotional, instrumental, informational, and appraisal. The literature on social support suggests that OHCs mainly feature four types of social support: informational support, emotional support, companionship (a.k. a., network support), and instrumental support [11, 12].

Users involved in OHCs designed for different health issues may need different types of social support. In OHCs for health promotion, such as communities interested in weight loss, informational support is more frequently expressed in initial posts of threads or in public channels, while emotional support is more popular in comments of threads or in private channels [13, 14]. By contrast, social support is exchanged differently among users suffering from chronic health conditions. For example, informational support is emphasized more in a diabetes group [15, 16], while network support is more frequent in an Amyotrophic Lateral Sclerosis OHC, a disease characterized by stiff muscles, resulting in difficulty speaking, swallowing, and eventually breathing [17]. Moreover, the geographical locations can also differentiate users in exchanging social support: urban users act more as suppliers of social support, while rural participants are recipients [18]. Therefore, social support exchanged in the community depends on the nature of both users and OHCs.

2.2 Cross-Cultural Comparison

Cross-cultural Studies are set to examine the scope of human behaviors and test hypotheses about human behavior and culture. The study set up the difference between human behavior as constant, while the culture as impact factor, to explore the behavior difference across different cultures. The past cross-cultural studies are conducted from various aspects, such as linguistic behavior, advertisements and even healthcare. For example, Ren [19] proposed that the cultural difference of healthcare are shown in five parts – belief of health, religion, social status of males and females, eating habits and human species. These cultural differences lead to the various reactions of people facing the identical health problems [20].

When the Internet becomes an important element for individuals seeking health related information, researchers found that the American and Chinese behave differently in searching information. For example, such variance reflects both in the seeking content and the seeking channels [21]. In terms of seeking social support, people from different regions also have opposite opinions. The eastern people may worry the negative emotions will impact the others in the same group and therefore seeking emotional may lead to the feeling of embarrassing [22, 23]. While the western people believe seeking social support is a correct way of pressure relief [24].

2.3   Research Question

Since cultural difference may lead to the different behavior of users in OHCs, our research goal is to measure such variance. Do users from different countries discuss similar content? Do they have similar demands in different types of social support? To answer the questions, we collected data from OHC for breast cancer in both USA and China as a case study.

3   Data Collection

3.1   An OHC in USA

In this research, we used Breastcancer.org as the American OHC, which is a very popular peer-to-peer website among breast cancer survivors and their caregivers. With more than 100 thousands registered users, the website provides various ways for its members to communicate. We designed a web crawler to collect data. Our dataset consists of more than 4.3 million public posts and user profile information from March 2007 to March 2018.

3.2   An OHC in China

Corresponding to Breastcanaer.org, we used Baidu Post Breast Bar as the Chinese OHC. There are two major reasons for selecting it as the research target. First, Baidu Post features the similar format as the Breastcancer.org, which is a peer-to-peer OHC. Second, as a popular forum in China, Baidu Post Bar contains large volume of data. With nearly 40,000 registered users, we collected posts and user information from March 2007 to March 2018, containing more than 186 thousands posts contributed by 36,180 users.

4   Preliminary Results and Discussion

To conduct the cross-cultural comparison, we summarized basic statistics on both individual and community level of two OHCs. First, Fig. 1 shows the user engagement, including number of posts users published and time span users being active, in two communities. The comparison suggests significant differences between users in the American and Chinese OHCs. Specifically, users from the American OHC contributed more posts and retained longer than the individuals from the Chinese OHC. Figure 2 shows the posts published over time. Note that, the Breastcancer.org was first launched at 2003, but the first post in Baidu Posts was published at 2007. To control other possible influential factors, such as breast cancer related events happened during 2003 to 2007, we keep consistency of the time range for two datasets. It is obvious that the average number of posts in the American OHC is higher than Chinese. The trend of contributions in American OHC reached the peak around 2011 and went down since 2012, while the posts in Chinese community increased steadily since 2015. It is very possible that the requirement of social support of American users is much higher than

Chinese, even if China has a much larger size of population and breast cancer patients, the penetration of the usage of online support group is not enough.

To understand what types of social support are most frequent, we implement LDA [25] on all posts within the time range in the two communities. Tables 1 and 2 provide the 10 topics and their corresponding distributions. For each topic, we summarize the theme based on 15 representative words. According to the literatures mentioned previously, social support in OHCs mainly contain informational support, emotional support and companionship [8]. We project the themes "Appointment", "Treatment", "Diagnosis", "Physical Appearance", "Payment", "Symptom" onto informational support, "Wishes" and "Emotions" onto emotional support, the "Daily topics" and "Off Topics" onto companionship. The distributions of social support across OHCs are shown in Fig. 3. It is obvious that the informational support topics are most frequent social support discussed in both communities. The emotional support is also discussed, holding more than 20% in both of them. While the companionship topics are more frequently in the American OHC than the Chinese one. It is very possible that, due to the close relationship with families influenced by the culture, Chinese people may have more offline channels to acquire social support than Americans.

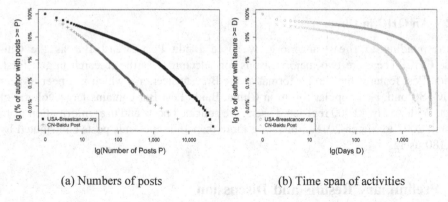

(a) Numbers of posts   (b) Time span of activities

Fig. 1. Complementary cumulative distributions of engagement metrics for the users

Since cultural difference may result in users' various behaviors in the OHCs, we conduct regression models to measure the correlation between users' social support behavior and their engagement. We collect users' time span (gap days from the first post to the last) as the dependent variables, their social support behaviors in three categories as independent variables. Table 3 shows the outcomes of OLS model. Apparently, posting informational support is positively correlated to a user's long-term involvement in the American OHC (1.16), which help oppositely in the Chinese OHC (−0.28). Therefore, Chinese users treat OHC as an information resource rather than sharing platform, in which they seek more informational support than provide. By Contrast, Companionship posts are positively contributed to the users' engagement in Chinese OHCs. A possible explanation is that Baidu Posts has a rewarding mechanism for user posting behavior. With such mechanism, the user login and post daily, especially most of the companionship posts are off-topic content.

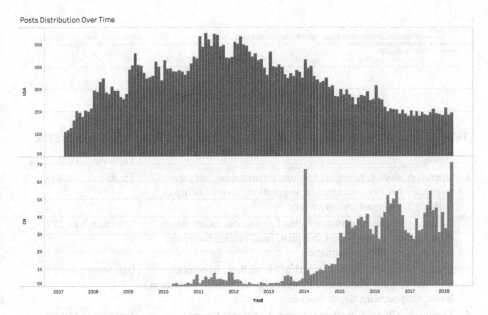

Posts Distribution Over Time

Fig. 2. Posts Distribution of Breastcaner.org and Baidu Post and Over Time

Table 1. 15 representative words of 10 topics of Breastcancer.org based on LDA.

No	Words	Topics	Percentage
1	Call don't time week wait'll didn't talk told check start phone month have doctor	Appointment	12.16%
2	Cancer breast treatment chemo rate stage women test age surgery node radiate BC diagnose cell	Treatment	11.52%
3	Hair red hot wear eye top ice color beach band pink dress clean black cream	Physical appearance	4.77%
4	Http pay people word post company American person site link study topic drug bill read	Payment	8.81%
5	Word mari tree star omg peace wind rose toe nut TV fast Ha plant fire	Daily topics	2.91%
6	False gonna tan arm ray lead ten earth hurt pound left lung mammogram male scar	Treatment	2.78%
7	Love hope lol day happy hug girl song glad sandy beauty deb fun nice tomorrow	Wishes	8.18%
8	Watch house eat rain car kid lol love favorite movie dog food DH cat play	Daily topics	13.08%
9	Person love time don life friend feel family people grate mom live god true care	Emotions	15.86%
10	Day time feel start night pain don sleep ducky week bad hope snow chemo tire	Symptom	19.94%

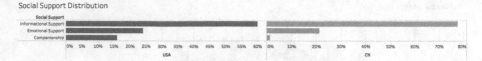

Fig. 3. Distribution of social support

Table 2. 15 representative words (translation) of 20 topics of Baidu Post based on LDA.

No	Words	Topics	Percentage
1	Operation, doctor, hospital, fibroma, examination, surgery, minimally invasive, recurrence, suggestion, review, benign, building Lord, mastectomy, worry.	Treatment	18.40%
2	Breast, hyperplasia, mammary gland, sensation, examination, mass, doctor, menstruation, hospital, hard block, discovery, nipples, pain, fibroma, situation	Symptom	11.27%
3	Breast, nodules, examination, echo, blood flow, hyperplasia, b ultrasound, color ultrasound, benign, signal, doctor, white aunt, lump, molybdenum target, boundary	Diagnosis	8.91%
4	Treatment, Chinese medicine, breast, traditional Chinese medicine, hospital, hyperplasia, effect, surgery, recuperation, recurrence, cure, method, medicine, doctor, no	Treatment	11.68%
5	Chemotherapy, treatment, breast cancer, mother, metastasis, surgery, white aunt, doctor, pathology, radiation, lymphatic, thank you, case, immunohistochemistry, excuse me	Treatment	11.56%
6	Mother, building Lord, refueling, blessing, 15, thank, the post, hope, white aunt, early recovery, mother, blessing, reply, auntie, peace	Wishes	12.00%
7	Chemotherapy, doctor, operation, mother, hospital, feeling, white blood cell, tomorrow night, wound, several days, uncomfortable, the first time, discharge, end	Treatment	7.86%
8	Experience, reply, check-in, 100, within, 25, 11, 200, bunker, copy, 30, 16, 50, 12, time	Off topics	1.21%
9	Mother, come on, mood, really, hope, good, mentality, breast cancer, children, strong, life, treatment, body, husband, cancer	Emotions	9.18%
10	Breast, hyperplasia, breast cancer, breast, underwear, women, disease, steel ring, diet, treatment, health, mood, normal, prevention, conditioning	Female health	7.92%

Table 3. Results of OLS regression.

Social support	Coefficients (USA)	Coefficients (CN)
Informational support	1.16***	−0.28***
Emotional support	0.31***	7.35***
Companionship	−1.12***	3.81**
Instances	73,610	34,490

**: $p < 0.01$, ***: $p < 0.001$

5 Conclusion and Future Direction

In this paper, we conduct a cross-cultural comparison on users' engagement in OHCs. It turns out that users indeed behave differently impacted by cultural backgrounds. Such difference reflects from various types of social support they published in the community. The current study features two limitations. First, we select breast cancer as a case study, which might limit the generalization of the conclusions. Second, we adopt LDA rather than text mining methods to assign social support labels to each post, which might decrease the accuracy. Even if we know users behave differently, how much is such variance related to cultural factors still needs our further effort to study. For the next step, we will analyze each post with text mining methods to explore specific cultural related clues. The outcomes will help us to better design OHCs across cultures.

References

1. Fox, S.: The social life of health information (2014). http://www.pewresearch.org/fact-tank/2014/01/15/the-social-life-of-health-information/
2. Rodgers, S., Chen, Q.: Internet community group participation: psychosocial benefits for women with breast cancer. J. Comput.-Mediat. Commun. **10**(4) (2005)
3. Wright, K.B.: Computer-mediated support for health outcomes. In: Sundar, S.S. (ed.) The Handbook of the Psychology of Communication Technology, pp. 488–506. Wiley, Hoboken (2015)
4. Gintis, H., Bowles, S., Boyd, R., Fehr, E.: Explaining altruistic behavior in humans. Evol. Hum. Behav. **24**, 153–172 (2003)
5. Dunkel-Schetter, C.: Social support and cancer: findings based on patient interviews and their implications. J. Soc. Issues **40**, 77–98 (1984)
6. Qiu, B., et al.: Get online support, feel better – sentiment analysis and dynamics in an online cancer survivor community. In: 2011 IEEE Third International Conference on Privacy, Security, Risk and Trust (PASSAT), 2011 IEEE Third International Conference on Social Computing (SocialCom), pp. 274–281 (2011)
7. Zhao, K., Yen, J., Greer, G., Qiu, B., Mitra, P., Portier, K.: Finding influential users of online health communities: a new metric based on sentiment influence. J. Am. Med. Inform. Assoc. **21**, e212–e218 (2014)
8. Wang, X., Zhao, K., Street, N.: Analyzing and predicting user participations in online health communities: a social support perspective. J. Med. Internet Res. **19**, e130 (2017)
9. Shumaker, S.A., Brownell, A.: Toward a theory of social support: closing conceptual gaps. J. Soc. Issues **40**, 11–36 (1984)
10. House, J.S.: Work Stress and Social Support. Addison-Wesley Longman, Boston (1981). Incorporated
11. Bambina, A.: Online Social Support: The Interplay of Social Networks and Computer-Mediated Communication. Cambria Press, Amherst (2007)
12. Keating, D.M.: Spirituality and support: a descriptive analysis of online social support for depression. J. Relig. Health **52**, 1014–1028 (2013)
13. Chuang, K.Y., Yang, C.C.: Interaction patterns of nurturant support exchanged in online health social networking. J. Med. Internet Res. **14**, e54 (2012)

14. Zhang, M., Yang, C.C.: Using content and network analysis to understand the social support exchange patterns and user behaviors of an online smoking cessation intervention program. J. Assoc. Inf. Sci. Technol. **66**, 564–575 (2015)
15. Greene, J.A., Choudhry, N.K., Kilabuk, E., Shrank, W.H.: Online social networking by patients with diabetes: a qualitative evaluation of communication with Facebook. J. Gen. Intern. Med. **26**, 287–292 (2011)
16. Zhang, Y., He, D., Sang, Y.: Facebook as a platform for health information and communication: a case study of a diabetes group. J. Med. Syst. **37**, 9942 (2013)
17. Loane, S.S., D'Alessandro, S.: Communication that changes lives: social support within an online health community for ALS. Commun. Q. **61**, 236–251 (2013)
18. Goh, J.M., Gao, G.G., Agarwal, R.: The creation of social value: Can an online health community reduce rural–urban health disparities? Manag. Inf. Syst. Q. **40**, 247–263 (2016)
19. 任梦梅: 论文化对医疗保健的影响. 西北医学教育. **15**, 845–848 (2007)
20. Mortenson, S.T.: Interpersonal trust and social skill in seeking social support among Chinese and Americans. Commun. Res. **36**, 32–53 (2009)
21. 李月琳, 刘冰凌: 中美网络用户信息搜寻行为比较研究:基于跨文化视角. 情报理论与实践. **38**, 116–121 (2015)
22. Matsumoto, D.: Unmasking Japan: myths and realities about the emotions of the Japanese. J. Jpn. Stud. **56**, 436–442 (1996)
23. Wellenkamp, J.C.: Everyday conceptions of distress. In: Russell, J.A., Fernández-Dols, J.M., Manstead, A.S.R., Wellenkamp, J.C. (eds.) Everyday Conceptions of Emotion, vol. 81. Springer, Dordrecht (1995). https://doi.org/10.1007/978-94-015-8484-5_15
24. Feng, B., Burleson, B.R.: Exploring the support seeking process across cultures: toward an integrated analysis of similarities and differences. Int. Intercult. Commun. Annu. **28**, 243–266 (2006)
25. Blei, D.M., Ng, A.Y., Jordan, M.I.: Latent Dirichlet allocation. J. Mach. Learn. Res. **3**, 993–1022 (2003)

Mobile Health

Development of Text Messages for Mobile Health Education to Promote Diabetic Retinopathy Awareness and Eye Care Behavior Among Indigenous Women

Valerie Onyinyechi Umaefulam[✉] and Kalyani Premkumar

University of Saskatchewan, Saskatoon, SK S7N 5E5, Canada
valerie.umaefulam@usask.ca

Abstract. Background: Diabetes is increasingly prevalent in Indigenous people along with associated ocular complications such as diabetic retinopathy, which is the most common cause of blindness in Canadian adults. Though the risk of diabetic retinopathy is higher particularly among Indigenous women, there is limited utilization of diabetic eye care services. Hence there is the need for studies and interventions that pursue an innovative and culturally appropriate way of providing relevant information to promote diabetes-eye knowledge and prompt eye care behavior among Indigenous women living with and at-risk of diabetes.

Aim: To develop diabetes-eye messages for a mobile health (mHealth) intervention to promote diabetic retinopathy awareness and eye care behavior among Indigenous women living with diabetes and at-risk of diabetes in Saskatoon.

Methods: In this study, we used a multi-stage content development approach to crafting text messages, informed by Self-determination theory. The authors carried out content development in four major phases: content selection, user input, review and refining of messages, and pre-testing of messages.

Result: Messages were selected via content analysis and literature search. The messages were informative/educational, reminders, motivational, and supportive. Important considerations in message development included: message prioritization, text message formatting, delivery, and dissemination plan.

Discussion and Conclusions: A collaborative approach with a multidisciplinary team was essential to develop a comprehensive, culturally pertinent and appropriate mHealth messaging. The study provided some key steps and considerations for the development of a mHealth text messaging initiative in an Indigenous population and may serve as a guide for similar health promotion interventions.

Keywords: Mobile health · Diabetic retinopathy · Indigenous

1 Introduction

1.1 Diabetes and Diabetic Retinopathy

Diabetes epidemic is acute among Canadian Indigenous populations and can be attributed to the social, cultural, and environmental changes Indigenous people have

© Springer Nature Switzerland AG 2018
H. Chen et al. (Eds.): ICSH 2018, LNCS 10983, pp. 107–118, 2018.
https://doi.org/10.1007/978-3-030-03649-2_11

undergone due to colonization. The First Nations, Metis and Inuit peoples make up the Canadian Indigenous people and the prevalence of diabetes is slightly higher in females within the 30–34 years age group [1]. Indigenous women (First Nations and Métis) are particularly prone to developing diabetes with more than four times the rate of non-Indigenous women, due to higher rates of obesity and gestational diabetes [2]. In addition, Indigenous women in Saskatchewan living with diabetes have higher rates of fetal macrosomia (children with birth weight >4,000 g), than non-Indigenous peoples [3].

Diabetic Retinopathy (DR) is a chronic eye complication of diabetes and the most common cause of blindness in developed countries including Canada, particularly among the working population (25–75 years of age) [4]. Few studies have assessed the prevalence of DR in Canada, particularly among Indigenous Canadians. However, Canadian Indigenous people have shown to have a higher rate of advanced DR changes compared to non-Indigenous populations which may be as a result of the early onset of diabetes, predisposing them to higher rates of DR complications [5]. A study that examined Indigenous peoples from Sandy Lake, in Northern Ontario, revealed a prevalence rate of 24% for non-proliferative DR, 5% for macular edema and 2% for proliferative DR [6].

It is theorized that women with myocardial ischemia and arteriosclerosis may be at greater risk of developing microvascular diseases such as retinopathy [7]. Also, DR tends to accelerate during hormonal changes such as pregnancy and puberty [8]. Accordingly, diabetes will lead to a significant burden of preventable vision loss in Indigenous communities, particularly in women if not addressed [9]. In addition, Indigenous women at risk of diabetes i.e. with family history of diabetes, gestational diabetes, pre-diabetes have greater risk of developing type 2 diabetes at an early age and increased risk of vision loss and associated ramifications that occur as a result of diabetic retinopathy blindness including; mental health conditions and poor quality of life. Hence, the authors focused on Indigenous women with diabetes and at-risk of diabetes in the study.

1.2   Mobile Health

mHealth is a term used to cover all mobile digital health technologies and health informatics such as personal digital assistants and mobile phones to improve health knowledge, behaviors and outcomes. mHealth has been widely applied to address health inequities in Indigenous communities which occurs due to economic, political and sociocultural factors and to mitigate some of these barriers [10]. Due to the ubiquity, affordability and ownership of digital technologies, mHealth has the potential to deliver preventative health services, and address disparities in diabetes complications between Indigenous and non-Indigenous communities [11].

1.3   Rationale

Diabetic retinopathy is a chronic eye complication of diabetes and the primary cause of blindness in Canada especially among adults. Almost all persons with diagnosed diabetes develop some stage of diabetic retinopathy over time and if poorly managed at critical periods, it can result in vision loss that subsequently impacts functional independence and productivity as well as increases the risk of physical and mental co-morbidities including falls, social isolation, and depression, thus making diabetic retinopathy a serious eye population health concern [12]. People living with diabetes can manage the onset and progression of diabetic retinopathy by adherence to diabetes medication, annual eye examination, and prompt retinopathy treatment where necessary. However, many people living with diabetes have inadequate understanding of diabetic eye complications, the importance of tight control of blood sugar, strict treatment adherence, and swift management of retinopathy signs/symptoms [4], resulting in low compliance with recommended annual screening [5].

Limited eye health literacy among other social determinants of health experienced by Indigenous people influence diabetic retinopathy awareness and eye care behavior leading to late diagnosis, poor management, poor prognosis, and vision loss. This is because, although Indigenous people are at high risk of diabetic eye complications, there are significant gaps in care, thus buttressing that interventions aimed at improving diabetes outcomes are essential [13]. Such interventions may empower Indigenous people with relevant knowledge that will influence their uptake of eye care services for early diabetic retinopathy identification, management, and the prevention of vision loss.

Indigenous women health risks, needs and preferences differ from men and non-Indigenous people, hence the gendered perspective in order to close the health/wellness gap [14]. Thus, with the increasing population of Indigenous people in cities such as Saskatoon and the population health impact of diabetic retinopathy in Indigenous women, it is vital to pursue an innovative, culturally relevant, and appropriate way of providing targeted diabetic eye care information to Indigenous women with diabetes and at-risk of diabetes in Saskatoon. To the best of our knowledge, there is no published report on the use of mHealth for diabetes-eye care among Indigenous women. Hence, this research process was part of a larger study that sought to evaluate the impact of the mHealth intervention in diabetic retinopathy awareness and eye care behavior among Indigenous women living with diabetes and at-risk of diabetes in the city of Saskatoon in Saskatchewan, Canada.

1.4 Purpose

To develop a relevant and culturally appropriate diabetes-eye content suitable for a mHealth intervention for Indigenous women living with diabetes and at- risk of diabetes in Saskatoon.

2 Literature Review

2.1 Diabetic Retinopathy

People living with diabetes have an increased risk of developing various eye complications at a younger age but, the main threat to vision due to diabetes is diabetic retinopathy (DR) which is a chronic eye condition. DR prevalence rate increases sharply after 5 years duration of type 1 diabetes in post pubertal individuals while in persons with type 2 diabetes, retinopathy may be present in about 21% soon after clinical diagnosis [15]. DR is often asymptomatic in its early stages but as it progresses, may cause irreversible vision loss.

2.2   Canadian Indigenous People

Canadian Indigenous people are the original inhabitants of Canada and constitute of First Nations, Inuit, and Métis people with unique languages, history, and cultures; and Saskatchewan has the second highest number of Indigenous people in Canada [16]. Generally, each of these Aboriginal groups have their own unique culture, way of life, language, food, beliefs, and are largely influenced by their natural environments. Large communities of Indigenous people live in Saskatoon and are the focus of this study.

2.3   Mobile Health

Initiatives to support the care and treatment of patients via mobile technology are emerging globally and mobile phone use is increasing rapidly with more than two thirds of the world's population now owning a mobile phone [17]. Hence, given the popularity of mobile phones, health professionals are increasingly using mobile phones to link people to health information and services across various settings. Research in high-income countries have shown that mHealth addresses numerous barriers in health care such as; access to medical services for vulnerable populations, enhanced communication among health care workers and patients, and improved health care delivery [18].

mHealth initiatives have thrived in both low and high-income contexts and mHealth technologies are contributing to a burgeoning number of novel health promotion, public, and population health interventions for numerous chronic disease management initiatives [19]. mHealth can support people in the management of chronic diseases during the interval between appointments and help reduce the risk of them developing complications that could have serious health consequences.

Text messaging (short message service or SMS) is now the most universal form of mobile communication and utilized to provide automated and tailored messaging [20]. Also, texts can be individually tailored for content and timing as well as for a range of variables, including language, age, gender etc. The development of health-related text messaging is on the other hand challenging in respect to the style, language, length of the messages, and quality of content in order to have maximal impact on recipients.

3   Methods

In this study, we used a multi-stage content development approach [21] to crafting text messages, informed by Self-determination theory. The authors carried out content development in four major phases: content selection, user input, review and refining of messages, and pre-testing of messages. Ethical approval was obtained from Research Ethics Board of the University of Saskatchewan.

3.1   Intervention Theory

Prior to developing the text message program, it was essential to have a prespecified framework for the focus of each information delivered. Health behavior theories can help guide the process of understanding underlying behavior change [22] and a theory driven mHealth intervention assists in providing certainty about its effectiveness. The authors used Self Determination Theory (SDT), which describes how behavior can be self-determined as a result of self-efficacy, intrinsic motivation, self-identity, needs fulfillment, and autonomy [23]. Theories of human behavior often account for the direction of behavior, but fail to account for what stimulates that behavior [24] thus, SDT posits that motivation for behavior can be self-determined when three needs are met; autonomy, competence, and relatedness.

SDT is particularly relevant to self-management of diabetes and its complications particularly as it relates to behavior change. Thus, the information on diabetes care should support the need for competence and relatedness which will prompt the feeling of autonomous integration and self-efficacy around this recommended health behavior change and may result in action planning, problem solving, and decision making.

This theory is an ideal guide for this study because it emphasizes the ways in which people actively cope with information about their health and make decisions regarding health behaviors. Also, engagement with Indigenous peoples should be respectful, supportive, and enhance self-efficacy to prompt behavior change. In addition, Schnall et al. [25] utilized self-determination theory to show how mHealth technology can be used as a social change agent to improve health via reminders and text alerts.

Focusing on beliefs and attitudes towards adherence and providing social support or social norms can strengthen motivation for engaging in behavior change [22]. Thus, we intend that the content should enhance competence (the knowledge of diabetes and its eye complications) and this will motivate and influence the ability of recipients to make autonomous and informed decisions regarding their eye care. This would be supported by relatedness which occurs via communication among family, friends, and health professionals who influence feelings about diabetes-eye risk and their eye care behavior.

3.2   Development Process

It is vital that mHealth applications align with health systems and services in the region, hence the need to involve stakeholders such as health care providers, patients, other groups addressing diabetes health care. The content development process brought together a multidisciplinary team of researchers, Indigenous people, information, communication and technology professionals; academics, health care workers and program coordinators to develop the mHealth diabetes-eye content for Indigenous women living with diabetes and at-risk of diabetes in Saskatoon. Five intended users of the mHealth initiative were also involved in the message development so as to enhance intrinsic value for the user [11] and incorporate their values and perceptions.

Content development occurred in four phases: content selection, User input, review and refining of messages, and pre-test of messages with a sample of the target audience.

Content Selection. During the first phase, the authors reviewed guidelines from Canadian Optometry and Diabetes organizations and conducted content analysis of patient directed diabetes-eye health educational materials via online searches from 2010–2017, using search terms: diabetic retinopathy and patient education. Major websites accessed included the Canadian Association of Optometrists, Canadian Diabetes Association, World Health Organization, National Eye Institute and secondary searches in diabetes organizations, support services such as Canadian National Institute for the Blind and provincial health organizations including, LiveWell Diabetes-Aim4Health program and Saskatchewan Optometric Association. The authors conducted searches until no new material was found and similar messages were deleted.

Identified relevant materials were considered and adapted to text messages. Materials such as complexity of treatments, graphics and photos were excluded since they were irrelevant or could not be used as text messages and would not be received by all phone types. The author (VU) who is an Optometrist prepared a library of 115 messages that aligned with the SDT constructs and incorporated various aspects, such as behavior change goals, clinical evidence and facts, and information from clinical guidelines. The messages were adapted for SMS to meet the 160 characters count limit. Field notes were maintained to document the process of content development.

User Input. In a preliminary study, the authors carried out four sharing circles [26] in the primary research which explored the information users would want to know about diabetes and eye care. The authors analyzed the transcripts of sharing circles and field notes to determine the type of information users would like to know or receive and what could motivate them to utilize eyecare services.

Four major themes emerged from the data: a. information on diabetes-eye care, b. etiology of diabetes, c. prevention and management, and d. Learning via images. Based on the themes, messages developed addressed: diabetic retinopathy related symptoms, the frequency of eye check, how to book an eye appointment, holistic information about diabetes. Users also requested for pictures of the eye, showing changes as the disease progresses, indicating that information communicated using images was helpful.

Review and Refining of Messages. A systematic approach with the engagement of end-users is important in developing mHealth content via involving input from a range of experts and users, evaluation and refinement, and pilot testing [27]. A multidisciplinary team of dieticians (n = 2), diabetes experts (n = 2), optometrists (n = 2), Indigenous community members (n = 3), peer leaders from the community groups (n = 2), Indigenous Elders (n = 2), researchers (n = 2), and potential participants (n = 5) (hereafter referred to as team) examined the library of messages via a community engaged workshop wherein team members reviewed each message and shared feedback during discussions on each of the messages ranging from "like it", "don't understand" and "not appropriate". The authors asked follow-up or clarifying questions as needed during the discussions and compiled notes on the feedback. The content was modified based on the feedback and recommendations, used plain language to ensure that the mHealth intervention was suitable for the targeted women.

Pre-testing of Messages. The content underwent pre-testing with five recipients for three days to ensure the delivery of the text messages to recipients on different mobile networks and sought feedback on real-time experiences in respect to message timing. Following the pre-testing, further minor modifications were incorporated. The authors developed the diabetic-eye content for mobile text messaging by ensuring that the messages aligned with the 160-character limit for a text message. Figure 1 shows an outline of the content development process.

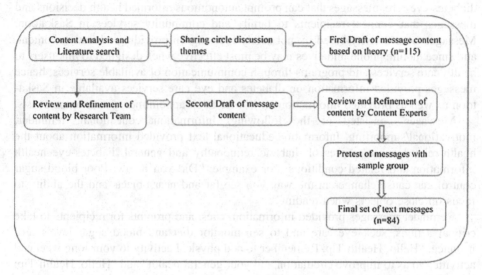

Fig. 1. Process of developing and refining text message content

4 Results

Key considerations in message development for the diabetes-eye mHealth intervention included: message prioritization, text message formatting, message delivery, and dissemination plan.

4.1 Message Prioritization

The authors prioritized selected message content based on the information provided by the intended recipients from prior formative study, key messages considered important by team members from feedbacks, and messages addressed the three constructs of the underlining theory. Based on these recommendations we included content on diabetes-eye care, information on diabetes, and prevention and management. Such as: "Health Tip: Do you know what you weigh? Maintaining a healthy body weight helps with your general health and reduces your risk of eye diseases. Check your weight today!"

Several themes emerged from the feedback from the review team, including language, positivity, and simplicity of messages. The team reported that the content of the motivational messages was acceptable due to the gentle, suggestive nature and suggested practical tips for adding necessary vegetables to traditional foods found in the city and some messages addressed this. The team shared that; a message that says, "Poor sugar control" was not positive and suggested it altered to "Unhealthy blood sugars". Again, "common sight threatening eye problems often have no warning signs. An eye exam is the only way to detect these conditions in their early stages" was too complex and team suggested it changed to, "An eye exam is the best way to find eye problems in the early stages. You can't always tell when your eyes are getting sick".

The authors included messages based on the theory that can increase knowledge of diabetes-eye care, messages that can prompt autonomous informed health decisions and messages that connect recipients to family and community services in Saskatoon. Messages were activity-based by not solely focusing on providing education content, and since mobile phone initiatives may be most effective when designed to link users to health care services and programs through communication of available services; hence messages provided information on diabetes and eye care services available in Saskatoon as well as provided information on how to book appointments with optometrists.

Messages consisted of the following: informational/educational, reminder, motivational/supporting. Information/educational text provided information about the health-related consequences of diabetic retinopathy and general diabetes-eye health information and related conditions. For example: "Did you Know: Poor blood sugar control can cause changes in the way you see far and near objects and the ability to focus on close objects when reading".

Reminder messages provided information, cues, and prompts for recipients to take critical actions, seek eye care and to self-monitor diet and blood sugar levels. For instance: "Hello. Health Tip: Remember to add physical activity to your long weekend activities so as to improve circulation and your general health" and "Hello. Health Tip: When was the last time you had an eye exam? If more than 1 year ago, and you are living with diabetes, you are due for an eye checkup".

Motivational/supporting text shared information that elicits engaging in activities that will enable recipients manage or prevent diabetes-eye conditions. For example: "Health Tip: Your daily habits and lifestyle such as exercising could seriously help your eyes without you knowing it. Keep up the good work".

4.2 Text Formatting

Messages were careful worded to ensure clarity and avoid misunderstandings. The author (VU) has experience in digital content development as such was responsible for shortening the messages to ≤ 160 characters while maintaining their meaning. In addition, we utilized a flexible approach thus, the content could be tweaked based on present conditions at the period of delivery.

4.3 Delivery

The authors considered cost, ease of messaging platform, ease of dissemination, applicability to devices and tracking of delivery when looking for messaging vendors.

The authors plan to deliver daily text messages to the target population's mobile devices (77 recipients) between 8.30am and 9am daily (as suggested by the intended recipients during review) by Telmatik a communications management and bulk messaging platform that supports personalized user outputs and inputs via text messaging and provides technological solutions [28].

4.4 Dissemination Plan

The authors designed a messaging sequence such that every week, messages provided information relating to: general eye care, information targeting those with diabetes, at risk of diabetes, action-based, and connecting with health/community services.

5 Discussion

The mHealth messages utilized evidence-based information and approaches for diabetes-eye prevention and management and it was informed by behavioral theory. Content analysis of diabetes educational material across various health organizations provided the team with an extensive list of message options. The theory helped organize messages and guided the choice of messages selected which was ideal in making message content development systematic and comprehensive [22]. The messages came from trusted sources, were informative, encouraging, reassuring, non-judgmental, and provided "cues to action'. In addition, the content gave information on availability of heath care services, not only focusing on the condition [29], and included information on co-morbidities associated with diabetes and the eyes, such as holistic information on diabetes and general eye care.

The community engaged feedback process enabled community members and intended users identify and address concerns such as the cultural appropriateness of the content. This aligns with a family-focused diabetes self-Care support mHealth intervention for diverse, low-income adults with type 2 diabetes that utilized community engagement in the development of the content and mHealth protocol [30]. In addition, it balanced bottom-up and top-bottom approaches in community health that often results in an acceptable and equitable intervention [11].

The messages did not focus on the negative health consequences of diabetes since it was not motivational and doesn't enhance self-confidence, rather the focus was on the benefits and opportunities for eye health. Morton and colleagues similarly indicated that messages on the benefits of physical activity rather than the impact of overweight in type 2 diabetes management was preferable [31]. In addition, a text message would prompt users to seek eye care if they are light-hearted, positive, supportive, and encouraging [31]. The authors added a personal greeting and encouragement in messages and this has shown to be useful in the design of text messaging content, as this may facilitate women's self-confidence and perceived self-efficacy [21], and may prompt them to utilize eye care services and manage their health.

6   Conclusion

This study supports the use of a collaborative approach in the development of mobile health messages. The approach involving multidisciplinary experts and community members resulted in a mHealth content that responded to participants needs, culturally appropriate and relevant. Messages were developed as a team, using an iterative process of writing, review, pre-testing and further modification until a final version was agreed upon. The diabetes-eye mHealth content was evidence based, flexible and aligned with the community needs, and the developed messages consisted of informational and educational, reminder, and motivating/supporting content as well as provided cues to making informed diabetes- eye care decisions. The mHealth intervention will provide evidence-based information about diabetes and eye care and ways that women can control and reduce their risk of the condition and improve diabetes-eye outcomes.

Mobile health applications are promising in addressing health disparities, particularly in Indigenous populations who disproportionately face barriers to self-management due to limited heath communication, cultural competency of health care workers, social support, and access to health care. This study provides some key steps and considerations for the development of a mHealth text messaging initiative that responds to community need in an Indigenous population. Future directions include testing the efficacy of the mHealth intervention in increasing diabetes knowledge and eye care behavior. Thus, the content is being evaluated among the targeted population to access the quality and reliability of this proposed approach and its impact is under analysis.

Strengths and Limitations. The authors developed the content specifically for Indigenous women living in Saskatoon as such reflects the needs of the population. Importantly, since a theory guided our process of crafting these messages, it can explain how the messages can potentially result in behavior change. Thus, the mHealth content and intervention may be adapted for use in other regions and in different contexts. Limitation includes the inability to provide pictorial content as requested by participants due to the text messaging platform chosen for content dissemination.

Acknowledgements. We would like to thank LiveWell-Aim4Health program Saskatoon, Saskatoon Indian and Metis Friendship Centre, Canadian Diabetes Association Saskatoon and Saskatchewan Optometric Association for their input in the content development.

Conflicts of Interest. The authors have no conflicts of interest to declare.

References

1. Saskatchewan Ministry of Health: Prevalence of Asthma, COPD, DIabetes, and Hypertension in Saskatchewan, 2010/11 (2013)
2. Dyck, R., Osgood, N., Lin, T.H., Gao, A., Stang, M.R.: Epidemiology of diabetes mellitus among First Nations and non-First Nations adults. Can. Med. Assoc. J. **182**(3), 249–256 (2010)
3. Harris, S.B., Bhattacharyya, O., Dyck, R., Hayward, M.N., Toth, E.L.: Type 2 diabetes in Aboriginal peoples. Can. J. Diabetes **37**(Suppl. 1), S191–S196 (2013)

4. Threatt, J., Williamson, F.J., Huynh, K., Davis, R.M.: Ocular disease, knowledge, and technology applications in patients with diabetes. Am. J. Med. Sci. **345**(4), 266–270 (2014)

5. Hooper, P., et al.: Canadian Ophthalmological Society evidence-based clinical practice guidelines for the management of diabetic retinopathy. Can. J. Ophthalmol. **47**(2), S1–S30 (2012)

6. Maberley, D., Cruess, A.F., Barile, G., Slakter, J.: Digital photographic screening for diabetic retinopathy in the James Bay Cree. Ophthalmic Epidemiol. **9**(3), 169–178 (2002)

7. Kelly, C., Booth, G.L.: Diabetes in Canadian women. BMC Womens Health **4**(Suppl. 1), S16 (2004)

8. Nentwich, M.M., Ulbig, M.W.: Diabetic retinopathy - ocular complications of diabetes mellitus. World J. Diabetes **6**(3), 489–499 (2015)

9. Chris, P.: Diabetes and Aboriginal vision health. Can. J. Optom. **72**(4), 8 (2010)

10. McBride, B., Nguyen, L.T., Wiljer, D., Vu, N.C., Nguyen, C.K., O'Neil, J.: Development of a maternal, newborn and child mHealth intervention in Thai Nguyen Province, Vietnam: protocol for the mMom project. JMIR Res. Protoc. **7**, e6 (2018)

11. Biagianti, B., Hidalgo-Mazzei, D., Meyer, N.: Developing digital interventions for people living with serious mental illness: perspectives from three mHealth studies. Evid.-Based Ment. Health **20**(4), 98–101 (2017)

12. Canadian Diabetes Association: Retinopathy. Can. J. Diabetes **37**(1), S1–S212 (2013)

13. Harris, S.B., Naqshbandi, M., Bhattacharyya, O., Hanley, A.J.G., Esler, J.G., Zinman, B.: Major gaps in diabetes clinical care among Canada's First Nations: results of the CIRCLE study. Diabetes Res. Clin. Pract. **92**, 272–279 (2011)

14. Halseth, R.: Aboriginal women in Canada: gender, socio-economic determinants of health, and initiatives to close the wellness-gap. Prince George, BC (2013)

15. Fong, D.S., et al.: Retinopathy in diabetes. Diabetes Care **27**(1), S84–S87 (2004)

16. Douglas, V.: Introduction to Aboriginal Health and Health Care in Canada: Bridging Health and Healing Springer, Secaucus (2014)

17. Pine, K.J., Fletcher, B.C.: It started with a text: an analysis of the effectiveness of mHeath interventions in changing behaviour and the impact of text messaging on behavioural outcomes. mHEALTH White Paper, pp. 1–9. Do Something Different Ltd., December 2015

18. Beratarrechea, A., Moyano, D., Irazola, V., Rubinstein, A.: mHealth interventions to counter noncommunicable diseases in developing countries: still an uncertain promise. Cardiol. Clin. **35**(1), 13–30 (2017)

19. Coughlin, S.S., Besenyi, G.M., Bowen, D., De Leo, G.: Development of the physical activity and your nutrition for cancer (PYNC) smartphone app for preventing breast cancer in women. mHealth. **3**(Feb), 5 (2017)

20. L'Engle, K.L., Mangone, E.R., Parcesepe, A.M., Agarwal, S., Ippoliti, N.B.: Mobile phone interventions for adolescent sexual and reproductive health: a systematic review. Pediatrics **138**(3), e20160884 (2016)

21. Odeny, T.A., Newman, M., Bukusi, E.A., McClelland, R.S., Cohen, C.R., Camlin, C.S.: Developing content for a mHealth intervention to promote postpartum retention in prevention of mother-to-child HIV transmission programs and early infant diagnosis of HIV: a qualitative study. PLoS ONE **9**(9), e106383 (2014)

22. Iribarren, S.J., Beck, S.L., Pearce, P.F., Chirico, C., Etchevarria, M., Rubinstein, F.: mHealth intervention development to support patients with active tuberculosis. J. Mob. Technol. Med. **3**(2), 16–27 (2014)

23. Deci, E.L., Ryan, R.M.: The "what" and "why" of goal pursuits: human needs and the self-determination of behavior. Psychol. Inq. **11**(4), 227–268 (2000)

24. Patrick, H., Williams, G.C.: Self-determination theory: its application to health behavior and complementarity with motivational interviewing. Int. J. Behav. Nutr. Phys. Act. **9**(1), 18 (2012)
25. Schnall, R., Bakken, S., Rojas, M., Travers, J., Carballo-Dieguez, A.: mHealth technology as a persuasive tool for treatment, care and management of persons living with HIV. AIDS Behav. **19**, 81–89 (2015)
26. Kovach, M.: Conversational method in Indigenous research. First Peoples Child Fam. Rev. **5** (1), 40–48 (2010)
27. Thakkar, J., et al.: Design considerations in development of a mobile health intervention program: the TEXT ME and TEXTMEDS experience. JMIR mHealth uHealth **4**(4), e127 (2016)
28. Telmatik: Company profile (2018). http://centredappels.telmatik.com/qui-sommes-nous/profil-de-lentreprise/. Accessed 16 Mar 2018
29. Evans, C., Turner, K., Suggs, L.S., Occa, A., Juma, A., Blake, H.: Developing a mHealth intervention to promote uptake of HIV testing among African communities in the conditions: a qualitative study. BMC Public Health **16**(1), 1–16 (2016)
30. Mayberry, L.S., Berg, C.A., Harper, K.J., Osborn, C.Y.: Development and feasibility of a family-focused mhealth intervention for low-income adults with type 2 diabetes. J. Diabetes Res. **65**, A213 (2016)
31. Morton, K., Sutton, S., Hardeman, W.: A text-messaging and pedometer program to promote physical activity in people at high risk of type 2 diabetes: the development of the PROPELS follow-on support program. JMIR mHealth uHealth **3**(4), e105 (2015)

Why People Are Willing to Provide Social Support in Online Health Communities: Evidence from Social Exchange Perspective

Tongyao Zhao(✉) and Rong Du

Xidian University, Xi'an 710126, China
tyzhao@stu.xidian.edu.cn

Abstract. More and more people in china are increasingly using Internet as a major source of health-related information in recent years. Online healthcare communities (OHCs) are interesting in this regard, appearing to serve as virtual communities for people to provide social support. However, the development of OHCs requires the active participation of its members to create and share knowledge. How to improve community members' provision of social support becomes a key issue for community managers. To address this issue, utilizing social exchange theory, we propose a benefit-cost model to study the incentive factors and inhibiting factors of the social support in OHCs. In the model, the benefits are extended to the psychological rewards in social exchange, including sense of belongings, reputation and sense of self-worth. Costs are divided into cognitive costs and executional costs. We study the moderation effect of psychological distance. Data will be collected from more than 300 users of well-known OHCs in China and analyzed by SmartPLS. The research findings can provide managerial implications for community managers.

Keywords: Online healthcare community (OHC) · Social exchange theory
Psychological distance · Social support

1 Introduction

In present era, the high-intensity fast-paced work and life are demanding more efforts from the people. According to the survey data of Linkip monitoring system, up to 60% of white-collar workers work over 8 h, 25% over 10 h, and 15% over 12 h. The average weekly exercise time for Chinese white-collar workers is less than 3 h. Long hours of overloaded work and the compressed exercise time have led more and more white-collar workers out of healthy 'tracks' [1]; With the advent of various electronic products, staying up at night playing mobile phones has become the norm for young people, which cause increasing concern about health. More than 40% of Internet users are in sub-healthy status [2].

In August 2017, eyeballs were attracted by a photo of Zhao Mingyi, a 50-year-old rock star from the iconic 1990s rock band Black Panther, holding a Thermoswent iral. The image sparked conversations about the dreaded midlife crisis and fears of the future. 'Thermoswent iral + Chinese wolfberry' and 'fitness' have become hot topics in microblogging. 'Thermoswent iral + Chinese wolfberry' is not only the choice of the

© Springer Nature Switzerland AG 2018
H. Chen et al. (Eds.): ICSH 2018, LNCS 10983, pp. 119–129, 2018.
https://doi.org/10.1007/978-3-030-03649-2_12

elderly, college students and young people at work also join the trend of healthcare. Therefore, online healthcare communities (OHCs) are paid more and more people's attention. The application of smart phones, WeChat subscriptions, friend circles, tweets and mobile APPs on healthcare have appeared one after another, which meet people's growing concern for health and provides important platforms for people to seek healthcare knowledge and discuss health experiences [3]. However, there are still many problems in the OHCs. Active members of the community tend to be a minority, and many people are in the silent state of consuming knowledge [4]. However, users are major components of the OHCs, and their contributions are driving force for OHCs' sustainable growth. Therefore, this study starts from the perspective of the provision of social support in OHCs.

Social support refers to using certain material and spiritual means to provide unpaid help to vulnerable groups in the society. In the healthcare field, social support refers to the provision of unpaid help to the groups with health problems [4]. "Social support is an exchange of resources between two individuals perceived by the provider or the recipient to be intended to enhance the well- being of the recipient" [5]. Therefore, considering the specific background and current problems of OHCs, we will study the factors that influence social support from the perspective of social exchange.

Social exchange theory seeks to explain individual behavior in the social resources exchange activities [6]. Social exchange theory suggests that individual behavior is guided by relatively simple principles, i.e., increasing the positive results and reducing the negative outcomes they expect [7]. Some scholars use the theory to study the motivation of members to contribute toward the knowledge [7], and some use it to address the restraining factor in the research of knowledge contribution [8]. Kankan-halli et al. construct the cost-benefit model of enterprise knowledge based on the social exchange theory [9]. Yan et al. establish a benefit-cost model for knowledge sharing of online medical communities [10]. Social exchange theory is also used to explain why students add their teacher as a Facebook friend [11], why individuals tweet and retweet [12]. In other words, social exchange theory can explain a wide range of user behavior with respect to information systems. The theory of social exchange provides a fundamental research framework for the research of social support in this study. The benefit-cost model [3] is constructed according to the "benefits gained" and "the costs paid" in the process of resource exchange, which could be translated to motivation and inhibition of social support behavior.

In social exchange theory, there are two kinds of rewards—material rewards and psychological rewards. Psychological rewards are the psychological gains arising during social exchange, e.g., interest, respect, recognition, etc. The rewards originating from providing social support for virtual communities are mainly caused by psychological satisfaction. Therefore, the 'benefit' will be extended to psychological rewards.

Thus, the first research question in this study is:

RQ1: How do the psychological rewards and costs impact on the provision of social support in OHCs?

Consider the particularity of the OHCs, where people seeking health information are sensitive and have relatively high requirements for information quality, this requires social support providers to have appropriate psychological feelings to provide timely and appropriate feedback. According to social cognitive theory, people's interpretation of an event will change with the perception of the psychological distance of the event (such as time distance, space distance, society distance, hypotheses distance, etc.), hence affect people's reactions.

The second research question in this study is:

RQ2: How does the psychological distance moderates the impact of psychological rewards on the provision of social support in OHCs?

The rest of the paper is organized as follows: We present the related work in the next section. Then, we propose a research model and relevant hypotheses. After that, we introduce our methodology. In the concluding part, we give discussions and extensions for further study.

2 Related Work

2.1 Online Health Community

Online health communities are valuable platforms for people to search for health information and discuss their experiences with medical treatments [10]. A number of online communities have emerged in recent years, thus making it easier than ever for users to find timely and personalized health information online [13].

Extensive studies have investigated the advantages and mechanisms of online health communities. Yan [10] studies the knowledge sharing in OHCs from the perspective of social exchange theory; Zhang [3] empirically examines the effects of extrinsic and intrinsic motivations on knowledge sharing intentions in OHCs; Wu [14] studies the channel effect in OHCs. Although a number of studies have investigated the online health communities, literatures that have focused on the motivations and inhibitions of provision on social support in OHCs are not much. To fill this research gap, we aim to explore the factors that influence social support in OHCs from the perspective of social exchange.

2.2 Social Support

Social support is an exchange of resources between at least two individuals perceived by the provider or the recipient to be intended to enhance the well-being of the recipient. The inclusion of the term exchange of social support makes our assumption as explicit that support necessarily involves at least two individuals and that there are potential costs and benefits associated with the exchange for both participants [5]. Therefore, in this study, researchers believe that social support will be affected by the benefits and costs.

Some scholars believe that social support is giving material help or directly providing assistance to those people indeed [15]. Some argue that social support is providing psychological and spiritual support to people in need [16]. Therefore, Provision of social support in this paper is defined as: material and spiritual aid to the people in OHCs.

Many studies have examined the social support provided via online communities for various health-related problems and topics, and these studies have provided an ample evidence that social support has clear benefits for participants in OHCs [17–19]. For those who experience many stress factors in life, such as serious diseases, social support becomes a contributing factor that has important effects on health recovery and daily coping [20, 21]. Especially in the case of chronic diseases, social support is not only beneficial to patients but also beneficial to their caregivers and families [19].

Some researchers study the behavior of online support. For example, in the online community, social identities influence social support seeking behavior, however, none of these studies involve research that affects the provision of online social support providers. The most relevant to this article are the studies of Lin [22] and Lee [4] et al. In study of Lin, action-facilitating support and nurturant support may directly or indirectly determine individuals' willingness to offer support. Lee [4] analyzes the provision of social support from the perspective of social cognitive theory, showing that psychological distance will negatively affect the provision of social support, while empathy will adjust the relationship between them.

As a kind of exchange behavior, social support will inevitably be affected by both benefit and cost factors. From this point of view, we starts from the perspective of social exchange theory and proposes that how the psychological reward and cost impact provision of social support. Combining with the characteristics of the healthcare and characteristics of the virtual platform, psychological distance is proposed as a moderator to study their relationships.

3   Research Model and Hypothesis

The "benefits" in social exchange theory tend to explain the motivation of people to participate in social activities [23]. Social exchange theory is also an important perspective for understanding relationships, which emphasizes that people in the process of interpersonal exchange will exchange valuable things, including material and psychological (eg, support, reputation, self-esteem, etc.) [24]. The members of the OHCs mainly want to receive non-monetary rather than monetary benefits. This is different from some online communities in which people benefit from monetary rewards or enjoyment [25]. As an online community of higher social value, OHC helps people to promote their health and well-being by providing and acquiring unique information, treatment options, and experiences with specific diseases [26]. People can get sense of belongings easily under this atmosphere, and will feel respected when the knowledge they contribute is recognized by others. Sense of self-worth is the highest level of social needs [27]. The psychological rewards are divided into three levels: sense of belongings, reputation and sense of self-worth.

Sense of belongings (SB) is also called attachment, identity, and sense of membership [28]. Studies found that sense of belonging could maintain and promote members' participation in the virtual community. Members of OHCs consult and get help when they encounter health-related issues. They also provide their own or their friends' healthcare experiences and knowledge to those in need, communicate with other members, get feedback, and even become friends with them. Sense of dependence, identity and membership are generated across the process. With this emotion, community members will be more concerned with the community and are willing to participate in knowledge sharing activities, answer questions more seriously [29].

In our study, reputation (R) refers to the respect and achievement that members of OHCs receive through knowledge sharing. However, the article is aimed at healthcare communities in China, so the impact of culture is taken into account. The behavior of individuals in the community is influenced by national culture [30]. Chinese reputation is "face". Faces are the respect, self-esteem and dignity of personal achievement and practice [31]. An important way to protect and gain face is to express yourself and show your strengths [10]. Members in OHCs share expertise, answer questions for help seekers, demonstrate their generosity and benevolence [10], receive feedback and praise, gain face or honor, which further motivate them to share knowledge.

Sense of self-worth (SSW) describes the extent to which people recognize themselves and provide value to the community through knowledge sharing [32]. In this study, sense of self-worth is the self-perceived self-esteem and self-efficacy gained by members of OHCs through sharing healthcare knowledge. Sense of self-worth could affects individual behavior [32]. The stronger the sense of self-worth gained through providing social support, the more positive the attitude. Accordingly, we make the following assumptions:

H1. Psychological rewards positively influence provision of social support in OHCs.

The "cost" of social exchange theory is defined as the negative result of exchange behavior [24], thus reducing the frequency of exchange behavior. Costs are divided into cognitive costs and executional costs [23]. Cognitive costs focus on psychological feelings such as unpleasantness, fatigue and pain experienced during the exchange of information. In order to contribute knowledge to an OHC, members must work hard to recall their previous healthcare experiences, a process that will make them remember the painful experiences. This negative impact will undermine members' provision of social support and thus reduce social support behavior. Execution costs are used to explain the time, money and effort spent on social support [9]. This process is considered a contribution, for a lot of time and effort can be used to do other things to get rewards or benefits [23]. Previous studies have shown that when knowledge sharing takes a great deal of time and effort, knowledge sharing behavior is often suppressed [11] therefore, we put forward the hypothesis:

H2. Cost negatively affect provision of social support in OHCs.

Psychological distance generally includes four major dimensions: temporal, spatial, social, and certainty-related distance. Taking the characteristics of the OHCs into account, we added two developing dimensions to the psychological distance: informational distance and experiential distance [33]. Information distance is the gap between the information required by the poster and the information actually held by the provider. A user in the OHC wants to answer the question from the poster, awkwardly finds that the knowledge he/she has is not sufficient, and thus is unable to provide social support. Experience distance is, whether the available information, whatever its amount, is based on first-hand information (e.g., the consumer's own prior experience) or second-hand and third-hand information (based on communication from other people, literature, or media). If the replier happens to have experience in this area, quickly replying detailed and real content, it is easy to resonate with the poster, thus providing better social support.

Events or objects are directly stripped from the psychological distance, affecting the perception and evaluation of events, and thus affecting individuals' motivations and preferences for behaviors [34]. If the distance to the incident is far, the motivation for people to take action is less intense [4]. A large number of studies have shown that psychological distance can affect individual judgment and behavior [4, 33, 35–37]. Knowledge providers will not provide social support when realizing that they have insufficient information or feel less relevant to the events, even if they have sufficient motivation to provide information. This is caused by excessive psychological distance. Therefore, we believe that psychological distance will moderate the relationship between psychological rewards and the provision of social support. We propose the following assumptions:

H3. Psychological distance negatively moderates the relationship between psychological rewards and provision of social support in OHCs.
Based on the assumptions above, we propose a research model shown in Fig. 1.

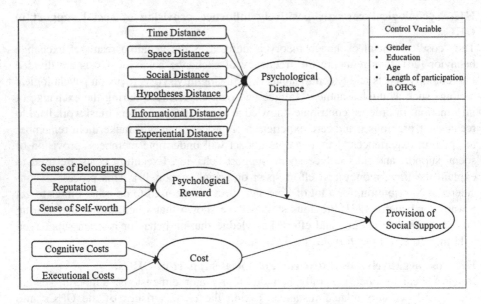

Fig. 1. Provision of social support model in online healthcare communities

4 Methodology

We plan to test our hypotheses with a questionnaire surveys after interviewing people who have spending long time in OHCs. After that, a pilot study needs to be conducted among these people to help us do some adjustments.

4.1 Instrument Development

Based on our research model, we developed a survey questionnaire to measure the proposed constructs that may contribute to provision of social support in OHCs. To measure each construct, questions were compiled and adapted from validated instruments used in the prior literature, and the wording was modified to fit the Chinese OHCs context. Specifically, we adapted items for sense of belongings (SB) from Zhao et al. [6]; Reputation (R) items from Yan; items for sense of self-worth (SSW) from Yan et al.; Cognitive cost (CC) and executional cost (EC) items from Yan et al. Items for psychological distance from Spence et al.; Items for provision of social support (PSS) from Lee et al. We conducted a backward translation process to ensure consistency between the Chinese and English versions of the instrument [10], and rated all items using a seven-point Likert scale, with 1 indicating "strongly disagree" and 7 indicating "strongly agree". As our construct measures are shown in Table 1.

Table 1. Construct measures

Constructs	Items	Sources
Sense of belongings	SB1: Through posting or replying in online healthcare communities, I feel a strong sense of belongings to the communities	Modified from Zhao et al. (2012)
	SB2: Through posting or replying in online healthcare communities, I feel I am a member of the communities	
	SB3: Providing healthcare knowledge for other members in the community, I feel other members are my close friends	
Reputation	R1: Providing healthcare knowledge for other members in the online healthcare community will make me gain face	Modified from Yan et al. (2017)
	R2: I care about others' attitudes toward me	
	R3: I will gain face if I have latest healthcare knowledge	
Sense of self-worth	SSW1: The healthcare knowledge I provided would help other members in the online healthcare community solve problems	Modified from Yan et al. (2017)
	SSW2: My healthcare knowledge would bring positive influence on other members in the online healthcare community	
	SSW3: My knowledge sharing would bring all my facilities into full play and make me more confident	
Executional costs	EC1: I cannot seem to find the time to share knowledge in the open healthcare knowledge community	Adopted from Yan et al. (2017)
	EC2: It takes me too much time to write a post or reply in the online healthcare community	
	EC3: It is laborious to share knowledge in the open healthcare knowledge community	
	EC4: The effort is high for me to share knowledge in the open healthcare knowledge community	

(continued)

Table 1. (*continued*)

Constructs	Items	Sources
Cognitive costs	CC1: It is annoying to recall every detailed aspect of my or others' healthcare experience in order to provide healthcare knowledge in the online healthcare community	Adopted from Yan et al. (2017)
	CC2: It is not enjoyable to recall my or others' medical treatment procedure in order to provide healthcare knowledge in the online healthcare community	
	CC3: It is costly to organize my or others' healthcare experiences cognitively for social support in the open healthcare knowledge community	
	CC4: It is hard for me to recollect healthcare experience and treatment solution	
Space distance	SD1: The people and things mentioned in the post are far away from me	Modified from Spence et al. (2012)
Time distance	TDI: The people and things mentioned in the post are far from now	
Social distance	SCD1: I am willing to become a neighbor with the person on the post	
	SCD2: I am willing to become friends with the person on the post	
Hypotheses distance	HDI: The people and things mentioned on the post are very unlikely to happen to me	
Informational distance	ID1: For the people and things mentioned on the post, I have little relevant information and knowledge	
Experiential distance	ED1: I have never personally experienced the things mentioned on the post	
Provision of social support	PSS1: After seeing the post, I will do my best to give the posters information or emotional support	Adopted from Lee et al. (2017)

4.2 Data Collection

To validate our research hypothesis, we need to work with OHCs to encourage OHCs users to participate in the survey. We searched the top ten healthcare communities from the website of China webmaster (http://top.chinaz.com) and selected the communities involved in the study. According to the characteristics of health care and integration with Chinese tradition, we finally selected three major OHCs: Sanjiu overall health net (Baidu estimated traffic of 1,699,600, Google included 2,140,000), Sanjiu Yang-shengtang (Baidu Estimated traffic of 19,300, Google 410,000), China Health Network (Baidu estimated traffic of 481,100, Google included 211,000).

We will ask the website administrators of these three OHCs to post and highlight our survey questionnaire and an invitation to participate. In order to inspire OHCs members' involvement, we would offer a gift valued at $2 to each respondent. Furthermore, ten respondents will be randomly selected to be awarded a $20 cash bonus. The data collection procedure will last three months.

5 Discussion and Planned Extensions

This paper has proposed a conceptual model to explore the relationship among psychological rewards, costs, provision of social support, and psychological distance within the context of online healthcare communities. We are using questionnaire survey to do the research. Future work will mainly focus on the collection and analysis of the data. Hopefully the findings of this research can provide implications not only for managers of OHCs to better improve community social support and sustain their development, but also for OHCs users to better exchange healthcare information and improve their health conditions.

References

1. LINKIP: Survey on sub-health conditions of white collar (2018). http://yq.linkip.cn/user/sjbg.do. Accessed 04 May 2018
2. iReseach (2017). http://report.iresearch.cn/report/201603/2561.shtml. Accessed 26 Apr 2017
3. Zhang, X., Liu, S., Deng, Z., Chen, X.: Knowledge sharing motivations in online health-communities: a comparative study of health professionals and normal users. Comput. Hum. Behav. **75**, 797–810 (2017). https://doi.org/10.1016/j.chb.2017.06.028
4. Lee, J., Liu, M., Liu, X., Zhang, P., Chen, Z.: Research on willingness to provide online social support: based on the perspective of the theory of interpretation level. J. Inf. Syst. **2**, 82–97 (2016). (in Chinese)
5. Shumaker, S.A., Brownell, A.: Toward a theory of social support: closing conceptual gaps. J. Soc. Issues **40**(4), 11–36 (1984). https://doi.org/10.1111/j.1540-4560.1984.tb01105.x
6. Song, C., Park, K.R., Kang, S.-W.: Servant leadership and team performance: the mediating role of knowledge-sharing climate. Soc. Behav. Pers.: Int. J. **43**(10), 1749–1760 (2015). https://doi.org/10.2224/sbp.2015.43.10.1749
7. Luo, Y.: Research on knowledge sharing motivation of virtual community members: based on the perspective of social network location. Doctoral dissertation, Fudan University (2013). (in Chinese)
8. Chen, S.: Research on influencing factors of users' knowledge sharing intention in online community. New Media Res. **1**(19), 1–2 (2015). (in Chinese)
9. Kankanhalli, A., Tan, B.C.Y., Wei, K.K.: Contributing knowledge to electronic knowledge repositories: an empirical investigation. MIS Q. **29**(1), 113 (2005). https://doi.org/10.2307/25148670
10. Yan, Z., Wang, T., Chen, Y., Zhang, H.: Knowledge sharing in online health communities: a social exchange theory perspective. Inf. Manag. **53**(5), 643–653 (2016). https://doi.org/10.1016/j.im.2016.02.001
11. Sheldon, P.: Understanding students' reasons and gender differences in adding faculty as Facebook friends. Comput. Hum. Behav. **53**, 58–62 (2015). https://doi.org/10.1016/j.chb.2015.06.043
12. O'Leary, D.E.: Modeling retweeting behavior as a game: comparison to empirical results. Int. J. Hum.-Comput. Stud. **88**, 1–12 (2016). https://doi.org/10.1016/j.ijhcs.2015.11.005
13. Ba, S., Wang, L.: Digital health communities: the effect of their motivation mechanisms. Decis. Support Syst. **55**(4), 941–947 (2013). https://doi.org/10.1016/j.dss.2013.01.003

14. Wu, H., Lu, N.: Online written consultation, telephone consultation and offline appointment: an examination of the channel effect in online health communities. Int. J. Med. Inform. **107**, 107–119 (2017). https://doi.org/10.1016/j.ijmedinf.2017.08.009

15. Pearlin, L.I.: Social structure and processes of social support (1985)

16. Hoffman, M.A., Ushpiz, V., Levy-Shiff, R.: Social support and self-esteem in adolescence. J. Youth Adolesc. **17**(4), 307–316 (1988). https://doi.org/10.1007/bf01537672

17. Atwood, M.E., Friedman, A., Meisner, B.A., Cassin, S.E.: The exchange of social sup-port on online bariatric surgery discussion forums: a mixed-methods content analysis. Health Commun. **33**(5), 1–8 (2017). https://doi.org/10.1080/10410236.2017.1289437

18. Loane, S.S., D'Alessandro, S.: Communication that changes lives: social support wi-thin an online health community for ALS. Commun. Q. **61**(2), 236–251 (2013). https://doi.org/10.1080/01463373.2012.752397

19. Yao, T., Zheng, Q., Fan, X.: The impact of online social support on patients' quality of life and the moderating role of social exclusion. J. Serv. Res. **18**(3), 369–383 (2015). https://doi.org/10.1177/1094670515583271

20. Coulson, N.S., Greenwood, N.: Families affected by childhood cancer: an analysis of the provision of social support within online support groups. Child Care Health Dev. **38**(6), 870–877 (2012). https://doi.org/10.1111/j.1365-2214.2011.01316.x

21. Chronister, J., Chou, C.-C., Liao, H.-Y.: The role of stigma coping and social support in mediating the effect of societal stigma on internalized stigma, mental health recovery, and quality of life among people with serious mental illness. J. Community Psychol. **41**(5), 582–600 (2013). https://doi.org/10.1002/jcop.21558

22. Lin, T.-C., Hsu, J.S.-C., Cheng, H.-L., Chiu, C.-M.: Exploring the relationship between receiving and offering online social support: a dual social support model. Inf. Manag. **52**(3), 371–383 (2015). https://doi.org/10.1016/j.im.2015.01.003

23. Liu, Z., Min, Q., Zhai, Q., Smyth, R.: Self-disclosure in Chinese micro-blogging: a social exchange theory perspective. Inf. Manag. **53**(1), 53–63 (2016). https://doi.org/10.1016/j.im.2015.08.006

24. Emerson, R.M.: Social exchange theory. Ann. Rev. Sociol. **2**(7), 335–362 (1976). https://doi.org/10.1146/annurev.so.02.080176.002003

25. Papadopoulos, T., Stamati, T., Nopparuch, P.: Exploring the determinants of knowledge sharing via employee weblogs. Int. J. Inf. Manag. **33**(1), 133–146 (2013). https://doi.org/10.1016/j.ijinfomgt.2012.08.002

26. Johnston, A.C., Worrell, J.L., Di Gangi, P.M., Wasko, M.: Online health communities. Inf. Technol. People **26**(2), 213–235 (2013). https://doi.org/10.1108/itp-02-2013-0040

27. Maslow, A.H.: Motivation and Personality. Harper, New York (1954)

28. Hagborg, W.J.: An investigation of a brief measure of school membership. Adolescence **33** (130), 461 (1998)

29. Zhao, L., Lu, Y., Wang, B., Chau, P.Y.K., Zhang, L.: Cultivating the sense of belonging and motivating user participation in virtual communities: a social capital perspective. Int. J. Inf. Manag. **32**(6), 574–588 (2012). https://doi.org/10.1016/j.ijinfomgt.2012.02.006

30. Siau, K., Erickson, J., Nah, F.F.-H.: Effects of national culture on types of knowledge sharing in virtual communities. IEEE Trans. Prof. Commun. **53**(3), 278–292 (2010). https://doi.org/10.1109/tpc.2010.2052842

31. Huang, Q., Davison, R.M., Gu, J.: Impact of personal and cultural factors on knowledge sharing in China. Asia Pac. J. Manag. **25**(3), 451–471 (2008). https://doi.org/10.1007/s10490-008-9095-2

32. Bock, G.M., Zmud, R.M., Kim, Y.M., Lee, J.N.: Behavioral intention formation in knowledge sharing: examining the roles of extrinsic motivators, social-psychological forces, and organizational climate. MIS Q. **29**(1), 87 (2005). https://doi.org/10.2307/25148669

33. Fiedler, K.: Construal level theory as an integrative framework for behavioral decision-making research and consumer psychology. J. Consum. Psychol. **17**(2), 101–106 (2007). https://doi.org/10.1016/S1057-7408(07)70015-3
34. Todorov, A., Goren, A., Trope, Y.: Probability as a psychological distance: construal and preferences. J. Exp. Soc. Psychol. **43**(3), 473–482 (2007). https://doi.org/10.1016/j.jesp.2006.04.002
35. Boothby, E.J., Smith, L.K., Clark, M.S., Bargh, J.A.: Psychological distance moderates the amplification of shared experience. Pers. Soc. Psychol. Bull. **42**(10), 1431–1444 (2016). https://doi.org/10.1177/0146167216662869
36. Hernández-Ortega, B.: Don't believe strangers: online consumer reviews and the role of social psychological distance. Inf. Manag. **55**(1), 31–50 (2018). https://doi.org/10.1016/j.im.2017.03.007
37. Puchalska-Wasyl, M.M.: The impact of psychological distance on integrative internal dialogs. Int. J. Psychol. **53**(1), 58–65 (2016). https://doi.org/10.1002/ijop.12266

Strategic Behavior in Mobile Behavioral Intervention Platforms: Evidence from a Field Quasi-experiment on a Health Management App

Chunxiao Li[1(✉)], Bin Gu[2], and Chenhui Guo[3]

[1] Shanghai Jiao Tong University, Shanghai, China
chunxiaoli@asu.edu
[2] Arizona State University, Tempe, AZ 85201, USA
[3] Michigan State University, East Lansing, MI 48824, USA

Abstract. In recent years, people have witnessed the growing popularity of mobile health applications, which represents a promising solution for health management. Developers of such mobile apps routinely deploy incentive programs, in which users receive financial rewards after achieving certain performance goals. In this paper, we seek to identify the effects of financial incentives, and to take a close examination at strategic behavior of users who self-report their performance. Drawing on the behavioral economics literature on incentives, we leverage a field quasi-experiment on a mobile health application to identify the effect of financial incentives. Using a difference-in-differences framework, we find that financial rewards lead to improvements in weight loss performance during the intervention period compared to the control group without financial rewards, but the performance difference does not persist after the removal of financial rewards at the end of the intervention period (i.e. no post-intervention effect). More importantly, we find evidence of strategic behavior: participants tend to over-report their initial body weight so as to increase the likelihood to reach performance goals and obtain the rewards. Further, we find that certain social networking features could possibly mitigate strategic behavior. In particular, participants who have more social connections and social activities are less likely to behave strategically. Our study contributes to the IS literature on leveraging economic incentives for online behavioral interventions and provides insights for the implementation of such incentives on digital health management platforms.

Keywords: Mobile health apps · Digital behavioral interventions
Financial incentives · Strategic behavior · Quasi-experiment
Difference-in-differences

1 Introduction

The rapid development of digital technology has facilitated innovations in health management, bringing in a variety of new applications in the healthcare industry [1]. With an expected market size of 31 billion U.S. dollars by 2020 [2], mobile health

H. Chen et al. (Eds.): ICSH 2018, LNCS 10983, pp. 130–141, 2018.
https://doi.org/10.1007/978-3-030-03649-2_13

applications have served as essential tools to enable cost-efficient health management and medical treatment, and have attracted considerable attention from both researchers and practitioners. As of 2017, mainstream mobile app stores contain more than 165,000 mobile health apps, and the total number of worldwide downloads had reached 3 billion. Despite the promising benefits such health apps have introduced, the effectiveness of them for health interventions is unclear, as previous studies have mixed results on their effect on users' health outcome. More importantly, the success of mobile health interventions not only depends on short-term progress but also requires changes to user behavior in the long run [3].

For the better design of mobile health apps, it is important to know how to stimulate user activity and enhance their performance. Although many forms of non-financial incentives have been designed for motivating users, money is still known as "one of the oldest and most reliable ways to motivate people [4]." While the use of financial incentives is widespread in the mobile health context, their impact remains unclear to researchers, since the findings in non-mobile settings may not apply to mobile settings [5]. On the one hand, financial incentives may have stronger effects when users take advantages of mobile features, such as mobility, flexibility [6], and social connectivity [7]. Specifically, mobile devices enable users to upload and download information anytime and anywhere and expand their social connections to people with similar interests or goals. Given that users are more exposed to mobile based information channel than traditional channels such as TV and prints [8], mobile enabled financial incentives could have stronger influences on users. On the other hand, financial incentives on mobile apps may induce unintended strategic behavior—it may encourage users to take "hidden" actions to increase their chances of receiving financial rewards, which may, in turn, lead to failure of incentives [9][1]. While previous literature has provided the foundation for understanding the impact of a variety of economic incentives, they have seldom conducted any critical examinations on incentive-induced strategic behavior. Without any remedies, such strategic behavior may not only increase the cost of deploying incentive programs but also decrease the outcome of health intervention and even jeopardize the long-term health statuses of users. Therefore, a deeper understanding of incentive-induced strategic behavior is critical to the success of financial incentives on mobile health apps. With this regard, we explore online social networking features, to understand whether social connections and social activities moderate such behavior. In summary, this paper aims to examine the following research questions:

1. *Do financial incentives induce strategic behavior of users in mobile health apps?*
2. *If there is strategic behavior, what is the net effect of financial incentives on user health outcome?*
3. *What online social network factor can mitigate strategic behavior?*

We study the above questions by leveraging a field quasi-experimental design on one of the leading mobile-based weight management app in China. Since 2013, the

---

[1] Strategic behavior appears with majority of incentive contracts, which may cause moral hazard issues. In our context, since the users self-report their weight records before and after the campaigns, there are a plenty of ways to overstate their weight-loss performance.

mobile app has created several weight loss campaigns with "deposit contracts" to incentivize users to reduce their body weights. According to previous literature, such financial incentive should incentivize weight loss performance of participants [10]. However, knowing the exact schedule and the threshold of campaigns in advance, the participants can game the incentive program, by over-reporting (intentionally or unintentionally) their initial body weight so that it becomes easier to reach the four percent threshold. We leverage quasi-experiments conducted by the mobile app to assess the effect of financial incentives on user behavior. In the quasi-experiment, users in the treatment and control groups are identical before the official announcement of the campaigns, teasing out possible self-selection bias. Our identification strategy is to gauge the "additional increase/decrease" in the performance of users in the treatment group, compared to the performance of users in baseline control group. Using a fixed effects difference-in-differences (DID) model, we quantify the short and long-term impact of financial incentive and identify evidence for strategic behavior.

Our key findings are as follows. First, we find evidence that financial incentives have short-term positive effect in digital weight interventions. The results suggest that users in the treatment group lose more weight than users in the control group, with estimated marginal effects ranging from 0.92% to 1.46% of body weight in the four independent campaigns across four seasons of one year. The overall improvement in weight-loss progress remains after the campaign, although there is an increase in average body weight during the post-intervention period. More importantly, we find evidence that users who participate in the campaigns have a slowdown in weight-loss progress relative to users who do not participate in the campaigns between the campaign announcement date and the start of the campaign while the two groups of users have similar weight-loss progress before the announcement date. This finding indicates the existence of strategic behavior. Third, we further uncover that, interestingly, strategic behavior is less prevalent among users with more intensive social networking activities. This suggests that social activities such as tweeting and being mentioned by others may exert monitoring pressure on the users for reducing strategic behavior. Finally, we perform several robustness checks: utilize propensity score matching to form matched sample, replicate the analysis with weekly panel data, and use alternative control group settings. All the results are consistent with to the previous analyses.

2   Methodology

2.1   Institutional Background and Data

We investigate one of the largest digital fitness & weight management apps in China that has a total of 40 million registered users as of June 2016. The mobile app has been widely known as the leading digital community for users who are looking for weight intervention or fitness on mobile devices. The platform offers various weight control instructions and diet plans, in addition to user profiles. More specifically, users have visualized dashboards demonstrating daily records of body weight, calories taken from food etc. Moreover, the mobile platform adopts social networking features.

The mobile app holds several weight loss campaigns with financial incentives (i.e., incentive programs) called "I bet I will be slimmer" since 2013. All the users are informed of the campaigns through notifications. To participate in the campaigns, users register by providing required information and depositing a fixed amount of money (i.e., 50 RMB) into a money pool. The campaigns require participants to reach the goal of losing four percent of body weight within 28 days. Participants who have eventually reached the threshold will share the money in the pool and receive additional gifts (such as a T-shirt) from the company that runs the platform, while who have not reached the threshold cannot get a refund. The platform creates a strict validation process to filter out unqualified users or potential frauds. It requires participants to take high-resolution photos of themselves standing on a weight scale from different angles with clear numbers on the scale, both before and after the campaigns. The incentive program provides us the opportunity to test both the short-term and long-term effects of monetary reward on health-related behavior.

More importantly, there is potential strategic behavior among the participants, because of the nonlinear nature of the compensation scheme. Imagine a participant who knows the schedule of the campaigns and the four percent threshold rule for getting the reward, in advance to the campaigns. The participants may want to maximize the probability of winning by adopting the following strategy: hold their weight loss progress or even gain some weight before the campaign and boost it during the campaign. Since this strategic behavior may hinder the users' social image, we suspect that social activities may moderate such strategic behavior: when the participant has intensive exposure in the social network, there should be a weaker motivation for such strategic behavior.

To conduct the study, we obtain the complete data from Oct 2013 to July 2016. Our dataset includes daily records on a population of users' demographics, personal weight, diet, and calorie records, social network structures, and social activities. Furthermore, we have a list of users who have attempted to participate in the campaigns and further merge the data with their characteristics. We build a social network of users based on their following relationship and social interactions. Eventually, we establish a panel dataset from these records.

2.2   Identification Strategy

We aim to identify the impact of financial incentives and the potential strategic behaviors associated with them in a mobile environment. One of the major identification challenges of the study is the self-selection bias in participation decisions. We resolve it by a field quasi-experimental design. As we are known, causal inference requires high similarity between observations in the treatment and control groups. Since in our context, users sign up for the incentive programs, introducing a non-random selection bias and endogeneity issue. Specifically, it is possible that unobserved user characteristics, such as opportunity costs of users, would simultaneously lead to participation in the campaigns and a certain level of weight-loss performance. We take advantage of the registration process to deal with the self-selection issue. We define the users who participated in the campaign as the incentive group (treatment group) and users who initiated the registration but did not eventually join the campaigns as the control group. This is better than using the users how have never initiated the registration process to form the control group since the two groups would have similar interests in losing weight, and population sizes of the two groups are more balanced.

While the remaining difference between two groups was the completion of registration, our quasi-experimental setting makes the unobserved characteristics of the incentive and control groups similar. Nevertheless, there is still a possibility that it suffers from the selection bias since the incentive group eventually attend the program. For instance, users who trust the system may be more likely to deposit money to the platform, and they may also have better weight loss performance. To mitigate the remaining resource of self-selection, we further apply *propensity score matching* (PSM) to match treatment group users with control group users and conduct the same analyses.

We exploit timing assumption for quasi-experiment design. Since the campaign lasts four weeks, we use four weeks as one period and finally define in total four periods. In the *Pre-Announcement* period, the campaign has not yet been announced; users in both treatment and control groups use the mobile app as usual. Therefore, there should be little differences between the two groups. In the *Pre-Intervention* period, the platform announces about the campaign users are allowed to register for the campaign. Practically, there are still no external incentives given to either of the group; there should be still no differences between the two groups. However, since the users in the treatment group know about the threshold rule of the incentive program, they may undertake specific behavior to "game" the incentive contract. During the *Intervention Period*, the treatment group has the chance to receive the reward by achieving the goal—losing four percent of body weight; the control group does not receive any monetary rewards, even if they reach four percent, and their weight loss effort purely depends on intrinsic or social motivations. In the *Post-Intervention Period*, for the treatment group, no matter whether they get the monetary reward or not, the financial incentive is removed, and there are no other rewards assigned to them. We keep track of *percentage change in body weight* of the two groups along the four periods so that the performance difference in the *Intervention* period reflects the short-term effect of financial incentive, and the performance difference in the *Post-Intervention* period reflects the long-term (post-intervention) effect. Moreover, the performance difference between the two groups in the *Pre-Intervention* period indicates the strategic behavior effect. We illustrate the timeline of the quasi-experiment in Fig. 1, for the third campaign.

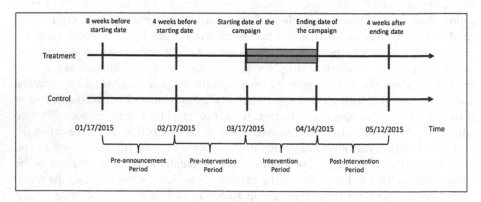

Fig. 1. Timeline of quasi-experimental design (the 3rd campaign)

3   Empirical Analyses

In this section, we report the steps and results of econometric analyses. Among all the "I bet I will be slimmer" campaigns, we utilize the first four campaigns in our main analysis because all four campaigns have the same deposit requirement, intervention time window, and threshold. Campaigns are held in the four seasons respectively (i.e., fall 2014, winter 2014, spring 2015, and summer 2015), providing season-specific results throughout one calendar year. We further split the entire panel dataset into treatment and control groups, and present summary statistics of the main variables by the group, as shown in Table 1.

Table 1. Summary statistics (four campaigns)

Variable	Mean	SD	Min	Max
	Treatment (54,364 Obs.)			
$Weight_{it}$	62.464	10.460	40.100	130.271
$DiffWeight_{it}$	−0.268	1.557	−9.900	9.884
$PercentWeightChange_{it}$	−0.332	2.421	−17.662	17.673
$LogFollowee_{it}$	3.140	1.238	0.000	7.639
$LogFollower_{it}$	2.278	1.937	0.000	14.906
$LogPost_{it}$	1.467	1.282	0.000	6.457
$LogMention_{it}$	0.652	1.138	0.000	7.305
	Control (125,503 Obs.)			
$Weight_{it}$	62.414	11.038	40.000	140.000
$DiffWeight_{it}$	−0.198	1.414	−9.921	10.000
$PercentWeightChange_{it}$	−0.203	2.167	−20.056	18.888
$LogFollowee_{it}$	2.846	1.236	0.000	9.814
$LogFollower_{it}$	1.622	1.896	0.000	16.267
$LogPost_{it}$	0.693	1.140	0.000	6.863
$LogMention_{it}$	0.381	0.920	0.000	8.762

3.1   The Effect of Incentive Program

We then turn to regression analysis to verify the effect of incentive programs in weight management. Our identification strategy relies on comparing the difference in *percentage weight change* between treated users and untreated users, before, during, and after each campaign. In addition, since social network measures and social activities may have impacts on their weight loss performance as well, they are included in the regression as control variables. In particular, we apply panel data difference-in-differences fixed effects regression model to estimate the impact of a financial incentive on weight loss performance.

$PercentWeightChange_{it}$

$$= \beta_1 PeriodDummies_t + \beta_2 Treatment_i \times PeriodDummies_t$$
$$+ \beta_3 LogNumFollowee_{it} + \beta_4 LogNumFollower_{it} + \beta_5 LogNumPost_{it}$$
$$+ \beta_6 LogNumMention_{it} + \alpha_i + \epsilon_{it}$$

The dependent variable $PercentWeightChange_{it}$ measures the weight loss performance of individual i at time t. In the main analysis, we adopt percentage change in weight as the measure ($PercentWeightChange_{it} = \frac{Weight_{it} - Weight_{it-1}}{InitialWeight_i} \times 100$), where initial weight is the users' body weight at the beginning of the campaign's pre-intervention period. One potential issue with the weight data is sparsity. For users with at least two weight records, we apply a MatLab-based interpolation algorithm to fill in missing daily weight records between two existing records. As a robustness check, we apply "left" interpolation method, in which we use previous weight record values until a new value enters, and the results are highly consistent.

We include *period dummies* to reflect one of the four periods in which the observation has made. *Treatment* is the binary variable that equals to *1* if the individual is in the treatment group and *0* otherwise. Hence, the coefficients of *period dummies* capture the percentage weight change of users in the control group, while the coefficients of *interactions between period dummies and treatment* capture the impact of the incentive program on percentage weight change in certain periods. Regarding social network measures, we include log-transformed *number of followees and number of followers* user i has until time t, which are equivalent to out-degree and in-degree of the user in the social network. Moreover, log of *number of tweets and mentions* reflect the intensity of social activities user i has made at time t. Notice that they reflect different social activities, since posting is action taken by the focal users and mention is action taken by their peers. We also include user fixed effects α_i in the model to control for unobserved individual heterogeneity. As a result, the estimated effect of the incentive program is free of time-invariant confounding factors, and the inclusion of other regressors further mitigates the impact of time-varying confounders. More importantly, we only include users in the quasi-experimental design we mentioned before, therefore our identification strategy provides valid causal inference.

Short-Term Effect of Incentives

Result 1 (Short-Term Effect): Individuals who have participated in financial incentive based campaigns have significantly better weight loss performance in the intervention period.

We present the estimates of the difference-in-differences model upon four campaigns in Table 2. In all specifications, the coefficients of period dummies reflect the weight loss patterns of users in the control groups, which vary across different campaigns. Relying on the DID setting, the coefficients of interaction terms represent the additional effect of an incentive program on weight loss performance of users in the treatment groups. We verify the short-term effect since the coefficients of *Period3 × Treat* in all campaigns are statistically significant (coefficients range from −0.92 to −1.46, p-values are smaller than 0.001). The marginal effect is an additional reduction of body weight from 0.9 to 1.5% in users who are incented by a reward, which is a considerably large magnitude since the weight loss target is 4%.

Table 2. Estimation result of DID

Campaign	Fall	Winter	Spring	Summer
Pre-interv.	0.259***	−0.023	−0.188***	0.160***
	(0.031)	(0.043)	(0.030)	(0.042)
Intervention	0.349***	−0.074	−0.806***	0.569***
	(0.035)	(0.046)	(0.035)	(0.046)
Post-interv.	0.499***	0.187***	−0.565***	0.628***
	(0.037)	(0.048)	(0.036)	(0.047)
Pre-interv. × Treat	0.541***	0.519***	0.570***	0.322***
	(0.066)	(0.073)	(0.070)	(0.068)
Interv. × Treat	−1.057***	−1.455***	−0.920***	−1.305***
	(0.073)	(0.076)	(0.073)	(0.073)
Post-interv. × Treat	0.532***	0.473***	0.388***	0.445***
	(0.071)	(0.075)	(0.071)	(0.071)
$LogFollowee_{it}$	0.125+	0.026	−0.000	0.183+
	(0.065)	(0.087)	(0.070)	(0.097)
$LogFollower_{it}$	0.354***	0.398***	0.288***	0.426***
	(0.048)	(0.057)	(0.048)	(0.072)
$LogPost_{it}$	−0.414***	−0.337***	−0.433***	−0.409***
	(0.021)	(0.026)	(0.024)	(0.023)
$LogMention_{it}$	−0.127***	−0.170***	−0.186***	−0.297***
	(0.024)	(0.033)	(0.031)	(0.031)
Observations	43,019	30,654	40,065	33,025
Number of users	12,244	8,703	11,107	9,161
R-squared	0.087	0.116	0.111	0.119

Note. The dependent variable is *PercentageWeightChange*. Robust standard errors are under the coefficients. ***significant at 0.001, **significant at 0.01, *significant at 0.05

Evidence of Strategic Behavior

Result 2 (Strategic Behavior Effect): Individuals who have participated in incentive based campaigns undertake strategic behavior to "game" against the incentive contract by retaining their body weight in the pre-intervention period.

We find that the coefficients of *Period2 × Treat* are positive and statistically significant for the four seasons (coefficient varies from 0.32 to 0.57, significant at 0.001 confidence level). It indicates that in the pre-intervention period, percentage weight change increases more (or reduces by a smaller amount) among the users who are incentivized by the reward program compared with the users without incentive. It suggests that the incentive program may already influence the participants before the campaigns start. The estimated effect should be attributed to strategic behavior for two reasons. First, as the quasi-experimental design is valid, there should be no difference in intrinsic and social motivation between the two groups of users. Second, since the weight loss performance in the pre-intervention period is not counted for determining the rewards of incentive campaigns, the incentive group users should not be motivated to exert more effort. Hence, the remaining explanation is strategic behavior, for the participants tend to "postpone" weight loss performance to the intervention period when performance is counted for reward so that they have higher chance to reach the 4% threshold for the reward.

Post-intervention Effect of Incentives

Result 2 (Long-Term Effect): Individuals who have participated in financial incentive based campaigns have even worse weight loss performance in the post-intervention period, although the overall long-term effect is still positive.

In addition, we test the effect of the incentive rewards after the intervention period. In Table 2, the coefficients of *Period4* × *Treat* are significantly positive which represent a smaller reduction or even a larger regain (coefficient varies from 0.39 to 0.43, significant at 0.001 confidence level) in body weight of the incentive group users. These results indicate that the incentive rewards affect the performance in the opposite direction in the post-intervention period and delimit the beneficial impact of the incentives. Nevertheless, when we combine the effects in three periods, we still observe a positive long-term effect of a financial incentive on weight loss performance. We also have interesting findings on the control variables. The association between outgoing degree (number of followees) of the users (as nodes in the social network) and weight loss performance is insignificant. By contrast, incoming degree (number followers) of users is negatively correlated with weight loss performance (coefficient varies from 0.29 to 0.43, p-value < 0.001). In addition, we find users' posting behavior is positively related to weight loss performance—users who post more messages tend to have better performance (coefficient varies from -0.34 to -0.45, p-value < 0.001). Similarly, users who are more frequently mentioned by their peers have better performance (coefficient varies from -0.13 to -0.30, p-value < 0.001). However, since there may have endogenous network formation and social activities are not exogenous, we do not interpret the estimation results of control variable as causal relationships.

To further mitigate endogeneity, we construct propensity score matched (PSM) panel datasets and conduct the same fixed effects regressions. Due to the space limitation, we cannot present tables showing the main effects with PSM data. Nevertheless, we also omit the table from regressions with weekly granular panel data. In general, both PSM results and weekly panel data results confirm our main findings of the strategic behavior in the pre-intervention period.

3.2   Moderators for Strategic Behavior

Result 4A: Users who have more social activities undertake less strategic behavior.

Result 4B: Users who have more social connections undertake less strategic behavior.

We next estimate the moderating effect of social networking features of the platform on the users' behavior toward incentives. We assume that there is an ignorable change in the user's the social network structure during the campaign time, so that we fix social network measures for each user-campaign pair at the beginning of the pre-intervention period. Consistent with the control variables, there are two sources of social networking measures in our setting: social activities measure such as number of tweets and number of mentions, and social network structure measure such as in-degree and out-degree of the users (i.e., number of followers and number of followees). We specify the moderators by whether users have a high or low social activities as well as a high or low number of social connections, to generate a binary variable (High = 1/Low = 0) for each social networking measure. We aggregate the four campaign data and conduct regression models with campaign fixed effects. In the model, each of the social networking measures is multiplied by $Treatment_i \times PeriodDummies_t$ to construct three-way interaction terms. We therefore identify the differential effect of incentive by variation in social networking measures.

$$PercentWeightChange_{it}$$
$$= \beta_1 TimeDummies_t + \beta_2 Treatment_i \times PeriodDummies_t$$
$$+ \beta_3 Moderator_i \times Treatment_i \times PeriodDummies_t$$
$$+ \beta_4 LogNumFollowee_{it} + \beta_5 LogNumFollower_{it} + \beta_6 LogNumPost_{it}$$
$$+ \beta_7 LogNumMention_{it} + \beta_8 CampaignDummies + \alpha_i + \epsilon_{it}$$

Figure 2(a) and (b) demonstrate the moderating effect of social activities in terms of number of tweets and mentions on the users' response toward incentives. In the pre-intervention period, there is less strategic behavior when users are active in either of the social activities. In the intervention period, intensive tweets or mentions results in a stronger positive effect of incentive on weight loss performance. Figure 2(c) and (d) show the moderating effect of social connections in terms of out-degree and in-degree on the users' response toward incentives. We observe a similar pattern in the pre-intervention period since strategic behavior is much smaller for users with high social connections. Nevertheless, the social network connections do not cause significantly different effects on weight loss performance during the intervention period.

Table 3 reports the detailed estimates of the difference-in-differences model with the three-way interaction terms. From Spec. 1 and 2, we observe that participants who post more tweets and who are more frequently mentioned by others undertake less strategic behavior in the pre-intervention period, better weight loss performance in the intervention period, and regain more body weight in the post-intervention period. Probably, in pre-intervention period, users with more tweets and mentions are more monitored by the users in the online community, so that they are less motivated to "game." During the intervention period, users who post more tweets try to become popular in the community, and thus they have a stronger motivation to achieve the goal of the incentive campaigns. By contrast, users with more mentions are already popular and have lower motivation to do so. Interestingly, users with more social activities are more likely to get weight after the campaigns. Relatively, socially motivated users significantly lose motivation after the campaigns terminate. Likewise, Spec. 3 and 4 compare the estimation results for users with high and low number of followee and followers, the estimates also indicate smaller strategic behavior among the users with more social connections.

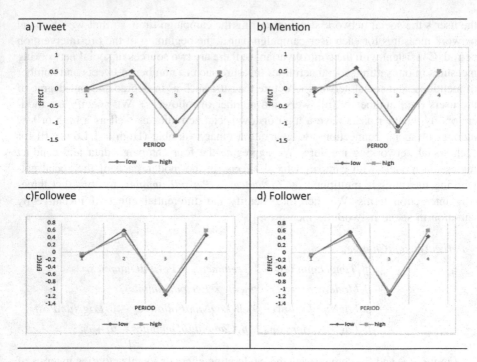

Fig. 2. Comparison between high and low social network characteristics.

Table 3. Estimation result of DID: differential effects by social networking features

Specification	1	2	Specification	3	4
Moderator	Tweet	Mention	Moderator	Followee	Follower
Pre-interv. × Treat × High Post	−0.186+ 0.070		Pre-interv. × Treat × High Followee	−0.144* 0.067	
Interv. × Treat × High Post	−0.394*** 0.076		Interv. × Treat × High Followee	0.102 0.072	
Post-interv. × Treat × High Post	0.116 0.075		Post-interv. × Treat × High Followee	0.118 0.073	
Pre-interv. × Treat × High Mention		−0.386*** 0.075	Pre-interv. × Treat × High Follower		−0.114+ 0.066
Interv. × Treat × High Mention		−0.140+ 0.080	Interv. × Treat × High Follower		0.075 0.072
Post-interv. × Treat × High Mention		0.019 0.080	Post-interv. × Treat × High Follower		0.163* 0.072
Campaign fixed effects	Yes	Yes	Campaign fixed effects	Yes	Yes
Observations	146,763	146,763	Observations	146,763	146,763
# of users	36,394	36,394	# of users	36,394	36,394

Note. The dependent variable is *PercentageWeightChange*. Robust standard errors are under the coefficients. ***significant at 0.001, **significant at 0.01, *significant at 0.05, +significant at 0.1.

4 Discussions and Conclusions

We examine the impacts of financial incentive and the associated strategic behavior in a mobile-based intervention practice. Our study provides evidence that financial incentive positively enhances weight loss progress in both short term and long term. However, it also leads to strategic behavior on the participants' performance in the pre-intervention period, before the incentive is deployed. Moreover, we find that intensive usage on the social networking features has a negative moderating effect on the strategic behavior. The participants who have more social connections or social activities are less likely to perform strategic behavior.

This study has various managerial implications. First, we provide insights to the practitioners about the implementation of financial incentives for health behavior intervention. It is very challenging to minimize strategic behavior while achieving successful behavioral interventions with high long-term user engagement. As a result, the design of incentive programs is the key to the question. Second, practitioners need to provide social networking features for users to build relationships, exchange information, and gain social support, to trigger social pressure. Our study demonstrates the importance of social networking features in mitigating strategic behavior. Therefore, the practitioners should come up with strategies to create social incentives to enhance performance.

Our study contributes to the literature on economic incentives for behavioral intervention under mobile-app-based settings. Moreover, we provide practical implications for mobile app developers for the design of the incentive programs.

References

1. Fox, S., Duggan, M.: Mobile health 2010. Pew Internet & American Life Project, Washington, DC (2010)
2. Statista (2017). https://www.statista.com/statistics/387867/value-of-worldwide-digital-health-market-forecast-by-segment/
3. Charness, G., Gneezy, U.: Incentives to exercise. Econometrica 77(3), 909–931 (2009)
4. Park, A.: The New Science of How to Quit Smoking. TIME Health (2015)
5. Kwon, H.E., So, H., Han, S.P., Oh, W.: Excessive dependence on mobile social apps: a rational addiction perspective. Inf. Syst. Res. 27(4), 919–939 (2016)
6. Ghose, A., Han, S.P.: An empirical analysis of user content generation and usage behavior on the mobile internet. Manag. Sci. 57(9), 1671–1691 (2011)
7. Yan, L., Tan, Y.: Feeling blue? Go online: an empirical study of social support among patients. Inf. Syst. Res. 25(4), 690–709 (2014)
8. Ghose, A., Goldfarb, A., Han, S.P.: How is the mobile internet different? Search costs and local activities. Information Systems Research 24(3), 613–631 (2013)
9. Mayer, C., Morrison, E., Piskorski, T., Gupta, A.: Mortgage modification and strategic behavior: evidence from a legal settlement with Countrywide. Am. Econ. Rev. 104(9), 2830–2857 (2011)
10. Gneezy, U., Meier, S., Rey-Biel, P.: When and why incentives (don't) work to modify behavior. J. Econ. Perspect. 25(4), 191–209 (2011)

How Using of WeChat Impacts Individual Loneliness and Health?

Meng Yin[1], Qi Li[2], and Xiaoyu Xu[3(✉)]

[1] School of Logistics and E-Commerce,
Henan University of Animal Husbandry and Economy, Zhengzhou, China
[2] School of Economic and Finance, Xi'an Jiaotong University, Xi'an, China
[3] School of Economic and Finance, Xi'an Jiaotong University,
No 74, Yanta Road, Yanta Direct, Xi'an City 710061, Shaanxi, China
xiaoyuxuec@126.com

Abstract. WeChat has been developed as the popular social media in China, and enables people to break the limits of time and space, give and obtain variety of social supports. In order to research the influence of social support on individual health, this study constructed a research model based on social support theory and loneliness. Data were collected through questionnaire and analyzed by SPSS and Smart PLS. Research results showed that informational support and network support during the WeChat usage can significantly influence users' perceived health. In addition, informational support, emotional support, and network support can significantly reduce the perceived loneliness. Network support exerts the strongest influence on perceived loneliness. Finally, the perceived loneliness significantly reduces the perceived health.

Keywords: WeChat · Social support · Loneliness · Perceived health

1 Introduction

WeChat has been developed as the popular social media in China, which provides multiple social functions such as instant message and moments. WeChat enables people to break the limits of time and space, share their opinions and emotions freely, and obtain various useful information. Hence, increasing the social interaction and communication, WeChat as a social media has satisfied the users' utilitarian gratification and costumer value. The user behavior in WeChat has attracted the increasing interests from both researchers and practitioners.

Prior literatures mainly focus on investigating the user behavior, such as social behavior, usage, and consumption behavior in social media such as WeChat. Theories in information systems science, social science, social psychology have been widely applied to studies kinds of user behavior in WeChat. However, the prior research mainly focus on the user adoption, continuous usage, social disclosure, information sharing behavior, and social commerce. Little research has explored how the usage of WeChat influences the user perceived health.

Social support theory is widely applied to study user behavior in social media, which indicates that the informational support, emotional support and network support

H. Chen et al. (Eds.): ICSH 2018, LNCS 10983, pp. 142–153, 2018.
https://doi.org/10.1007/978-3-030-03649-2_14

derived from the social media are critical factor in influencing the user attitude, perceived value, and usage behavior. As the typical social media, WeChat also offers multiple functions and service to provide informational support, social support, informational support and network support. Hence, the customer needs can be gratified, such as needs for various information, emotional communication and relationship development and maintain. Consequently, the free and instant communication has largely reduce the perceived loneliness. Moreover, prior studies have indicate that the perceived loneliness can significantly reduce the users' perceived health. Hence, it is interesting to investigate whether the usage of WeChat can reduce the users' perceived loneliness and improve the user perceived health. This study aims to investigate the following research question: How the social support and perceived loneliness impact the perceived health.

2 Literature Review

2.1 Usage of WeChat

Social media has broken the limits of time and space, and deeply changed individual communication. As a typical social media, WeChat is free to download, install, use and support different kinds of terminal and operating systems including smartphone, Pad and Computer involving ISO, Android and Windows. WeChat users can communicate and interact with friends through test messaging, hold-to-talk voice messaging, WeChat group, play games, and can share their video, photo, location, news and article to other uses, and users also can pay the bill, transfer money to others [1]. As shown in a report from Tencent, WeChat global active users have exceeded 1 billion in 2018. WeChat has become the most widely used social media in China and an important communication platforms for user's life and work.

With the rapid development of WeChat, scholars began to pay attention to WeChat user behavior research. According to previous information system researches, user behavior of information system can be divided to parts [2], the first is adoption which include usage intention and usage behavior [1, 3], the second is postadoption including information sharing [4], continuance intention [5–7] and purchase behavior [8]. Initial usage behavior and continuance usage behavior are two main research area. Motivation theory, Theory of Planned behavior [4, 6], Expectation disconfirmation theory [5, 7], consumer value and social theory [6] are applied in WeChat usage behavior research. Entertainment, sociality and information from WeChat usage have significant influence on users' attitudes has been confirmed by Lien et al. [1]. In order to explore impact of satisfaction and stickiness on users' usage intention, Lien et al. constructed a research model based on expectation disconfirmation theory, and confirmed interaction, environment and outcome of WeChat have significant effect on increasing users' satisfaction and usage intention [3].

How to enable users to continue using WeChat is very important for WeChat service provider, and it is also a research hotspot in usage behavior research. Zhang et al. researched users' continuance intention of WeChat based on consumer perceived value and confirmed that social value and hedonic value have significant influence on continuance intention [5]. Besides perceived value, social factors, information system related factors all have significant influence on continuance intention, Chen integrated guanxi into technology acceptance theory to research continuance intention of WeChat, and confirmed guanxi, perceived usefulness, perceived ease of use and perceived enjoyment have significant impact on continuance intention [6]. And perceived enjoyment, information sharing and media appeal are all significant influence factors of continuance intention, which was confirmed by Gan et al. based on Use and Gratification [7].

From above literature analysis, we can see usage behavior of WeChat is research hotspot in nowadays. However, many scholars focus on user initial usage behaver and continuance usage behaver while neglecting the influence effect of WeChat usage on users. Because of the rapid development of society and people's busy work, human is much more easy to perceive loneliness which is not good for health. WeChat can increase interpersonal commutation, which can reduce user loneliness. Therefore we want to explore the influence of WeChat usage on user through the perspective of health.

2.2 Social Support Theory

Social support theory was first proposed by Cobb in 1976 [9], and it was proposed as a central concept for health and well-being [10], which refers to an individual's experiences of being cared for, being responded to, and being helped by people in that individual's social group based on resources or aid exchanged [9, 11]. Social support is a multi-dimensional construct [12, 13] and is generally classified into three types including information support, emotion support and network support in the context of social media [14].

Social support theory was first applied to the field of psychiatry and then introduced into sociology, psychology, and management. With the development of social media technology, scholars have given considerable attention to the influence of social support in online communities [12]. Facebook, LinkedIn, Twitter, Weibo and WeChat are typical social media which were researched to examine the influence of social support on user behaviors including usage behavior [14], shopping [11, 15] and etc. Lin et al. [14] classified social support into three types including information support, emotion support and network support in the context of social media, and confirmed three kinds of social supports all have influence on the relationship commitment and usage behavior of social media. Besides usage behavior, social commerce is another point of research in the context of social media. Liang et al. [11] and Hajli et al. [15] both have confirmed the significant influence of social support on consumer social commerce intention, found information support and emotion support are two important support in social media.

Besides the influence of social support on usage behavior and purchase behavior, social support has also been widely researched as one of key determinants influencing individual's health [16]. And studies have witnessed positive effects of social support on various health outcomes [17, 18], such as increasing psychological health and physical health. Social support has been studied as a moderator or a direct influence factor which can improve health through increasing subject wellbeing [17] or health-related self-efficacy [16, 18] and reduce negative influence factors including stress and loneliness [19]. Oh et al. [16] researched health information seeking behavior on Facebook and confirmed that emotion support has significant influence on health-related self-efficacy which will improve user's perceived health. Davis et al. collected user data from Facebook, proved that social media is an important way to get social support and social supports have significant influence on improving of personal health [20].

WeChat provides information support, emotion support and network support to users through text message, public accounts, circle of friends, applet of WeChat and etc. previous studies have confirmed the significant influence of social support on usage behavior, social commerce, and health, but there is limitations in the research of user usage, social commerce, health in the context of WeChat, especially the influence of WeChat usage behavior on user's health. Therefore, examining the influence effect of WeChat usage behavior on health is significant and available based on social support theory.

2.3 Loneliness and Health

Loneliness can be defined as an individual experience associated with different levels of pain, suffering, and disengagement because of bonds with other individuals are lacking or the expectation of social relationships are not satisfied [21]. Loneliness is a common and important health related issue which not only exists in old age but also in other groups [22]. And it can be classified social loneliness and emotion loneliness [21, 23], social loneliness is result of a lack of insertion or relation within social groups or community that can provide a sense of belonging and companionship [24, 25], and the emotion loneliness results from lack of a significant loss, or the lack of intimate partner [24, 25].

In order to decrease the loneliness offline, individual begin to use internet and social media to construct their own online community and exchange with other online users [26]. But there are two consequences of using of internet and social media, increasing loneliness and decreasing loneliness, which depend on variety of influence factors of satisfaction of individual expectation. Some influence factors of loneliness can be summarized, some factors have positive impact and lead to or increase individual perceived loneliness, some factor have negative influence and decrease individual perceived loneliness and some factors have different influences because of different demographics [21], personality [27] and etc. Demographics, perceived health, social satisfaction [21] and shyness, self-esteem [28] all have been confirmed that they have positive significant influence on individual loneliness and lead to loneliness. Social support and positive social activities increase individual's satisfaction of social relationship and quality of life, and decrease individual loneliness directly or indirectly [26, 29].

Loneliness is regard as negative feeling and it has positive and negative outcomes in human physical health and human mental health [21]. Because of loneliness, some people will try their best to build relationship with others and sharing their feelings and life with others, which is good for their health. On the contrary, loneliness also can causes physical health problems for human, such as sleeping disorders, blood pressure

[30], physical inactivity, daily smoking [31], onset of dementia and cardiovascular disease [32, 33] and etc. [34]. Of course, it is also confirmed loneliness is associated with individual perceived health, depression, mortality [21] and motivation decreasing [29]. In short, loneliness has influence on human behaviors and individual perceived health.

3 Hypotheses Development

In order to examine the influence of different dimensions of social support on perceived health and loneliness. This study develops the research model based on the social support theory, perceived loneliness and perceived health. According to the literature review analysis, the research model proposes that the social support, including informational support, emotional support and network support derived from the usage of WeChat are able to significantly reduce the perceived loneliness and increase the perceived health (Fig. 1).

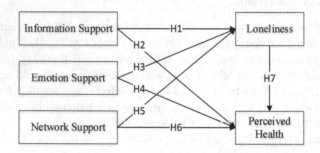

Fig. 1. Research model of social support

3.1 Influence of Information Support

Information support refers to the provision of advice, factual input, and feedback regarding actions [35], and include practical resources such as objective information, suggestions, advice, and appraisals of situations that helped receivers reduce uncertainty and cope with illness [14]. WeChat Group, WeChat message and WeChat Official Account provide variety of information for users including health information, exercise information and information of friends and family and etc. Individual can get immediate information on health protecting, exercise, and activities, which motivate individual do exercise, protect their health and take part in social activities, and all those behaviors reduce loneliness and increase individual health perceived. As Oh et al. [16] confirmed social support has significant influence on individual health related perceived, and increasing psychological health and physical health [17, 18], and reduce perceived loneliness [26, 29]. Hence, hypotheses were proposed as below:

H1: Information support has significant negative influence on loneliness.
H2: Information support has significant positive influence on perceived health.

3.2 Influence of Emotion Support

Emotion Support refers to expressions of caring, concern, encouragement, empathy and sympathy to reduce stress, loneliness or negative affect [14, 35], such as happiness, failure, sadness, and etc. individual posts information, pictures, videos about their work and life through WeChat group, and WeChat messages to share their emotions, and individual can get replying, retweeting, liking and get emotion support from these feedbacks. Emotion support from friends increase individual confidence, self-esteem, and self-efficacy [16, 17] and reduce individual stress, nervous and loneliness [26, 29], which then motivate individuals take themselves better [18]. The influence of social support on loneliness and health related perceived have confirmed in the context of social media by prior researches, hence it is available for emotion support in the context of WeChat. Hypotheses were proposed as below:

H3: Emotion support has significant negative influence on loneliness.

H4: Emotion support has significant positive influence on perceived health.

3.3 Influence of Network Support

Network support refers that WeChat enables the users to meet other users with similar interest and develop the network, and people can perceive the presence of companions with others to engage in the shared social activities [14]. People can find different kinds of friends through WeChat, such as business friends, family numbers, and high school classmates and etc. the building of social network on WeChat will enhance the exchange between individuals and the sharing of similar interest, which will increase the sense of community belonging and reduce the personal loneliness. As one dimension of social support, network support inherits the influence effect of social support on loneliness and perceived health [17, 18]. Network support from the WeChat reduce the individual loneliness [26, 29] and has positive influence on perceived health. Hence, hypotheses were proposed as below:

H5: Network support has significant negative influence on loneliness.

H6: Network support has significant positive influence on perceived health.

3.4 Influence of Loneliness on Health

As a negative feeling, loneliness has different negative outcomes which related to personal health [21, 34], and mortality [36] and health related issues [21]. And many scholars have confirmed that loneliness has negative impact on perceived health through different ways including physical health, mental health, and unhealthy behaviors and etc. Such as, loneliness may give rise to the anxiety generating thoughts which inhibit relaxation and affect sleep quality, and the nervous and sleeping disorder are bad for personal health. And loneliness is also associated with smoking, alcohol abuse, physical inactivity, and being overweight which engage in risky health [31, 34]. Another mechanism is the stress which may line loneliness and poor health [34]. Hence, hypothesis was proposed as below:

H7: Loneliness has significant negative influence on perceived health.

4 Methodology

4.1 Design of Questionnaire

Survey research is adopted as the research method in this study. Questionnaire is developed to collect empirical data for statistical analysis. Data are processed and analyzed by SPSS, and hypotheses are tested by Smart PLS. The questionnaire consists three parts: the first part includes the description of questionnaire. The second part is the basic information survey of participants involve gender, age, education and etc. The third part are measures of latent variables. Measures of latent variables are all from prior researches and adapted based on the research context. And Five-point Likert scale with anchors of strongly disagree one to strongly agree five for all items in our study is used. Information support, emotion support, and network support are adapted from Oh et al. [16] and Lin et al. [35], loneliness is adapted from Pittman et al. [37], and Perceived health is adapted from Stewart [38]. As survey is conducted in China, measures of latent variables from previous researches are translated into Chinese firstly and then translated into English by two e-commerce scholars, and the questionnaire is confirmed after modifying many times.

4.2 Data Collection

We collect pre-test data through WeChat and QQ, and then modify item descriptions of questionnaire based on the analysis of pre-test data, and then collect data through a questionnaire service website (www.sojump.com). 180 questionnaires are collected. In order to eliminate the impact of external trauma on perceived health, 59 respondents are excluded from the overall respondents. Eventually, 121 valid respondents are collected, the effective rate of questionnaires is 67.2%.

Table 1. Demographic characteristics

Variable	Frequency	Percent	Variable	Frequency	Percent
Gender			Live alone or not		
Male	59	48.2	Yes	23	19.0
Female	62	51.2	No	98	81.0
Age			Education		
17 years old and below	0	0	Junior high school and below	2	1.7
18-24 years	13	10.7	High school	4	3.3
25-44 years	94	77.7	junior college	24	19.8
45-59 years	12	9.9	undergraduate college	81	66.9
60 years old and above	2	1.7	Graduate and above	10	8.3
Usage time of WeChat					
0-2 years	3	2.5	4-6 years	54	44.6
2-4 years	47	38.8	6 years and above	17	14.0

As shown in Table 1, 51.2 of participants are women, and most of all are living with others. The main age group is between 18 and 45 years old, and account for 88.4%. The main education degree is undergraduate, and account for 66.9%. There are 7 years since WeChat appeared in 2011, and 83.4% participants have used for 2 to 6 years.

5 Data Analysis

5.1 Measurement Model

Reliability, convergent validity and discriminant validity are tested through SPSS and Smart PLS. first of all, Cronbach's α of the whole data is measured through SPSS, and the value is 0.615 which is close to 0.7, because of limitation of sample, we think it can be accepted in this research. And the value of KMO is 0.782 which means data can be used for factor analysis. The mean, standard deviation (S.D.), factor loading and composite reliability (CR) are used for assessing the internal consistency of various measuring items, and Cronbach's α is used to measure the reliability of various measuring items. When the values of CR and Cronbach's α are all above 0.7, it means measurement model has good internal consistency. As shown in Table 2, the factor loading, Cronbach's α and CR are all above 0.7 except the network support and perceived health which are close to 0.7. Hence, we think the reliability and internal consistency have met the basic standard.

Table 2. Reliability, Variance, and Confirmatory Factor Analysis

Construct	Items	Mean	S.D.	Loading	α	CR	AVE
Information support	InSp1	3.80	0.770	0.817	0.761	0.862	0.675
	InSp2	4.01	0.935	0.817			
	InSp3	3.72	0.906	0.831			
Emotion support	EmSp1	3.63	0.867	0.823	0.703	0.829	0.620
	EmSp2	3.91	0.856	0.868			
	EmSp3	3.45	1.000	0.656			
Network support	NeSp1	4.08	0.862	0.633	0.599	0.796	0.671
	NeSp2	3.85	1.005	0.971			
Loneliness	Lons1	2.35	1.256	0.818	0.787	0.876	0.702
	Lons1	2.02	1.064	0.871			
	Lons1	1.83	1.054	0.823			
Perceived health	PHea1	4.33	.925	0.716	0.655	0.810	0.587
	PHea2	4.18	.885	0.819			
	PHea3	3.92	.862	0.761			

Convergent validity and discriminant validity are tested through AVE, and convergent validity is good when the value of AVE is above 0.5, and the discriminant validity is good when the square root of AVE values are greater than the correlation between variables. As shown in Table 2, AVE of each variable is above 0.5, which indicates the data have good convergent validity. As shown in Table 3, the square root of each AVE value is on the diagonal and the rest are the correlation coefficients, and the square root of each AVE value is higher than correlation coefficients which indicates the data have good discriminant validity.

Table 3. Discriminant validity of measurement model

Construct	InSp	EmSp	NeSp	Lons	PHea
InSp	**0.822**				
EmSp	0.484	**0.787**			
NeSp	0.320	0.497	**0.819**		
Lons	−0.268	−0.329	−0.341	**0.838**	
PHea	0.335	0.321	0.359	−0.359	**0.766**

5.2 Hypotheses Testing

Hypotheses were tested and structural equation model was constructed through the Smart PLS software, and the research results were shown in Fig. 2. Information support, emotion support and network support all have significant negative impact on loneliness, and H1, H3, and H5 are accepted. Information support, emotion support and network support explain 16.1% of the variance in loneliness together. Information support and network support have significant influence on perceived health and explain 23.1% of the variance in perceived health with loneliness. As we proposed in hypothesis 7, Loneliness has significant negative impact on perceived health, and H7 is accepted.

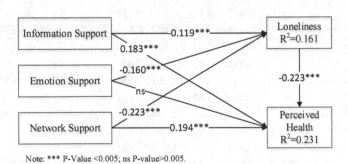

Note: *** P-Value <0.005; ns P-value>0.005.

Fig. 2. Results of research model

6   Discussion and Conclusions

6.1   Summary of Key Findings

Accordingly, the research results suggest that the informational support and network support during the WeChat usage can significantly influence users' perceived health. In addition, informational support, emotional support, and network support can significantly reduce the perceived loneliness. Network support exerts the strongest influence on perceived loneliness. Finally, the perceived loneliness significantly reduces the perceived health.

6.2   Contributions

This study aims to provide the following theory implications. Firstly, the research results suggest that social support can significantly increase the perceived health. Hence, this study aims to expand the generalization of social support theory in investigating the perceived health in the social media context. Secondly, the social support derived from the social media usage can significantly reduce the perceived loneliness, and loneliness can decrease the perceived the perceived health. The research results suggest that the loneness is a critical factor in determining the perceived health in social media.

Accordingly, this research aims to provide several practical implications to facilitate the perceived health. Firstly, in order to improve the effect of social support on perceived health, practitioners in social media can enhance the interactivity of the functions to induce the emotional and informational share behavior. Secondly, in order to reduce the perceived loneliness, practitioners can design different social media to meet the users' various social needs. Specifically, the practitioners should focus on designing the informational, emotional and network functions of the social media.

6.3   Limitations and Future Researches

There are some limitations can be deeply researched in the future though many hypotheses are confirmed. The first, besides the information support, emotion support and network support which provide by social media, there are many other dimensions of social support can be applied in this research context, such as esteem support, tangle support and etc. Second, social support can not only reduce the loneliness, but also improve the individual's subjective well-being. Subjective well-being can improve individual perceived health significantly which has been confirmed by previous scholars. Hence, the influence of subject well-being on perceived health and the mediating effect of subject well-being on the social support and perceived health should be deeply researched in the future. Third, because of the certain gap between the actual health and perceived health, there is a certain limitation that perceived health is used to measure the actual health condition to research the social support on health. Individual actual health can be divided into physical health and mental health, which can be applied in the future research, and tested the social support of social media on physical health and mental health.

References

1. Che, H.L., Cao, Y.: Examining WeChat users' motivations, trust, attitudes, and positive word-of-mouth: evidence from China. Comput. Hum. Behav. **41**, 104–111 (2014)
2. Venkatesh, V., Morris, M.G., Davis, G.B., et al.: User acceptance of information technology: toward a unified view. MIS Q. **27**(3), 425–478 (2003)
3. Lien, C.H., Cao, Y., Zhou, X.: Service quality, satisfaction, stickiness, and usage intentions: an exploratory evaluation in the context of WeChat services. Comput. Hum. Behav. **68**, 403–410 (2017)
4. Chen, Y., Liang, C., Cai, D.: Understanding WeChat users' behavior of sharing social crisis information. Int. J. Hum.-Comput. Interact. **34**(3), 1–11 (2018)
5. Zhang, C.B., Li, Y.N., Wu, B., et al.: How WeChat can retain users: roles of network externalities, social interaction ties, and perceived values in building continuance intention. Comput. Hum. Behav. **69**, 284–293 (2016)
6. Chen, L., Goh, C.F., Sun, Y., et al.: Integrating guanxi, into technology acceptance: an empirical investigation of WeChat. Telematics Inform. **34**, 1125–1142 (2017)
7. Gan, C., Li, H., Gan, C., et al.: Understanding the effects of gratifications on the continuance intention to use WeChat in China: a perspective on uses and gratifications. Comput. Hum. Behav. **78**, 306–315 (2018)
8. Cobb, S.: Social support as a moderator of life stress. Psychosom. Med. **38**(5), 300–314 (1976)
9. Cohen, S., Hoberman, H.M.: Positive events and social supports as buffers of life change stress. J. Appl. Soc. Psychol. **13**(2), 99–125 (2010)
10. Liang, T., Ho, Y., Li, Y., et al.: What drives social commerce: the role of social support and relationship quality. Int. J. Electron. Commer. **16**(2), 69–90 (2011)
11. Zhu, D.H., Sun, H., Chang, Y.P.: Effect of social support on customer satisfaction and citizenship behavior in online brand communities: the moderating role of support source. J. Retail. Consum. Serv. **31**, 287–293 (2016)
12. Chiu, C.M., Huang, H.Y., Cheng, H.L., et al.: Understanding online community citizenship behaviors through social support and social identity. Int. J. Inf. Manag. J. Inf. Prof. **35**(4), 504–519 (2015)
13. Lin, X., Zhang, D., Li, Y.: Delineating the dimensions of social support on social networking sites and their effects: a comparative model. Comput. Hum. Behav. **58**, 421–430 (2016)
14. Hajli, M.N.: The role of social support on relationship quality and social commerce. Technol. Forecast. Soc. Chang. **87**(1), 17–27 (2014)
15. Oh, H.J., Lauckner, C., Boehmer, J., et al.: Facebooking for health: an examination into the solicitation and effects of health-related social support on social networking sites. Comput. Hum. Behav. **29**(5), 2072–2080 (2013)
16. Lakey, B., Adams, K., Neely, L., et al.: Perceived support and low emotional distress: the role of enacted support, dyad similarity, and provider personality. Pers. Soc. Psychol. Bull. **28**(11), 1546–1555 (2002)
17. Williams, K.E., Bond, M.J.: The roles of self-efficacy, outcome expectancies and social support in the self-care behaviours of diabetics. Psychol. Health Med. **7**(2), 127–141 (2002)
18. Arora, N.K., Rutten, L.J.F., Gustafson, D.H., et al.: Perceived helpfulness and impact of social support provided by family, friends, and health care providers to women newly diagnosed with breast cancer. Psycho-Oncology **16**(5), 474–486 (2010)
19. Davis, M.A., Anthony, D.L., Pauls, S.D.: Seeking and receiving social support on Facebook for surgery. Soc. Sci. Med. **131**, 40–47 (2015)

20. Ferreira-Alves, J., Magalhães, P., Viola, L., et al.: Loneliness in middle and old age: demographics, perceived health, and social satisfaction as predictors. Arch. Gerontol. Geriatr. **59**, 613–623 (2014)
21. Ponzetti, J.J.: Loneliness among College Students. Fam. Relat. **39**(3), 336–340 (1990)
22. Weiss, R.S.: Loneliness: the experience of emotional and social isolation. Contemp. Sociol. **25**(25), 39–41 (1975)
23. Russell, D., Cutrona, C.E., Rose, J., et al.: Social and emotional loneliness: an examination of Weiss's typology of loneliness. J. Pers. Soc. Psychol. **46**(6), 1313–1321 (1984)
24. Ditommaso, E., Spinner, B.: Social and emotional loneliness: a re-examination of Weiss' typology of loneliness. Pers. Individ. Differ. **22**(3), 417–427 (1997)
25. Song, H., Zmyslinskiseelig, A., Kim, J., et al.: Does Facebook make you lonely?: a meta analysis. Comput. Hum. Behav. **36**(36), 446–452 (2014)
26. Ryan, T., Xenos, S.: Who uses Facebook? An investigation into the relationship between the Big Five, shyness, narcissism, loneliness, and Facebook usage. Comput. Hum. Behav. **27**(5), 1658–1664 (2011)
27. Zhao, J., Kong, F., Wang, Y.: The role of social support and self-esteem in the relationship between shyness and loneliness. Pers. Individ. Differ. **54**(5), 577–581 (2013)
28. Kang, H.W., Park, M., Wallace, J.P.: The impact of perceived social support, loneliness, and physical activity on quality of life in South Korean older adults. J. Sport. Health Sci. **7**(2), 237–244 (2018)
29. Hawkley, L.C., Hughes, M.E., Waite, L.J., et al.: From social structural factors to perceptions of relationship quality and loneliness: the Chicago health, aging, and social relations study. J. Gerontol. **63B**(6), S375–S384 (2008)
30. Perissinotto, C.M., Cenzer, I.S., Covinsky, K.E.: Loneliness in older persons: a predictor of functional decline and death. Arch. Intern. Med. **172**(14), 1078–1083 (2012)
31. Momtaz, Y.A., Hamid, T.A., Yusoff, S., et al.: Loneliness as a risk factor for hypertension in later life. J. Aging Health **24**(4), 696–710 (2012)
32. Christiansen, J., Larsen, F.B., Lasgaard, M.: Do stress, health behavior, and sleep mediate the association between loneliness and adverse health conditions among older people? Soc. Sci. Med. **152**, 80–86 (2016)
33. Stickley, A., Koyanagi, A., Leinsalu, M., et al.: Loneliness and health in Eastern Europe: findings from Moscow, Russia. Public Health **129**(4), 403–410 (2015)
34. Lin, T.C., Hsu, S.C., Cheng, H.L., et al.: Exploring the relationship between receiving and offering online social support. Inf. Manag. **52**(3), 371–383 (2015)
35. Luo, Y., Hawkley, L.C., Waite, L.J., et al.: Loneliness, health, and mortality in old age: a national longitudinal study. Soc. Sci. Med. **74**(6), 907–914 (2012)
36. Pittman, M., Reich, B.: Social media and loneliness: why an Instagram picture may be worth more than a thousand Twitter words. Comput. Hum. Behav. **62**, 155–167 (2016)
37. Stewart, A.L., Hays, R.D., Ware, J.E.: The MOS short-form general health survey: reliability and validity in a patient population. Med. Care **26**(7), 724–735 (1988)

Smart and Connected Health Projects: Characteristics and Research Challenges

Jiangping Chen[1](✉) ⓘ, Minghong Chen[2] ⓘ, Jingye Qu[3] ⓘ,
Haihua Chen[1] ⓘ, and Juncheng Ding[4] ⓘ

[1] Department of Information Science, University of North Texas, Denton,
TX 76203, USA
Jiangping.Chen@unt.edu
[2] School of Information Management, Sun Yat-sen University,
Guangzhou 510006, China
[3] School of Information Technology and Media, Beihua University,
Jilin 132013, China
[4] Department of Computer Science, University of North Texas, Denton,
TX 76203, USA

Abstract. The Smart and Connected Health (SCH) program at the National Science Foundation (NSF) has been established as a stand-alone solicitation since 2012. This article reviews and analyzes the 100 projects that have been funded since 2012 to understand their characteristics and the research challenges they have addressed in SCH. Descriptive analysis, topic analysis based on Latent Dirichlet Allocation (LDA), and comparative content analysis were performed. Our study indicated that NSF SCH projects, featured with collaborative and multidisciplinary research endeavor, have been exploring more than 36 diseases or health problems, and five major research challenges including electronic health record (HER) data processing, system design or computational model building, personalized or patient-centered medicine, training and education, and privacy preserving. Much more research projects are needed to investigate algorithms, devices, and impacts of smart health on diseases and communities.

Keywords: Smart and connected health · NSF projects · Text analysis
Data analysis

1 Introduction

With the rapid development of the infrastructures and technologies of smart cities that reconstruct the thinking behind existing healthcare systems and telemedicine, a new and ubiquitous concept called smart health, or smart and connected health (SCH) has emerged [1], leading the innovation of health care service mechanism. Although SCH has not been precisely defined, it refers to any digital healthcare solutions or systems that can operate remotely with integration of innovative computational and engineering approaches to support the transformation of health and medicine services [2, 3]. According to Clancy [3], SCH defines not only information communication technology

H. Chen et al. (Eds.): ICSH 2018, LNCS 10983, pp. 154–164, 2018.
https://doi.org/10.1007/978-3-030-03649-2_15

development, but also a state-of-thinking, a way of lifestyle, and a vow for connected entities to improve healthcare facilities in the home, city, country and globe with the aid of a number of intelligent agents. SCH as a field of study at the intersection of public health, information system, big data, cloud computing, deep learning and artificial intelligence, has received a lot of attention from academia and industry.

U.S. National Science Foundation (NSF), as the most influential research and management organization in the world, has supported numerous scientific research projects that have led to global economic growth and the improvement of the quality of people's lives and health. Since 2012, NSF has supported the Smart Health and Wellbeing (SHB) Program. Later, it transfers to the Smart and Connected Health (SCH) program. As specified by SCH program solicitation [1], SCH program aims to "develop next generation healthcare solutions and encourage existing and new research communities to focus on breakthrough ideas in a variety of areas of value to health, such as sensor technology, networking, information and machine learning technology, decision support systems, modeling of behavioral and cognitive processes, as well as system and process modeling". There are 100 SCH projects that have been funded by NSF. Compared to scientific publications, the funded projects provide much more valuable information, which contribute to the hot themes and research challenges.

The purpose of this study is to adopt text analysis and text mining methods to analyze SCH projects funded by NSF, including what have been funded, characteristics of funded projects, and health problems and research challenges addressed by these projects. This study helps SCH researchers to understand the scope and characteristics of current NSF funded SCH projects so they can better prepare their NSF proposals. It also provides a case study to data science students and educators on how text analysis can be conducted for specific purposes.

2   General Characteristics: A Descriptive Analysis

We collected data from NSF website using its advanced ward search page [4] with NSF program element code 8018 (the code for smart and connected health program) on March 31, 2018. As a result, we retrieved 146 records that include the metadata of 100 SCH projects funded by NSF from 2012 to 2017. One project may have more than one record, as NSF allows different institutions to file their proposals separately even they are collaborating on the same project. The 146 records were retrieved and downloaded into an Excel file. The 25 metadata of the records include: Award Number, Title, NSF Division, Program(s), Start Date, Last Amendment Date, Principal Investigator (PI), State, Organization, Award Instrument, Program Manager, End Date, Awarded Amount to Date, Co-principal Investigators (Co-PI), PI email address, Organization Information (street, city, state, zip code, phone), NSF Directorate, Program Element Code(s), Program Reference Code(s), ARRA Amount, and Abstract. For the purpose of our study, we conducted analysis on 10 of the metadata elements of the records. Table 1 is a sample NSF project record with the 10 elements. Below we report our general descriptive analysis of the 146 records.

Table 1. Selected metadata information of a sample NSF-funded project

Project Element	Example
Title	EAGER: Synthesizing Notes from Electronic Health Records to Make Them Actionable for Heart Failure Patients
Program(s)	Smart and Connected Health
Start Date	06/15/2017
PI	Jodi Forlizzi
Co-PI	Carolyn Rose, John Zimmerman
Organization	Carnegie-Mellon University
Awarded amount	$316,000.00
State	PA
End Date	05/31/2019
Abstract	This Early-concept Grant for Exploratory Research aims to help patients and caregivers have increased access to electronic health information. The research focuses on the Electronic Health Record (EHR). …. The research investigates new and more effective presentations of this information to patients (e.g., graphic, abstracted, actionable). …

2.1   Number of Funded Projects over Years

We found that the number of SCH funded records is increasing over years, from 4 records in 2012 to 48 records in 2017, as indicated in the dotted line showed in Fig. 1. The only exception is 2016 when there were 3 fewer records than year 2015, but still more records than year 2014. In 2017, the number of SCH records achieved 48, a growth of 65.52% over 2012. Note this calculation does not reflect the actual growth rate of the number of projects, because some projects have multiple records due to simultaneous filing of NSF proposals. As indicated by 2018 solicitation, 8-16 projects can be funded per year in the future [1].

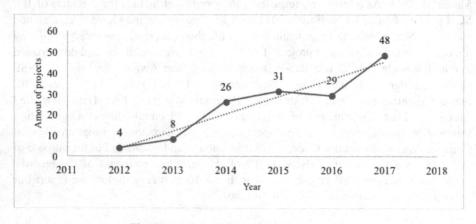

Fig. 1. Number of funded project over years

2.2   Geographical Distribution

The 146 records indicated that funded SCH projects were distributed in 35 states of the U.S. The top five states were Massachusetts, Texas, Pennsylvania, California and New York, all of which had more than 10 projects. Additionally, there were 4 states which had more than 5 projects, including Florida, North Carolina, Virginia and Maryland. Other states just had 1 or 2 projects. Some states, such as New Mexico and Hawaii did not have any project funded by NSF, however, that does not mean there were no researchers in these states involved in NSF funded SCH projects. Because NSF records only list PIs' states, it is very possible that some researchers participated as CO-PIs or major staff in SCH projects in those states are not listed.

2.3   Number of PI and CO-PIs

It is important to analyze the number of PI and CO-PIs to understand the situation of collaboration in SCH projects. The nature of SCH project demands that multidisciplinary teams work together to address multi-dimensional challenges ranging from fundamental science to clinical practice [1]. The distribution of the number of PI and CO-PIs were reported in Fig. 2.

NSF projects have only one PI, but can have multiple Co-PIs. In this study, we found that 51% of SCH records had two or more investigators. Among them, 34 records contain one PI and one CO-PI, 18 records having 2 CO-PIs, and 15 records having 3 CO-PIs. Furthermore, 5 records have 5 investigators (one PI and 4 CO-PIs) and 2 records have 6 investigators (one PI and 5 CO-PIs). The single PI projects may need more exploration. They may be part of a collaborative projects but filed the proposal separately, or maybe the PIs have a multidisciplinary research teams that have the required capabilities for conducting SCH projects.

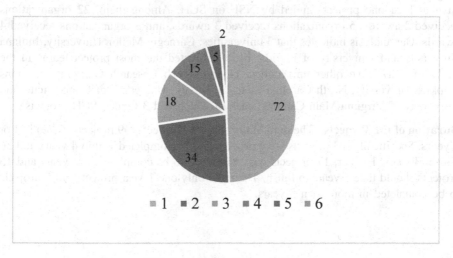

Fig. 2. Number of investigators

2.4   Amount of Funds

For amount of funds, 15% of the 146 records are more than $1,000,000, 30% between $500,001–$1,000,000, 46% between $100,001–$500,000, 2% between $50,001–$100,000, and 7% less than or equal to $50,000. The amount of funds is showed in Table 2.

Table 2. Amount of Funds for Each SCH Record

Award amount	Number of projects	Percent (%)
More than $1,000,000	22	15
Between $500,001–$1,000,000	44	30
Between $100,001–$500,000	67	46
Between $50,001–$100,000	3	2
Less than or equal $50,000	10	7

In addition, we found that the amount of funds increases year by year, except for 2015 and 2017. In 2015, the total award amount was $14,474,172, which is $2,719,603 less than that of 2014. And the total award amount of 2017 was $18,980,644, which is 1,525,830 less than that of 2016. However, the numbers of SCH records in 2015 and 2016 are more than the previous year respectively, which indicates that the fund for each project on average was reduced in these two years. For 2018, the anticipated Funding Amount will be $11,000,000 to $20,000,000 [1].

2.5   Other Features

Organizations. There were 105 organizations that received at least one SCH award, or have at least one project funded by NSF on SCH. Among them, 22 organizations received 2 awards, 5 organizations received 3 awards, and 3 organizations received 4 awards. Our analysis indicates that 3 universities: Carnegie-Mellon University, Indiana University and University of Florida, have cultivated the most project teams in the study of SCH. Five other universities: Georgia Tech Research Corporation, Johns Hopkins University, North Carolina State University, University of Connecticut, and University of Virginia Main Campus, each of which had 3 funded SCH projects.

Duration of the Projects. The duration of majority projects (99 projects, 68%) is 3 or 4 years. Specifically, 63 projects were proposed to be completed within 4 years and 36 within 3 years. Further, 17 projects were proposed to be completed in 2 years and 15 projects should take 5 years to finish. There are only one 1-year project, and 5 projects to be completed in more than 5 years.

3 Term Frequency and Topic Analysis

3.1 Term Frequency and Word Cloud

The records we downloaded about NSF SCH projects includes titles and abstracts. They are well developed by the investigators containing most valuable information regarding the purposes, methods, diseases/health problems, and activities of the projects. After a review of the 146 records, we found that there are actually only 100 projects. Thirty-two projects have multiple entries (2 to 7) in the downloaded file. As explained earlier, NSF allows different organizations to file their proposals separately even they work on the sample project. Therefore, for the content analysis in this section and after, we removed the duplicate titles and abstracts in the download project file, leaving 100 titles and 100 abstracts for analysis.

We conducted automatic term frequency analysis using NLTK, the natural language processing toolkit [5]. After automatic processing and manual review of the most frequent 500 words, we obtained a list of words with their term frequency. The top 50 words are listed in Table 3. Figure 3 is the word cloud of the top 403 content words. The word cloud was created using wordart.com – a free word cloud generator [6].

Table 3. Most Frequent Terms in Titles and Abstracts

Term	Frequency	Term	Frequency	Term	Frequency
Develop	257	Learning	97	Individual	64
Health	225	Disease	95	Algorithms	61
Patient	220	Provide	88	Behavior	61
Model	211	Approach	86	Advance	60
System	204	Improve	86	Novel	59
Technical	144	Healthcare	74	Sensor	59
Clinical	122	support	71	Potential	58
Student	119	Care	70	Collaborative	57
Medical	117	Integrate	70	Human	57
Monitoring	103	Information	66	Real-time	57

We can make sense of the projects by observing the term frequency table and the word cloud: Most of the SCH projects are developing something, whether that is new device, new models, new technologies, or new processes; funded projects are well aligned with NSF program solicitation that focus on patient, health, medicine, student and care; many projects involve develop and use of systems and models. To make an accurate term frequency table, it is important to conduct stemming, or to normalize the different forms of words. For example, different forms for "model" can be "modeling," "Modeling," "models\," and "Models" in the original abstract.

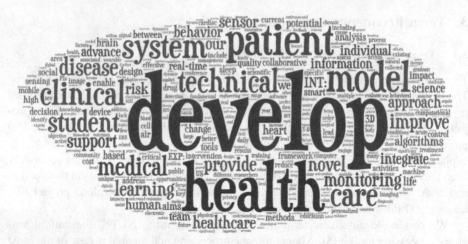

Fig. 3. Word cloud of SCH projects

3.2 Topic Analysis with Latent Dirichlet Allocation (LDA) Model

Latent Dirichlet allocation (LDA) model [7] has often been used to automatically identify the latent semantic topics in unstructured collections of documents. Giving a list of text documents, LDA model can identify topics in each document by a cluster of semantically related words [8, 9]. Since LDA model can represent the document in a topic space instead of a word space, it helps to deal with the synonymy and polysemy problem from the semantic perspective and at the same time reduce the dimensionality. LDA has therefore been used in many semantic analytical researches such as: identi-fication and monitoring the disruptive technologies [10], generating of the patent development maps [11], classification and pattern identification in patents [12] and so on. Specifically, Nichols [13] proposed a topic model approach to explore the inter-disciplinary of the NSF funding portfolio based on the NSF award and proposal database, which can help the NSF employees to better assess and administrate the funding portfolio, and the researchers to avoid duplicating others' research projects.

We conducted LDA analysis of the abstracts of the 100 projects. The purpose was to exam whether LDA could bring new insights to our understanding of the projects. Table 4 lists the word-level topics as identified by LDA. We used the open-source topic modeling tool gensim [14] for LDA analysis. Our program was configured to output 20 top terms for 20 topics.

It appears Table 4 displays a different set of important terms from what we could obtain for term frequency analysis in Sect. 3.1. For examples, disease names and health problem related terms such as "diabetes", "osteoporosis", "cardiac", and "cancer" are present in the list under different topics. Furthermore, we conducted LDA on bi-grams and tri-grams. More content terms were identified.

Table 4. The 20 topics generated by LDA analysis

Topic ID	Terms under each topic
1	Sleep, family, cpr, physical, feedback, therapy, child, researchers, obesity, evaluate
2	knowledge, behavioral, natural, sleep, smart, environmental, ontology, integration, researchers, transportation
3	Dynamics, cardiac, environmental, computer, stateoftheart, imaging, multiscale, schemes, dimension, analyzing
4	Management, gestures, sensors, user, specific, pis, researchers, behavioral, feedback, capacitive
5	Software, motor, computer, function, pd, inspire, dynamics, cardiac, challenges, simcardio
6	Detection, automation, physiological, early, clinicians, ad, methodologies, images, critical, education
7	Mobile, personalized, emerging, advanced, study, asthma, researchers, ii, critical, computer
8	Cancer, sleep, adaptive, intervention, effective, strategies, screening, breast, national, dynamic
9	Imaging, guidelines, cognitive, chronic, specific, efforts, ultrasound, objective, multiple, effective
10	Smart, imaging, mobile, diabetes, devices, ai, sensors, personalized, management, tools
11	Imaging, failure, cardiac, software, device, simcardio, surgical, driving, fibrillation, source
12	Postoperative, prosthesis, management, energy, agitation, family, smart, intervention, life, behavioral
13	Dyadic, conference, dynamics, wellbeing, forum, psychotherapy, behavioral, finegrained, indicators, power
14	Colon, mobile, education, imaging, aims, smart, behavioral, device, knowledge, undergraduate
15	Surgical, outcomes, connectomics, conference, services, natural, mobile, social, forecasting, university
16	Conference, dental, osteoporosis, informatics, international, services, doctoral, biomedical, collected, elderly
17	Goals, inspire, personalized, coaching, outcomes, physicians, alerts, smart, adolescent, significant
18	Sepsis, imaging, diagnostic, outcomes, cognitive, tests, enable, knowledge, ultrasound, cartilage
19	Mathematical, theory, intervention, social, emergency, devices, therapy, effective, smart, tools
20	Children, mobility, impairments, driving, agitation, dynamics, adhd, management, dyadic, imaging

4 Research Challenges Addressed by the Projects

One of the purposes of this study is to identify major research challenges that have been addressed by these SCH projects. Specifically, we would like to understand what diseases or health problems these projects have been tackling, and what popular research problems NSF investigators have been working on.

Two of the authors conducted a content analysis focusing on coding the projects (mainly the abstracts) on research problem/challenge, method/algorithm, disease, data, device, and other outcomes. The results of the analysis cannot be reported in this paper in detail due to the restriction on paper length. The content analysis helped us to achieve our purposes.

4.1 Diseases/Medical Problems Addressed by the Projects

The content analysis discovered that about 36 types of diseases or health problems have been tackled by the investigators, including respiratory diseases, infection plus systemic manifestations of infection, environmental public health issues, dementia, obesity, sickle cell disease, diabetes, cognitive disorders, mental trauma, heart problems, genetic diseases like cancer, sepsis, healthy life related problems, adolescent health, Attention-Deficit/Hyperactivity Disorder (ADHD) in teenagers and young adults, life threatening events in neonates, major complications following surgery, retinopathy of prematurity, strokes, epilepsy, depression, amputation, cardiovascular, traumatic brain injury, perioperative services, hepatitis C, alzheimer's disease, knee osteoarthritis, cognitive fatigue, psychotherapy, and children with mobility impairments. This list looks quite extensive. However, still many diseases or health problems are not included in these projects.

4.2 Research Areas and Challenges

Our analysis indicates that researchers are working in the following areas in smart and connected health:

(1) Create novel methods and tools for the analysis of large-scale Electronic Health Record (EHR) data and social medial data to help diseases diagnose accurately, to improve patient care and/or to reduce costs;
(2) Develop new or integrated methods, models, frameworks, and systems to help treat, monitor, or understand some diseases such as Asthma, Type-II Diabetes Mellitus (T2DM), Infection, and Heart Failure;
(3) Develop new devices, mostly wearable sensors for disease monitoring, environmental control, injuries prevention, and safety;
(4) Promote education in data science, training, and communication.

Understandably, different projects are dealing with different health problems. Based on the results of our term frequency analysis, topic analysis, and content analysis, we believe the following are the major research challenges investigated by these projects:

Electronic Health Record (EHR) data processing. At least 8 projects work on frameworks, integrating solutions, models, data mining approaches, and machine learning approaches to process EHR. Data processing is one of the major challenges in current big data environment and future smart health [15].

System design or computation model building. At least 22 projects emphasized system design and model building as one of their major objectives. Researchers work on developing systems and models to collect data and conduct data analysis.

Personalized or patient-centered medicine. At least 12 projects explore personalized or patient-centered medicine.

Training and education. At least 6 projects focus on student support for attending international conferences, institute support on global healthcare education.

Privacy preserving. At least 3 projects concentrate on exploring privacy preserving in EHR or other medical data.

5 Summary and Future Research

This paper analyzes 100 NSF projects that were identified as under the smart and connected health program based on their information retrieved from NSF website. Descriptive statistical analysis, topic analysis and content analysis were performed to understand the characteristics and research challenges tackled by these projects. SCH is a very important research area with many challenging research problems. Researchers who are interested in conducting SCH research will need to have collaborative spirit and be able to work as part of a team. We believe there are many opportunities for researchers to seek funding in NSF and other agencies in the area of smart and connected health.

This study is the beginning of our endeavor on smart and connected health. Our future research will be on two topics: One is to explore sophisticated text analysis techniques for effective and efficient understanding and mining of texts. The other is to initiate our NSF proposal application by tacking one of the interesting smart and connected health challenges.

References

1. Pramanik, Md.I., Lau, R.Y.K., Demirkan, H., Azad, Md.A.K.: Smart health: big data enabled health paradigm within smart cities. Expert. Syst. Appl. **87**, 370–383 (2017)
2. National Science Foundation: Smart and Connected Health (SCH): Connecting Data, People and Systems (2018). https://www.nsf.gov/pubs/2018/nsf18541/nsf18541.htm
3. Clancy, C.M.: Getting to "smart" health care. Health Aff. **25**(6), 589–592 (2006)
4. National Science Foundation: Awards advanced search (2018). https://www.nsf.gov/awardsearch/advancedSearch.jsp
5. Bird, S., Klein, E., Loper, E.: Natural language processing with Python – analyzing text with the natural language toolkit (2018). http://www.nltk.org/book/
6. WordArt.com. https://wordart.com/. Accessed 2018

7. Blei, D.M., Ng, A.Y., Jordan, M.I.: Latent Dirichlet allocation. J. Mach. Learn. Res. **3**(Jan), 993–1022 (2003)
8. Rosen-Zvi, M., Griffiths, T., Steyvers, M., Smyth, P.: The author-topic model for authors and documents. In: Proceedings of the 20th Conference on Uncertainty in Artificial Intelligence, pp. 487–494. AUAI Press (2004)
9. Steyvers, M., Smyth, P., Rosen-Zvi, M., Griffiths, T.: Probabilistic author-topic models for information discovery. In: Proceedings of the Tenth ACM SIGKDD International Conference on Knowledge Discovery and Data Mining, pp. 306–315. ACM (2004)
10. Momeni, A., Rost, K.: Identification and monitoring of possible disruptive technologies by patent-development paths and topic modeling. Technol. Forecast. Soc. Chang. **104**, 16–29 (2016)
11. Kim, M., Park, Y., Yoon, J.: Generating patent development maps for technology monitoring using semantic patent-topic analysis. Comput. Ind. Eng. **98**, 289–299 (2016)
12. Venugopalan, S., Rai, V.: Topic based classification and pattern identification in patents. Technol. Forecast. Soc. Chang. **94**, 236–250 (2015)
13. Nichols, L.G.: A topic model approach to measuring interdisciplinarity at the National Science Foundation. Scientometrics **100**, 741–754 (2014)
14. Gensim. https://radimrehurek.com/gensim/. Accessed 2018
15. Olshansky, S.J., et al.: The future of smart health. Computer **49**, 14–21 (2016)

Medical Big Data and Healthcare Machine Learning

Designing a Novel Framework for Precision Medicine Information Retrieval

Haihua Chen[1], Juncheng Ding[2], Jiangping Chen[1]([⊠]),
and Gaohui Cao[3]

[1] Department of Information Science, University of North Texas,
Denton, TX 76203, USA
Jiangping.Chen@unt.edu
[2] Department of Computer Science, University of North Texas,
Denton, TX 76203, USA
[3] School of Information Management, Central China Normal University,
Wuhan 430079, China

Abstract. Precision medicine information retrieval (PMIR) is about matching the most relevant scientific articles to an individual patient for reliable disease treatment. The corresponding Precision Medicine (PM) Track organized by 2017 Text REtrieval Conference [1] provides a test collection for evaluating the performance of PMIR techniques for finding reliable medical evidence. It significantly facilitates PMIR research and system development. However, the performance of current PMIR systems is still far from satisfactory. This study aims to investigate the application of the latest information retrieval and text mining techniques to PMIR. Based on a review of previous efforts and approaches, we propose three promising techniques: keyphrase extraction for indexing, hybrid query expansion including word embeddings, and retrieval results re-ranking with supervised regression analysis for PMIR. A novel framework for PMIR is therefore designed. A PMIR system based on this framework will be implemented and tested using 2017 and 2018 TREC Precision Medicine Track datasets.

Keywords: Precision medicine · Information retrieval · Keyphrase extraction
Query expansion · Supervised learning

1 Introduction

For many complex diseases, there are no "one size fits all" solutions for patients with a particular diagnosis, the proper treatment for a patient depends upon genetic, environmental, and lifestyle choices [2]. Therefore, personalize treatment in consideration of different factors is necessary. Precision medicine is introduced to enable clinicians to efficiently and accurately predict the most appropriate course of action for a patient [3]. However, the practice of precision medicine found that a large number of treatment options were usually produced [4], which increases the challenges for physicians to choose the most appropriate treatments for the patient. An information retrieval (IR) system might be able to help if it can quickly locate relevant evidences.

© Springer Nature Switzerland AG 2018
H. Chen et al. (Eds.): ICSH 2018, LNCS 10983, pp. 167–178, 2018.
https://doi.org/10.1007/978-3-030-03649-2_16

Precision Medicine Information Retrieval (PMIR) will benefit at least three groups of people [5]. The first group is patients. More reliable disease treatment strategies mean a higher possibility of treatment success, which can also save patients' time and money; The second group is physician or clinician. PMIR will make their treatment decisions easier and more reliable; The third group is IR researchers who can test their models and algorithms in the medicine domain.

Given the significance and the challenges of PMIR, 2017 Text REtrieval Conference has organized the Precision Medicine Track to bring together the biomedical IR community to explore effective solutions. The organizer provided a test collection and conducted manual IR evaluation to understand the performance of PMIR techniques for finding reliable medical evidence from millions of scientific abstracts. TREC evaluation has pushed forward PMIR system development and effectiveness. However, PMIR performance is still far from satisfactory. For examples, the best systems conducting medical scientific abstracts retrieval could only achieve 0.4593, 0.2987, and 0.6310 in terms of IR measures infNDCG, R-prec, and P@10 [2]. There is still much room for improvement.

This paper aims to explore effective and efficient computational solutions on PMIR. The three main contributions of this paper include:

- We survey various existing methods in terms of different stages of PMIR task and compare their advantages and disadvantages;
- We investigate several promising techniques that could be used to improve PMIR performance and discuss the mechanisms in detail;
- We propose a framework integrating these techniques for developing a new PMIR system.

The remainder of this paper is structured as follows. In Sect. 2, we give a brief overview of previous studies on PMIR and compare the advantages and disadvantages between different methods, especially those explored at TREC 2017 Precision Medicine Track. Section 3 presents the research questions and the framework. Next, we describe three techniques that have the potential to improve PMIR performance in the proposed framework in Sect. 4. Finally, in Sect. 5, we summarize this paper and discuss the next steps for this research.

2 Related Studies

Precision medicine is not a new concept [6]. However, it was paid greater attention after the new initiative announced by former President Barack Obama in 2015 on this subject [3]. Researchers and practitioners from different communities including medical information retrieval group have devoted significant efforts to this area since then. For example, TREC has sponsored for three consecutive years the Clinical Decision Support track (2014–2016), and the Precision Medicine track (in 2017). The latter focused on providing useful precision medicine-related information to clinicians treating cancer patients [1].

PMIR is considered a multiple-stage process: The document collections including MEDLINE Articles and conference proceedings are first indexed. Then queries generated from the topics are sent as input to a PMIR system to retrieve relevant documents from the index. The top N retrieved results are returned by the IR system as the relevant documents for each topic. These results are usually re-ranked based on different re-ranking strategies to achieve higher retrieval performance.

As described in TREC 2017 Precision Medicine Track [1], the objective of the PMIR task is to retrieve biomedical articles on existing knowledge, in the form of article abstracts (largely from MEDLINE/PubMed). Figure 1 shows the format of two scientific abstracts from PubMed and AACR Proceedings respectively in the TREC document collection. These documents contain important elements such as the title abstract, chemical list, mesh descriptor.

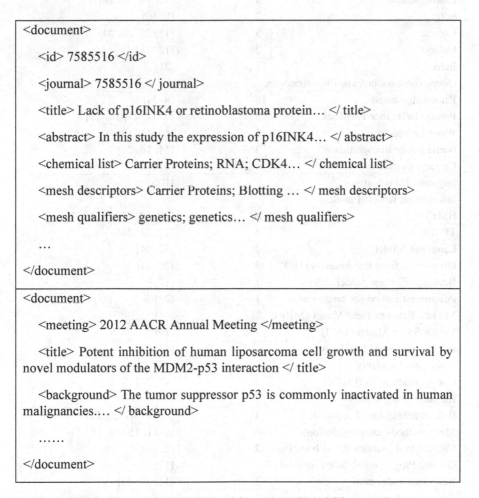

Fig. 1. Format of MEDLINE articles and AACR/ASCO proceedings

There were 32 groups participated in 2017 Precision Medicine Track. Only 17 groups published their reports on the scientific abstract task detailing their search methodologies and results [7]. Most of the groups followed the general process described above. By conducting a comparison on the methodologies of the 17 groups, we found a large overlap in terms of the methods used in each stage. Table 1 summarizes the methods used by TREC 2017 PMIR systems.

Table 1. Summary of TREC 2017 PMIR systems

Methods	Number of teams	References
IR platforms (for indexing and retrieval)		
Terrier	4	[17, 19, 22, 23]
Elastic Search	4	[13, 14, 16, 18]
Solr	2	[8, 10]
Lucene	5	[11, 20, 22, 24]
Galago	2	[12, 15]
Indri	1	[21]
Query construction/expansion strategies		
Knowledge-based	16	[8–24]
Pseudo Relevance Feedback	5	[9, 14, 17, 19, 23]
Word Embeddings	3	[10, 11, 19]
Name Entity Recognition	3	[14, 16, 20]
Concept Extraction	1	[21]
Negation Detection	1	[10]
Information retrieval models		
BM25	6	[10, 12, 13, 18, 19, 24]
TF-IDF	3	[11, 22, 24]
Language Model	2	[22, 24]
Divergence from Randomness (DFR)	3	[22–24]
Bernoulli-Einstein model (BB2)	1	[17]
Poisson estimation for randomness	1	[22]
Markov Random Field Model (MRF)	1	[14]
Vector Space Model (VSM)	1	[19]
Information-based Similarity	1	[24]
Axiomatic Similarity	1	[24]
Log-logistic model (LGD)	2	[17, 22]
Re-ranking algorithms		
Rule matching-based approach	4	[8, 14, 16, 20, 21]
Multi-methods merging (fusion)	10	[8–11, 15, 16, 18, 20–22, 24]
Clinical trial citations-based boosting	2	[8, 10]
Genetic Programming-based method	1	[12]
Relevance Judgement	3	[13, 19, 23]

The first step of the PMIR process is indexing, which will be largely depended on a good IR platform. Table 1 indicates that 11 groups have chosen Lucene (Solr and

Elasticsearch are also Lucene-based) for indexing and retrieval, as Lucene is considered efficient for indexing large document [25]. Another fact is that Lucene has become the de facto platform in industry for building search applications [26].

The second step is query construction. In this stage, TREC topics (see an example in Fig. 2) were used to formulate queries and sent to the retrieval system to match the indexes of the document collection. Participants incorporated query expansion techniques to expand the topic terms in three aspects: gene aspects, disease aspects, and other aspects [10, 24]. Different kinds of knowledge bases such as NCI thesaurus, Mesh dictionary, and Wikipedia are frequently used in this process. Pseudo relevance feedback is another popular query expansion method [9, 14, 17, 19], in which terms from top retrieved documents were added to the original queries. Recently, word embeddings have also been proved to be effective in query expansion [10, 11, 19].

<topic number="1">

  <disease> Acute lymphoblastic leukemia </ disease>

  <gene> ABL1, PTPN11 </ gene>

  <demographic> 12-year-old male </ demographic></topic>

Fig. 2. A TREC PM topic

The next step is matching or retrieval applying one or more models implemented in the IR platforms. Popular models include BM-25, TF-IDF, and others, as indicated in Table 1.

The final and important component of PMIR process is re-ranking. Participants have explored different re-ranking strategies. Multi-methods fusion is the most widely implemented one [8–11, 15, 16, 18, 20–22, 24]. It combines the ranked list of documents obtained from each aspect or each matching model to produce a single ranked list of documents relevant to the topic, Reciprocal Rank Fusion [27] (RRF) and Generalized Document Scoring [28] (GDS) have been used as merging algorithms. Usually, participants also develop heuristic rules to filter out irrelevant documents. For example, Wang et al. [21] filtered the results based on the demographic information in the term-based representation, while Mahmood et al. set the rule that articles with target genes and diseases more frequent in title or conclusions sections of retrieved documents, received higher ranking [20].

In addition to systems participated in TREC 2017 Precision Medicine Track, other studies paid attention to the precision medicine information retrieval. Nguyen et al. proposed to create a benchmark for clinical decision support search to compare different techniques of leading teams, enhancing the ability to build on previous work [29]. Previde et al. developed a web-based information retrieval, filtering, and visualization tool – GeneDive, facilitating efficient PMIR mainly in gene aspect [30]. Gonzalez-Hernandez et al. held a session during Pacific Symposium on Biocomputing 2018 to bring together researchers in text mining, bench scientists, and clinicians to collaborate and develop integrative approaches for precision medicine [31]. Balaneshin-kordan and Kotov proposed to optimize the weight of explicit and latent concepts in the query to improve the performance [32], while Wang, Zhang and Yuan introduced a tensor factorization based approach, which beat the best results of TREC CDS 2014 [33]. Although significance efforts have been devoted to PMIR, the performance is still far from satisfactory.

3 Research Questions and Design

We would like to design our PMIR system based on the literature review of previous PMIR techniques and the advances in information retrieval techniques. It seems promising that a combination of approved approaches with carefully selected new techniques could improve the performance of PMIR. In this study, we plan to investigate the effectiveness of such strategy. Specifically, we seek to answer the following research questions:

- RQ1: What information can be added to the document to enhance indexing for information retrieval?
- RQ2: Which query expansion strategy or query expansion strategy combinations can generate more effective queries?
- RQ3: Can supervised learning methods which involve the relevance judgement results in the past as training data in the re-ranking stage improve PMIR performance?

To answer these research questions, we design a PMIR framework, as depicted in Fig. 3. This framework follows the general steps described in Sect. 2. It can be divided into four basic modules: Data preprocessing and indexing, query construction and expansion, matching, and re-ranking. Each is described in more detail below.

Data Preprocessing and Indexing. In Fig. 3, the left part on the top describes the data preprocessing and indexing. Specifically, NLTK [34] will be used to clean data, Metamap Lite's NegEX [35] to detect and remove negated terms, MAUI [36] to extract keyphrases in the abstracts or background text, and Lucene was used to index the generated keywords together with the original metadata values of the abstracts.

Query Construction and Expansion. The right part on the top in Fig. 3 is about query construction and query expansion. The first step is negation detection and removing, as Nguyen et al. have confirmed the positive effect of negation detection [29]. Then the topics are divided into two aspects: disease aspect and gene aspect. We can ignore the demographic aspect and other aspect in the topic because scientific articles do not refer to the demographics or comorbidities of patients [24]. For query expansion, we can apply multiple methods, including knowledge-based method, word embeddings, and topic modeling and combine them with pseudo-relevance feedback. Expansion can be conducted on both disease aspect and gene aspect. Furthermore, to avoid query drift during query expansion, we can use term frequency merging to reweight expansion terms to reduce the impact of spurious expansion terms being over represented in the modified query [37].

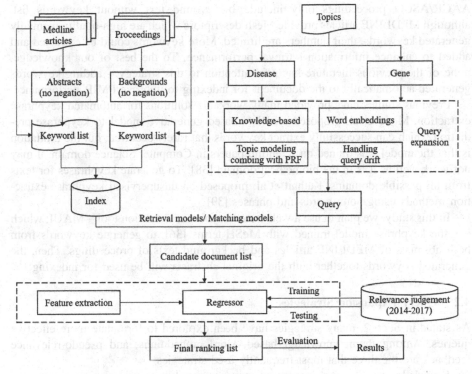

Fig. 3. The proposed framework

Matching. After the previous two steps, information retrieval models embedded in Lucene will be able to match the queries formulated against indexes of documents and output a list of ranked documents for each topic.

Re-ranking. This module evaluates the list of retrieved documents to make sure that relevant ones are ranked on the top of the list for each topic. In our framework, we will explore a supervised regression analysis method which takes previous relevance judgement results as training and validation data. A model that can predict the scores of the documents in the candidate list will be trained using a neural network.

To summarize, we will investigate three new techniques to improve PMIR system performance, including: keyphrase extraction for indexing, hybrid query expansion strategies including word embeddings, and re-ranking with supervised regression analysis. Next section will discuss how the three techniques should be used.

4 The Proposed Techniques

4.1 Keyphrase Extraction for Indexing

Keywords or keyphrases provide a concise representation of the topical content of a document, which can improve the efficiency of information retrieval [38]. However,

AACR/ASCO proceedings only include background text without keywords list, although MEDLINE articles provide Mesh descriptors which are high-quality manually generated keywords, their numbers are limited. More keywords could be extracted and added to enhance information retrieval performance. To the best of our knowledge, none of the previous literature has paid attention to this strategy – adding keywords generated automatically to the document for indexing to improve PMIR performance.

Previous studies have provided many workable solutions for automated keyphrase extraction. Meng et al. proposed an RNN-based generative model to keyphrase prediction which can successfully extract keywords that rarely occurred, but the limitation is that the model was trained on scientific papers in Computer Science domain, it may not work well as it is in the biomedical domain [38]. To generate keyphrases for texts from all possible domains, Kathait et al. proposed an unsupervised keyphrase extraction methods using noun words and phrases [39].

In this study, we plan to use a well-tested keyphrase extraction tool – MAUI, which has the keyphrase model trained with MeSH terms [36], to generate keywords from both abstracts of MEDLINE articles and background texts of proceedings. Then, the generated keywords together with the original abstracts will be used for indexing.

4.2   Query Expansion Strategies

As stated in Sect. 2, many strategies have been explored to formulate more effective queries. Among them, knowledge-based, word embeddings, and pseudo-relevance feedback are the three that most frequently used strategies.

Knowledge-based query expansion strategies apply various synonyms extracted from external resources to enrich the query. Table 2 summarizes the common external resources used in disease aspect query expansion and genetic aspect query expansion respectively by TREC 2017 Precision Medicine Track participants.

Table 2. External resources for knowledge-based query expansion

	External resource	Description
Disease aspect	NCI thesaurus	It contains information for nearly 10,000 cancer and related diseases
	Mesh dictionary	It is the NLM controlled vocabulary thesaurus used for indexing articles for PubMed
	Disease Ontology	It semantically integrates disease and medical vocabularies through extensive cross mapping of DO terms to MeSH, ICD, NCI's thesaurus, SNOMED and OMIM
Genetic aspect	UniProtKB	It contains high-quality synonyms for both protein and gene names
	dbSNP	It is a public repository for genetic variation
	NeXtProt	It is a human protein-centric knowledgebase

Word embeddings is a state-of-the-art technique which captures semantic similarities between words (cosine similarities between their high dimension vectors) that are not visible on the surface [40]. The synonyms of a word can be easily captured based on a well-trained embeddings. As suggested by Nguyen et al., word embeddings in precision medicine could be created by a combination of Wikipedia and Medline abstracts using Gensim [29].

Pseudo-relevance feedback-based query expansion is based on the assumption that the top N documents in the initial retrieval results are a good feedback of the query [19]. Thus, the keyphrases extracted from these documents can be treated as supplementations of the original query. In this study, we will use topic modelling to train the topic distribution for each query based on the top 10 pseudo-relevance feedback documents.

However, query expansion may lead to query drift, especially the pseudo-relevance feedback-based method, as the top 10 documents can include many irrelevant terms to the original query [37]. For example, the query expansion results based on pseudo-relevance feedback of the 10th topic (disease: Lung adenocarcinoma, gene: KRAS/G12C) of TREC 2017 precision medicine track are shown in Table 3. Obviously, among the expansion terms with pseudo-relevance feedback, *"pancreatic carcinoma" and "BRAF"* are not related to the original query terms, which may negatively affect IR performance. Therefore, to reduce the negative influence, we will merge the term frequencies with the original query term instead of directly add the expansion terms to the query term list. Low-frequency terms will be filtered out when formulating the final query.

Table 3. Query expansion results of the 10th topic of TREC-17-PM

Original terms	Some expansion terms
Lung adenocarcinoma	Pulmonary adenocarcinoma, non-small cell lung cancers, NSCLC, *pancreatic carcinoma*
KRAS (G12C)	GTPase, p21, C-Raf, RALGDS, *BRAF*

4.3 Re-Ranking with Supervised Regression Analysis

Recently, supervised learning methods have been proven effective with enough high-quality training data [41]. Fortunately, TREC precision medicine track provides this dataset (2017 PM labelled data and 2014-2016 CDS labelled data). Moreover, since the ranking process involves scoring the candidate documents based on their relevance to the query, which inspires us to conduct a regression analysis. By using supervised regression analysis to re-rank the candidate document list, we can balance the model complexity, the labelled data size, and the prior knowledge to achieve maybe better results through a unified model.

Two modules can be considered at this stage: the feature extraction module and the regression analysis module. Basically, the complexity of features depends on how much prior knowledge we can obtain from the training data. Our statistics show that nearly 100,000 labelled abstracts or background texts in the past four years that can be used as training data. Therefore, we will use a simpler feature set (such as tf-idf) but a more complicated regression analysis model (such as neural network) to avoid the bias of the model [42].

Given an input query q and a candidate document list $\mathbf{D} = \{d_1, d_2, \ldots, d_n\}$, the feature extraction module will generate a set of features $\mathbf{F} = \left\{ \vec{f_1}, \vec{f_2}, \ldots, \vec{f_n} \right\}$ based on $\{d_1, d_2, \ldots, d_n, d\}$, the goal is to calculate the score of each candidate document $\mathbf{S} = \{s_1, s_2, \ldots, s_n\}$, with linear regression analysis, $s = \vec{f} . \vec{w} = w_0 + w_1 f_1 + w_2 f_2 + \ldots + w_l f_l$, neural network analysis in each layer can be indicated as $y = \sigma(\vec{x} . \vec{w})$. Based on the training data: $\vec{t} = \{q, d_1, s_1, d_2, s_2, \ldots, d_n, s_n\}$, $\mathbf{T} = \left\{ \vec{t_1}, \vec{t_2}, \ldots, \vec{t_n} \right\}$, N represents the labelled query number, we will come up will a model predicting the score of each document in the candidate list of a coming query, and final ranked list is generated based on the score of each document. The final ranked list will be evaluated by the measurement of infNDCG, R-prec, P@10, which are widely used in the IR community.

5 Summary and Future Work

This paper presents a novel framework for conducting PMIR based on our analysis of participating systems of TREC 2017 Precision Medicine (PM) Track and latest literature of IR and data mining. We propose three promising techniques that may boost PMIR system performance: Keyphrase extraction for indexing, hybrid query expansion including word embeddings, and retrieval results re-ranking with supervised regression analysis for PMIR. Our next step will be implementing these techniques in our PMIR system and test it with TREC 2017 PM track test collection. The research will inform IR community the applicability of these techniques and help the community to develop effective solutions to precision medicine information retrieval.

References

1. TREC Precision Medicine/Clinical Decision Support Track. http://www.trec-cds.org/2017. html. Accessed 09 Apr 2018
2. Roberts, K., et al.: Overview of the TREC 2017 precision medicine track. In: TREC, Gaithersburg, MD (2017)
3. Collins, F.S., Varmus, H.: A new initiative on precision medicine. N. Engl. J. Med. **372**(9), 793–795 (2015)
4. Frey, L.J., Bernstam, E.V., Denny, J.C.: Precision medicine informatics. J. Am. Med. Inform. Assoc. **23**(4), 668–670 (2016)
5. Aronson, S.J., Rehm, H.L.: Building the foundation for genomics in precision medicine. Nature **526**(7573), 336–342 (2015)
6. National Research Council: Toward precision medicine: building a knowledge network for biomedical research and a new taxonomy of disease. National Academies Press, Washington DC (2011)

7. The Twenty-Sixth Text REtrieval Conference (TREC 2017) Proceedings. https://trec.nist. gov/pubs/trec26/trec2017.html. Accessed 09 Apr 2018
8. Paschea, E., et al. Customizing a variant annotation-support tool: an inquiry into probability ranking principles for TREC precision medicine. In: TREC, Gaithersburg, MD (2017)
9. Jo, S.H., Lee, K.S.: CBNU at TREC 2017 precision medicine track. In: TREC, Gaithersburg, MD (2017)
10. Nguyen, V., Karimi, S., Falamaki, S., Molla-Aliod, D., Paris, C., Wan, S.: CSIRO at 2017 TREC precision medicine track. In: TREC, Gaithersburg, MD (2017)
11. Foroutan Eghlidi, N., Griner, J., Mesot, N., von Werra, L., Eickhoff, C.: ETH Zurich at TREC precision medicine 2017. In: TREC, Gaithersburg, MD (2017)
12. Wu, J., Ma, X., Fan, W.: HokieGo at 2017 PM task: genetic programming based re-ranking method in biomedical information retrieval. In: TREC, Gaithersburg, MD (2017)
13. García, P.L., Oleynik, M., Kasáč, Z., Schulz, S.: TREC 2017 precision medicine - medical university of Graz. In: TREC, Gaithersburg, MD (2017)
14. Wang, Y., Komandur-Elayavilli, R., Rastegar-Mojarad, M., Liu, H.: Leveraging both structured and unstructured data for precision information retrieval. In: TREC, Gaithersburg, MD (2017)
15. Yin, T., Wu, D.T., Vydiswaran, V.V.: Retrieving documents based on gene name variations: MedIER at TREC 2017 precision medicine track. In: TREC, Gaithersburg, MD (2017)
16. Przybyla, P., Soto, A.J., Ananiadou, S.: Identifying personalised treatments and clinical trials for precision medicine using semantic search with thalia. In: TREC, Gaithersburg, MD (2017)
17. Cieślewicz, A., Dutkiewicz, J., Jędrzejek, C.: POZNAN contribution to TREC PM 2017. In: TREC, Gaithersburg, MD (2017)
18. Ling, Y., et al.: A hybrid approach to precision medicine-related biomedical article retrieval and clinical trial matching. In: TREC, Gaithersburg, MD (2017)
19. Li, C., He, B., Sun, Y., Xu, J.: UCAS at TREC-2017 precision medicine track. In: TREC, Gaithersburg, MD (2017)
20. Mahmood, A.A., et al.: UD_GU_BioTM at TREC 2017: precision medicine track. In: TREC, Gaithersburg, MD (2017)
21. Wang, Y., Fang, H.: Combining term-based and concept-based representation for clinical retrieval. In: TREC, Gaithersburg, MD (2017)
22. Noh, J., Kavuluru, R.: Team UKNLP at TREC 2017 precision medicine track: a knowledge-based IR system with tuned query-time boosting. In: TREC, Gaithersburg, MD (2017)
23. Viswavarapu, L.K., Chen, J., Cleveland, A., Chen, H.: UNT precision medicine information retrieval at TREC 2017. In: TREC, Gaithersburg, MD (2017)
24. Goodwin, T.R., Skinner, M.A., Harabagiu, S.M.: UTD HLTRI at TREC 2017: precision medicine track. In: TREC, Gaithersburg, MD (2017)
25. Azzopardi, L., et al.: The lucene for information access and retrieval research (LIARR) workshop at SIGIR 2017. In: Proceedings of the 40th International ACM SIGIR Conference on Research and Development in Information Retrieval, Shinjuku, Tokyo, Japan, pp. 1429–1430. ACM (2017)
26. Yang, P., Fang, H., Lin, J.: Anserini: enabling the use of lucene for information retrieval research. In: Proceedings of the 40th International ACM SIGIR Conference on Research and Development in Information Retrieval, Shinjuku, Tokyo, Japan, pp. 1253–1256. ACM (2017)
27. Cormack, G.V., Clarke, C.L., Buettcher, S.: Reciprocal rank fusion outperforms condorcet and individual rank learning methods. In: Proceedings of the 32nd International ACM SIGIR Conference on Research and Development in Information Retrieval, Boston, MA, USA, pp. 758–759. ACM (2009)

28. Li, P.V., Thomas, P., Hawking, D.: Merging algorithms for enterprise search. In: Proceedings of the 18th Australasian Document Computing Symposium, pp. 42–49. ACM, New York (2013)
29. Nguyen, V., Karimi, S., Falamaki, S., Paris, C.: Benchmarking clinical decision support search. arXiv preprint arXiv:1801.09322 (2018)
30. Previde, P., et al.: GeneDive: a gene interaction search and visualization tool to facilitate precision medicine. In: Proceedings of the Pacific Symposium on Biocomputing, pp. 590–601. World Scientific, Kohala Coast (2018)
31. Gonzalez-Hernandez, G., Sarker, A., O'Connor, K., Greene, C., Liu, H.: Advances in text mining and visualization for precision medicine. In: Proceedings of the Pacific Symposium on Biocomputing, pp. 590–601. World Scientific, Kohala Coast (2018)
32. Balaneshin-kordan, S., Kotov, A.: Optimization method for weighting explicit and latent concepts in clinical decision support queries. In: Proceedings of the 2016 ACM International Conference on the Theory of Information Retrieval, Newark, Delaware, USA, pp. 241–250. ACM (2016)
33. Wang, H., Zhang, Q., Yuan, J.: Semantically enhanced medical information retrieval system: a tensor factorization based approach. IEEE Access 5, 7584–7593 (2017)
34. Bird, S., Loper, E.: NLTK: the natural language toolkit. In: Proceedings of the ACL 2004 on Interactive poster and demonstration sessions, Barcelona, Spain. Association for Computational Linguistics (2004)
35. Demner-Fushman, D., Rogers, W.J., Aronson, A.R.: MetaMap Lite: an evaluation of a new Java implementation of MetaMap. J. Am. Med. Inform. Assoc. 24(4), 841–844 (2017)
36. Medelyan, O., Frank, E., Witten, I.H.: Human-competitive tagging using automatic keyphrase extraction. In: Proceedings of the 2009 Conference on Empirical Methods in Natural Language Processing, Singapore. Association for Computational Linguistics (2009)
37. Crimp, R., Trotman, A.: Automatic term reweighting for query expansion. In: Proceedings of the 22nd Australasian Document Computing Symposium, Brisbane, QLD, Australia. ACM (2017)
38. Meng, R., Zhao, S., Han, S., He, D., Brusilovsky, P., Chi, Y.: Deep keyphrase generation. arXiv preprint arXiv:1704.06879 (2017)
39. Kathait, S.S., Tiwari, S., Varshney, A., Sharma, A.: Unsupervised key-phrase extraction using noun phrases. Int. J. Comput. Appl. 162(1), 1–5 (2017)
40. Habibi, M., Weber, L., Neves, M., Wiegandt, D.L., Leser, U.: Deep learning with word embeddings improves biomedical named entity recognition. Bioinformatics 33(14), i37–i48 (2017)
41. Holzinger, A.: Interactive machine learning for health informatics: when do we need the human-in-the-loop? Brain Inform. 3(2), 119–131 (2016)
42. Allison, P.D.: Change scores as dependent variables in regression analysis. Sociol. Methodol. 20, 93–114 (1990)

Efficient Massive Medical Rules Parallel Processing Algorithms

Xin Li[1]([⊠]), Guigang Zhang[2], Chunxiao Xing[3,4,5,6], and Zihan Qu[7]

[1] Department of Rehabilitation, Beijing Tsinghua Changgung Hospital,
Beijing 100084, China
horsebackdancing@sina.com
[2] Institute of Automation, Chinese Academy of Sciences, Beijing 100190, China
[3] Research Institute of Information Technology, Beijing, China
[4] Beijing National Research Center for Information Science and Technology,
Beijing, China
[5] Department of Computer Science and Technology, Beijing, China
[6] Institute of Internet Industry, Tsinghua University, Beijing 100084, China
[7] Tinghua University High School, Beijing 100084, China

Abstract. Massive rules processing will play a very important role in the ad hoc computing. In this paper, we first give the massive KOA medical rules processing framework. We propose two kinds of massive rules processing algorithms: Massive Rules processing algorithm without and with external communication. In the Knee Osteoarthritis medical area, lots of rules can be set, our algorithms can be used to process rules set by all kinds of Knee Osteoarthritis rules systems.

Keywords: Knee Osteoarthritis (KOA) · Rules · Massive rules
Parallel processing · Algorithms

1 Introduction

With more and more applications such as the Internet of Things and the Internet of Things, more and more sequential big data streams continue to emerge. For example, timing big data flow from the Internet of Things (timing monitoring data sent from time to time when thousands of sensors of aircraft engines, etc.); various applications from the Internet (such as e-commerce trading sites) continue to conduct various transactions Generated timing data stream; various timing data streams from physiological and psychological monitoring of millions or even tens of millions of patients monitored from the wearable system in real time; behavioral time series of large data streams from various users of social networks. These temporal big data flows are rule trigger conditions that establish the dynamics of various decision support systems. For example, once the monitoring data of the aircraft engine changes, it is possible to trigger the rules of various failure modes so that it can be judged in a timely manner what kind of failure the aircraft has, how the engine maintenance personnel should take decision-making measures and so on.

However, the exits rule processing algorithm such as RETE [1], TREAT [2] and LEAPS [3] algorithms cannot process massive rules real time, especially when the rules

© Springer Nature Switzerland AG 2018
H. Chen et al. (Eds.): ICSH 2018, LNCS 10983, pp. 179–184, 2018.
https://doi.org/10.1007/978-3-030-03649-2_17

numbers arrive at millions. In order to overcome the shortcomings of RETE, TREAT and LEAPS algorithms, we developed these two massive rules processing algorithms in this paper.

The rest of this paper is arranged as follows, we begin with background and related work in Sect. 2. In Sect. 3, we give the massive KOA medical rules processing framework. In Sect. 4, we propose two kinds of dfficient massive KOA medical rules parallel processing algorithms. We conclude this paper and give the future work in Sect. 5.

2 Related Work

The core of rule processing system is the rule processing algorithm. The traditional rule processing algorithms have RETE, TREAT and LEAPS and later RETE2 [4]. The most famous rule processing algorithm is RETE algorithm. This algorithm is designed by Charles L. Forgy, a student of CMU. RETE algorithm is very effective in the expert system [5–7]. Almost of rule engines tools use the RETE as their processing algorithms [8–10] such as the Drools, ILOG and HAL etc. This algorithm has gained a very big successful.

The study of rules processing theory and algorithms is basically toward the development of an active rule engine and the ability to handle big data in both directions. In order to improve the processing efficiency of the rule engine, the rule set is often used to perform rule optimization before processing. Sometimes faced with some complex event processing requirements, the rules after processing, the use of association rules and various effective algorithms for further rule mining and processing. For complex large-scale rule processing, especially when dealing with big data, the current research is mainly through pattern mining for complex rules, optimization of templates, optimization of rule processing processes using various machine learning algorithms, and automatic establishment of processing mechanisms. And use the parallel processing mechanism to complete.

The optimization of mass-rule rules is a very complex problem. Optimization here refers to finding the solution with the least time complexity or space complexity from the description of the semantic rules given by the user. However, the most natural language description is used to find out the most Even though excellent solutions are extremely difficult to see today, human understanding of things is hierarchical, and it is unrealistic to expect to automatically obtain deeper understanding from the language descriptions of shallow understanding of things. The more feasible approach is to capture features from the problem description, and then select the most appropriate one from the first defined optimal solution based on the problem features. Therefore, the optimization task is how to let the system automatically choose the best solution to solve the user's problem. One possible solution is similar to the object-oriented method overloading. That is, storing the universal abstract solution into the system in advance and then describing the problem. The input conditions given by the user are used to judge which solution the system should use to solve, and different input conditions correspond to different solving methods. Therefore, in order to achieve this goal, we must design a not only semantic richer rule description language, but also need to design a rule description language with semantic optimization performance and a corresponding solution rule model.

3 Massive KOA Medical Rules Processing Framework

Once the number of massive KOA medical rules reaches a mass scale of tens or even hundreds of millions, the requirements for the processing technology of rules will become higher and higher. How to make so many rules can be processed in time is that all users are also rules Executive engine designers are most concerned with the issue. At this point, how to optimize a rule network to improve the processing efficiency of the rule network has become increasingly important. The framework adopts a rule network optimization method based on rule consolidation and its equivalent replacement based on rules modules. The architecture design tries to merge the duplicate rule nodes in different rules to achieve the goal of rule consolidation or partial consolidation. At the same time, the rule module that calculates the function is replaced by the rules module that calculates the cost, and the rule that has high computational cost is replaced by the rule module with low computation cost. Modules to achieve the purpose of regular module optimization (Fig. 1).

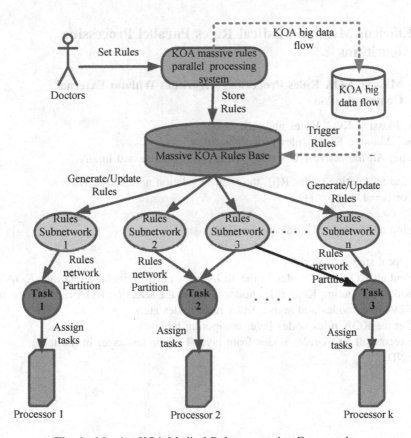

Fig. 1. Massive KOA Medical Rules processing Framework

The massive KOA medical rules processing framework, based on the analysis of existing various rule processing algorithms, addresses the defects of existing rule processing algorithms, and tries to adopt a mass-rule rule pattern matching model suitable for massive rule processing. Through this matching model, Quickly find the various rules that need to be processed and put them into the execution plan. When the rules are executed, the execution of mass rules can be implemented quickly and efficiently according to the massive rules runtime execution method of the massive KOA medical rules framework.

The last architecture uses a massive rule parallel processing mechanism. Mainly include: The rules of the mass to generate independent rules subnet method. Task preallocation method. Study the rational division method of subnets. The balanced segmentation method, the equilibrium-dependent minimum-cost segmentation algorithm, and the balance dependence cost and the minimum communication cost segmentation algorithm are proposed. Regular subnet internal communications and external communications between processors. Map the task specifically to the corresponding handler's methods, and so on.

4   Efficient Massive Medical Rules Parallel Processing Algorithms

4.1   Massive KOA Rules Processing Algorithm Without External Communication

Input: Massive KOA Rules network.
Output: Massive KOA Rules processing plan.
Assume: All the active KOA rules nodes will be processed finally.

1 Find all relation nodes R[i], the total of relation nodes have r.
2 For (i = 1, i <= r; i++)
3 {
4 Find all the layer 1's rule nodes R[i]
5 }
6 Repeat step 2 to step 5
7 Find all KOA rules nodes in the KOA rules network include relations KOA rules nodes, computing KOA rules nodes (such as the selection KOA rules nodes, union KOA rules nodes and active KOA rules nodes etc.)
8 Get the KOA rules nodes layer computing table
9 Execute all KOA rules nodes from layer 1 to the last layer in the table.
10 END.

4.2   Massive KOA Rules Processing Algorithm with External Communication

Input: KOA Rules network.
Output: Massive KOA rules processing plan.
Assume: All the active KOA rules nodes will be processed finally.

The step 1 to the step 8 is the same with the massive KOA rules processing algorithm without external communication.

1   Find all relation KOA rules nodes R[i], the total of relation KOA rules nodes have r.
2   For (i = 1, i <= r; i++)
3   {
4   Find all the layer 1's KOA rules nodes R[i]
5   }
6   Repeat step 2 to step 5
7   Find all KOA rules nodes in the KOA rules network include relations KOA rules nodes, computing KOA rules nodes (such as the selection KOA rules nodes, union KOA rules nodes and active KOA rules nodes etc.)
8   Get the KOA rules nodes layer computing table 1

The following is the key steps which are used to reduce the external communication cost.

9   Find these KOA rules nodes which need to communicate with the other processors.
10   Find all these step 9's rule nodes' former KOA rules nodes
11   Move the step 9's all KOA rules nodes in the front of the table.
12   Move the step 10's all KOA rules nodes in the front of the table.
13   Execute all KOA rules nodes from layer1 to the last layer in another table
14   END.

5   Conclusion and Future Work

In this paper, we give the massive KOA medical rules processing framework firstly. Then, we propose two kinds of massive KOA medical rules processing algorithms. We will use these two kinds of algorithms into the Knee Osteoarthritis (KOA) medical application systems in the future.

Acknowledgment. This work was supported by NSFC (91646202), Research/Project 2017YB142 supported by Ministry of Education of The People's Republic of China, the 1000-Talent program.

References

1. Forgy, C.L.: Rete a fast algorithm for the many pattern/many object pattern match problem. Artif. Intell. **19**, 17–37 (1982)
2. Mirankerm, D.P.: TREAT: a better match algorithm for AI production systems. In: Proceedings of AAAI 87 Conference on Artificial Intelligence, pp. 42–47, August 1987
3. Cheng, A.M.K., Fujii, S.: Self-stabilizing real-time OPS5 production systems. IEEE Trans. Knowl. Data Eng. **16**(12), 1543–1554 (2004)
4. Rete II (2018). http://www.pst.com/rete2.htm
5. Cadonna, B., Gamper, J., Böhlen, M.: Sequenced event set pattern matching. In: Proceeding of EDBT2011. 22–24 March, Uppsala, Sweden, pp. 33–44 (2011)
6. Wang, P., Wang, H., Liu, M., Wang, W.: An algorithmic approach to event summarization. In: Proceeding of SIGMOD, pp. 183–194 (2010)
7. Marcus, A., Bernstein, M.S., Badar, O., Karger, D.R., Madden, S., Miller, R.C.: Tweets as data: demonstration of TweeQL and Twitinfo. In: Proceeding of SIGMOD, pp. 1259–1262 (2011)
8. Sheykh Esmaili, K., Sanamrad, T., Fischer, P.M., Tatbul, N.: Changing flights in mid-air: a model for safely modifying continuous queries. In: Proceeding of SIGMOD, pp. 613–624 (2011)
9. Gordin, D.N., Pasik, A.J.: Set-oriented constructs: from rete rule bases to database systems. In: Proceedings of the 1991 ACM SIGMOD International Conference on Management of Data, p. 60 (1991)
10. Gaudiot, J.-L., Sohn, A.: Data-driven parallel production systems. IEEE Trans. Softw. Eng. **16**(3), 281–293 (1990)

Intelligent Diagnosis and Treatment Research of Knee Osteoarthritis Based on Big Data

Xin Li[1(✉)], Guigang Zhang[2], Chunxiao Xing[3,4,5,6], and Yong Zhang[3,4,5,6]

[1] Department of Rehabilitation, Beijing Tsinghua Changgung Hospital, Beijing 100084, China
horsebackdancing@sina.com
[2] Institute of Automation, Chinese Academy of Sciences, Beijing 100190, China
[3] Research Institute of Information Technology, Beijing, China
[4] Beijing National Research Center for Information Science and Technology, Beijing, China
[5] Department of Computer Science and Technology, Beijing, China
[6] Institute of Internet Industry, Tsinghua University, Beijing 100084, China

Abstract. Knee Osteoarthritis (KOA) is a common and frequently-occurring chronic disease. The traditional KOA diagnosis lacks personalized and systematic diagnosis and treatment models, and lacks high-quality and large-sample randomized controlled clinical studies. In this paper, we propose a kind of intelligent diagnosis and treatment method for KOA based on big data and artificial intelligence.

Keywords: Knee osteoarthritis (KOA) · Big data · Artificial intelligence

1 Introduction

Knee osteoarthritis is a common, multiple, disabling, and costly chronic degenerative disease. Incidence of the disease is relatively hidden. Grass-roots medical personnel have insufficient awareness of osteoarthritis prevention and control. They are easily overlooked in the early and middle stages of the disease. Due to the lack of continuous observation and effective treatment of diseases, many patients suffer from disease progression and lead to severe disability; Patients with knee osteoarthritis need joint replacement surgery, which greatly increases the patient's pain and financial burden. At present, there are many methods for the treatment of knee osteoarthritis at home and abroad. Due to the lack of a unified and clear treatment path guidance, patients can not get standardized assessment, diagnosis and treatment, rehabilitation and management when they are treated by doctors of different disciplines or professions. It is the conservative treatment of patients with a large number of diseases in the early and middle stages, and lost the best time for treatment.

In the Sect. 2, we will do some reviews for the related work. And we will introduce the architecture of intelligent diagnosis and treatment research for knee Osteoarthritis based on big data in Sect. 3. In Sects. 4,5,6 and 7, we will have some descriptions for the detail of each part of the architecture.

H. Chen et al. (Eds.): ICSH 2018, LNCS 10983, pp. 185–190, 2018.
https://doi.org/10.1007/978-3-030-03649-2_18

2   Related Work

In decision support systems, the effective handling of rules is crucial. In the processing of rules, the rules engine plays an indispensable role. The rule engine [1] includes three stages in making fact judgments: matching, selecting, and executing. Traditional rule pattern matching processing algorithms are most typical with RETE [2], TREAT [3], LEAPS, and RETE2.

In recent years, studies on dynamic assisted examinations have focused on the relationship between knee OA prognostic scores and biomechanical gait parameters. Gait analysis and predicting models can effectively identify individuals at high risk of knee joint OA screening and are cost-effective. Evaluation of Osteoarthritis Methods [4]. In a multicenter cross-sectional study in Japan, changes in forefoot function were closely related to the onset and progression of knee osteoarthritis [5].

Currently, in the KOA classification, the mainstream deep learning algorithm is a convolutional neural network (CNN). Joseph Antony used a 128-layer convolutional neural network, VGG, to classify KOA. The accuracy of KOA classification for normal X-ray pictures KL = 1, 2, and 3 was 64.7%, 77.6%, and 92.9%, respectively. Later, Antony made further improvements on this basis, which improved the accuracy by about 30% over the Wndchrm method and improved the speed of operation. In addition to mainstream CNN, Luca Minciullo also made improvements to traditional machine learning algorithms to improve the accuracy of the KOA classification, with an AUC of 0.88. In addition to the influence on the choice of algorithm, Antony pointed out that the diversity of data is also conducive to the improvement of model performance: Compared to the model of single database training, the model that is trained by combining the data of the above two databases can obtain higher accuracy.

Knowledge maps originated from the Google Knowledge Graph and are essentially a semantic network. The node represents the entity (Entity) or concept (Concept), and the edge represents various semantic relationships between entities/concepts.

At present, the entity sets of internationally famous knowledge maps are generally constructed based on existing term sets, encyclopedias, and other established and regular data sets. The entity sets such as YAGO [6] and DBpedia [7] are directly derived from Wikipedia. Using existing authoritative data sets to construct the entity set of the knowledge map, a more reliable set of entities can be obtained. However, for a specific field, the coverage of existing dataset entities is still insufficient, and the granularity of entities is also coarser and less satisfactory than the target. On the other hand, existing mature data sets may miss some less popular long-tailed words and new terminology nouns that have emerged in recent years because of the relationship between version updates and insufficient human resources. Therefore, knowledge maps such as NELL [8] and UMLS [9] also attempt to use natural language processing techniques to extract new entities from the text data of the Internet and continue to iterate to improve the knowledge map.

Traditional data fusion is to map multi-source heterogeneous data to a unified data model. There are many mature methods and systems. The focus of this project is to study data fusion in knowledge maps. The data fusion of knowledge map refers to how to construct a complete knowledge map after acquiring the entity and entity relationships in the knowledge map. What is mainly involved in the medical and health field is the disambiguation of the relationship between entities and entities.

There are many words or entities in natural language that have multiple meanings. The purpose of disambiguation algorithm is to distinguish the meaning of these words or entities in the specific context. The most direct basis for disambiguation is the context, but traditional disambiguation methods use the Bag of Words model to represent contexts, ignoring the semantic relationships between context words, ambiguous words and context. Using the knowledge base, this problem can be solved to some extent. At present, knowledge bases such as WordNet and Wikipedia are often used to disambiguate. In contrast, the advantage of Wikipedia lies in the large scale, but the disadvantage is less stringent than WordNet.

3 Architecture

As shown in Fig. 1, our research architecture will be divided into five areas for research: a big data computing platform that supports KOA's smart health management decisions, KOA's health knowledge maps and data fusion, KOA's health data's semantic analysis and knowledge discovery, and Process KOA smart health management decision model and rules, KOA intelligent diagnosis, treatment, rehabilitation and prediction system based on big data analysis.

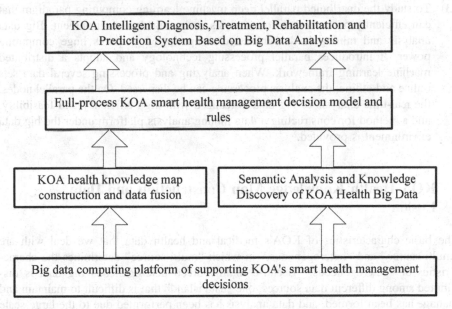

Fig. 1. Architecture of intelligent diagnosis and treatment research for knee osteoarthritis based on big data

4 Big Data Computing Platform of Supporting KOA's Smart Health Management Decisions

Faced with pre-hospital, intra-hospital and post-hospital multi-source and heterogeneous KOA health data, one urgent problem to be solved is how to construct a big data computing platform to effectively manage it, so that data can be efficiently retrieved and applied, and Further in-depth analysis and processing of large-scale linked data, mining multi-dimensional intrinsic knowledge to support smart health decisions. The research content of the computing platform is as follows:

(1) Build an open KOA health big data computing platform that supports decision analysis services. Use the existing cloud platform construction technology to build a lightweight cloud platform, and build a distributed cluster with parallel computing capabilities on this platform to support the complex analysis and processing of health data, and implement scalable high-performance big data storage and query.

(2) Research on management methods for KOA smart health big data in the cloud environment. KOA health data has significant multi-source and heterogeneous characteristics. The management of structured data, semi-structured data, and unstructured data across the entire platform must take into account the diversity of data storage, the operability of data interaction, and data. Perceived dynamic changes and data security and reliability.

(3) To study the distributed parallel deep machine learning computing paradigm that can efficiently perform decision analysis under big data environment. Big data analysis and mining is data-intensive computing. It requires huge computing power. It introduces parallel processing technology and adopts a distributed machine learning framework. When analyzing and processing several data sets online and offline, the analysis processing can be dispersed. On the parallel nodes, the real-time analysis of big data is realized with high efficiency and feasibility, and a method for constructing a data mining analysis platform under the big data environment is provided.

5 KOA Health Knowledge Map Construction and Data Fusion

The basic characteristics of KOA's medical and health data that we deal with are "multi-source" and "heterogeneous," in which "multi-source" determines the characteristics of "heterogeneous." Because multi-sourced heterogeneous big data is distributed among different data sources, one "data island" that is difficult to maintain and manage has been formed, and data analysis has been performed due to the large-scale data, various types, high speed, and high timeliness. Excavation cannot be carried out using traditional methods, and the knowledge contained in the data is difficult to extract effectively. Specifically, the health knowledge map we have constructed is composed of different data sources through data fusion. The diversity of data sources determines that the data sources themselves have different structures. For example, some data exist in the form of a relational table. For example, the ICD-10 data in a case contains a rich subtype relationship of the disease, and the Internet inquiry data is a document and so on.

6 Semantic Analysis and Knowledge Discovery of KOA Health Big Data

Traditional health big data modeling, using patient event sequences, clinical feature-time matrix methods, etc., does not directly utilize medical knowledge accumulated over many years. This project is based on KOA's health knowledge maps, performs semantic analysis of case health data, uses knowledge of diseases and medical fields, and conducts in-depth knowledge discovery of patient case health data. In this paper, the KOA health knowledge map constructed from multi-source heterogeneous KOA disease health data was integrated as a hidden knowledge to perform semantic analysis on case health data and a case-concept heterogeneous information network was established. With this heterogeneous information network as an auxiliary monitoring information, knowledge discovery of patient case health data is performed, and the effect of scientific problems such as classification, clustering, and similarity measurement based on patient cases is improved.

7 Full-Process KOA Smart Health Management Decision Model and Rules

It mainly includes the following three aspects:

(1) Research on a model library for the whole process KOA smart health management decision.

In the KOA smart health management, the relevant medical health decision models are various, so it is necessary to study an extensible system to effectively manage these models. We use the basic idea of the service component library in software engineering to build a model library that is oriented to the whole process KOA smart health management decision. It defines the basic principles and processes that need to be followed when a new decision model is added to the model library, including the description of the model and how to call it. According to the granularity, we divide the model into atomic model and combined model. For the combined model, we will study the combination of models. These models should follow the characteristics of high cohesion, weak coupling, easy combination, high efficiency of operation and convenience of invocation.

(2) Research on expression and generation of semantic rules for decision-making of full-process KOA smart health management.

A prerequisite for the management decision model to be able to effectively provide decision services is the need for a set of rules to handle the system. This section examines the expression of semantic rules and the generation of semantic rules for the full-process KOA smart health management decision. In order to enhance the flexibility of the rules, a kind of natural language-based regular expression method (satisfying IF (NLP: natural language-like) THEN (NLP: NLP-like natural language) mode) and establishing various rule nodes for generating various semantics rule.

(3) Research on the Generation, Optimization and Processing of Semantic Rule Networks for Decision-making KOA Smart Health Management.
Complex decision-making for full-process KOA smart health management requires many atomic semantic rule services to be combined, and these service combinations are accompanied by the generation of a regular network. This section mainly studies the semantic rule network generation method, the semantic rule network optimization and processing methods (rule merging, rule integration, rule conflict resolution, etc.).

Acknowledgment. This work was supported by NSFC (91646202), Research/Project 2017YB142 supported by Ministry of Education of The People's Republic of China, the 1000-Talent program.

References

1. Bhargavi, R., Pathak, R., Vaidehi, V.: Dynamic complex event processing — adaptive rule engine. In: International Conference on Recent Trends in Information Technology (ICRTIT), pp. 189–194 (2013)
2. Forgy, C.L.: RETE: a fast algorithm for the many pattern/many object pattern match problem. Artif. Intell. **19**, 17–37 (1982)
3. Miranker, D.P.: TREAT: a better match algorithm for AI production systems. In: proceedings of AAAI 87 Conference on Artificial Intelligence, pp. 42–47 August 1987
4. Long, M.J., Papi, E., Duffell, L.D., McGregor, A.H.: Predicting knee osteoarthritis risk in injured populations. Clin. Biomech. (Bristol, Avon) **47**, 87–95 (2017)
5. Uritani, D., Fukumoto, T., Myodo, T., Fujikawa, K., Usui, M., Tatara, D.: The association between toe grip strength and osteoarthritis of the knee in Japanese women: a multicenter cross-sectional study. PLoS ONE **12**(10), e0186454 (2017)
6. Hoffart, J., Suchanek, F.M., Berberich, K., et al.: YAGO2: exploring and querying world knowledge in time, space, context, and many languages. In: International Conference on World Wide Web, WWW, Hyderabad, India, 28 March–April, pp. 229–232 (2011)
7. Auer, S., Bizer, C., Kobilarov, G., Lehmann, J., Cyganiak, R., Ives, Z.: DBpedia: a nucleus for a web of open data. In: Aberer, K., et al. (eds.) ASWC/ISWC -2007. LNCS, vol. 4825, pp. 722–735. Springer, Heidelberg (2007). https://doi.org/10.1007/978-3-540-76298-0_52
8. Carlson, A., Betteridge, J., Wang, R.C., et al.: Coupled semi-supervised learning for information extraction. In: ACM International Conference on Web Search & Data Mining, pp. 101–110. ACM (2010)
9. Bodenreider, O.: The unified medical language system (UMLS): integrating biomedical terminology. Nucleic Acids Res. **32**(Database issue), D267–D270 (2004)

Use of Sentiment Mining and Online NMF for Topic Modeling Through the Analysis of Patients Online Unstructured Comments

Adnan Muhammad Shah$^{(\boxtimes)}$, Xiangbin Yan, Syed Jamal Shah,
and Salim Khan

School of Management, Harbin Institute of Technology,
Harbin, People's Republic of China
adnanshah486@gmail.com

Abstract. Patients have posted thousands of online reviews to assess their doctors' performance. Mechanisms to collect unstructured feedback from patients of healthcare providers have become very common, but there are scarce researches on different analysis techniques to examine such feedback have not frequently been applied in this context. We apply text mining techniques to compare online physician reviews from RateMDs and Healthgrades, to measure the systematic similarities and differences in patient reviews between these two platforms. We use sentiment analysis techniques to categorize online patients' reviews as either positive or negative descriptions of their health care. We apply a customized text mining technique, ONMF topic modeling to identify the major topics on two platforms. Our text mining techniques revealed research area on how to use big data and text mining techniques to help health care providers, and organizations hear patient voices to improve the health service quality.

Keywords: Text mining · Sentiment analysis · Topic modeling
Physician reviews

1 Introduction

Recently, online physician reviews have become very important for patients in every country. A recent survey established that around 72% of web users had used internet for seeking health information in the past years, and out of every five one doctor has been rated and reviewed on physician-rating websites (PRWs) [1]. A survey on seven European countries indicated that, on average, more than 40% of people considered the information on web2.0 about of these eHealth services to be important when choosing a new physician. In Germany, 25% of survey respondents mentioned that they had used the Internet to search for a doctor. In Holland, out of one-third of the entire country population, searched for ratings of healthcare providers [2]. In the U.S., 19% of citizens consider online doctor ratings are "important" for them in deciding to choose a good doctor. All of these studies have analyzed that physician reviews have increasingly become popular and played a vital role among health consumers [3].

H. Chen et al. (Eds.): ICSH 2018, LNCS 10983, pp. 191–203, 2018.
https://doi.org/10.1007/978-3-030-03649-2_19

Health consumers are not only consuming online health information, but they are producing it as well in the form of ratings and textual reviews. This shift has generated a proliferation of patient-generated content, including online doctor reviews. It may be interesting to analyze large corpora of such reviews in consumer sentiment regarding their healthcare experiences [4]. PRWs also establish a new information platform for patients that can be used to compare patients' emotions and feelings about health care services across different channels, which can help both the physicians and organizations to improve their service delivery process [5]. RateMDs and Healthgrades etc. are few of the famous websites that allow patients to share their personal health experience with their doctors on a variety of medical aspects [1].

Qualitative analysis of online reviews can provide vital insights into the physician service quality, but it requires trained investigators to read and analyze text reviews [4]. While in previous studies data regarding customer perception of service quality have been collected via traditional approaches, e.g., survey or comment card, etc. [6]. However online customer feedback mechanisms have been incredibly gaining popularity in their purchase decision making. It has been suggested that online feedback mechanisms present a unique way to consider the technological delivery characteristics [7]. To further motivate this study, it is essential to explore the usability of PRWs. However, there are scarce researches that have made a direct comparison of online physician reviews across different platforms using machine learning approach. The present study intends to examine and compare online physician reviews from RateMDs and Healthgrades by addressing the following questions. First, what's the accuracy and precision of tones (sentiment) of patients' reviews from these two platforms about physician service quality? Second, what are the major topics among patients' reviews from these two platforms? Third, do these different classification algorithms accuracy and topics vary among both platforms? We utilize a machine learning classification algorithms that jointly captures sentiments; attribute terms and categories from online patients' comments. To detect the latent topics in the documents, we apply online nonnegative matrix factorization (ONMF) topic modeling algorithms.

To this end, our contributions in the study are as follows. First, we propose mechanisms to detect the sentiments in two platforms documents and then evaluate the performance of the proposed mechanism by using different machine learning classification algorithms. Second, we propose an efficient ONMF framework to detect, and elimination of latent topics in text streams. Third, we suggest the mechanism to find the similarities and differences between two platforms regarding machine learning algorithms performance and major topics. We organized our work as follows: Sect. 2 introduces the study related work. Section 3 describes the methodology and framework. Sections 4 and 5 discuss the experiments results, implications, and conclusions.

2   Related Work

There have been several studies concerning online reviews using machine learning approaches. Liu et al. [8] proposed a method on the basis of the sentiment analysis technique and the intuitionistic fuzzy set theory to rank the different products through online reviews. An algorithm was developed based on sentiment dictionaries to identify the positive, neutral or negative sentiments on the alternative products concerning the product's features in each review. Wallace et al. [4] analyzed a corpus comprising nearly 60, 000 online doctor reviews with a state-of-the-art probabilistic model of text. They presented a probabilistic generative model that captures latent sentiment across different aspects of care. Giatsoglou et al. [9] suggested a fast, flexible, generic methodology for sentiment detection out of textual snippets which express people's opinions in different languages. The proposed method took on a machine learning approach with which textual documents were represented by vectors, used for training a polarity classification model. Previous studies investigated how sentiment analysis (an artificial intelligence procedure that classifies opinions expressed within the text) can be used to design real-time satisfaction surveys. These studies predict, from free-text, a reasonably accurate assessment of patients' view about different performance aspects of physicians using machine learning classification algorithm [10, 11].

Regarding our second theme of study, Tu et al. [12] proposed an ONMF method. Unlike the existing online topic detecting methods, the generated topics in ONMF were organized in a hierarchical structure. Besides, the method can track the evolving process of the topic hierarchy, which was accomplished by adaptively adding emerging topics and removing fading topics. Klein et al. [13] applied a unique approach to study online conspiracy theorists who used NMF to create a topic model of authors' contributions to the main conspiracy forum on Reddit.com. They argued that within the forum, there are multiple sub-populations distinguishable by their loadings on different topics based on differences in users' background beliefs and motivations.

3 Methods and Data

This study focused solely on two PRWs, i.e. RateMDs.com and Healthgrades.com. RateMDs was founded in 2004 and was one of the first PRW in the U.S, while most other major competitors began rating services only after 2008. It has the largest number of user-submitted reviews with narratives by a large margin, based on the web traffic ranking website [14]. Patients submit textual reviews and ratings voluntarily on RateMDs, rather than online surveys [2]. We retrieved 422 physicians reviews consist of different disease risks specialties based on Centre for disease control & prevention.

Healthgrades is a U.S-based company that provides information about physicians and hospitals. Healthgrades has amassed information on more than 3 million U.S. physicians [15]. Patients can input their opinions in the online survey based on their

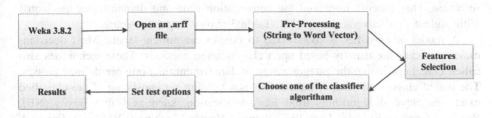

Fig. 1. Sentiment analysis framework: model building and sentiment prediction

experience with an individual physician, and view providers ratings at no charge. We scrapped 758 physician reviews of different disease specialties on Healthgrades.

3.1 Machine Learning from Unstructured Feedback

We applied data processing techniques to all the online free-text comments about physicians on the RateMDs and Healthgrades. Our purpose was to test whether we could automatically predict patients' views on a number of topics from their free-text responses. A machine learning classification approach was applied in which an algorithm convert patients comments into word vector format and then classify the comments into categories from a given set of examples, using open-source Weka 3.8 data mining software. Previous studies used it that provides accurate classification results, including in health care [11]. The algorithms in Weka were trained using all patients' comments and ratings about physicians left on the RateMDs from 2004–17 (5560 in a total of 422 physicians) and Healthgrades from 2010–17 (2916 in a total of 758 physicians) as a learning set. 70% and 30% reviews from both data sets were used as a train (labeled by experts) and test datasets to test the predicting accuracy of the model. We performed 5-fold cross-validation.

Pre-Processing and Classification through Machine Learning

There are two components of machine learning approach: (1) pre-processing, in which patients comments are split into string to word vector format to build a representation of the data [16], and (2) classification, that predicts categorical class labels and classifies data (constructs a model) based on the training set and the values (class labels) in a classifying attribute and uses it to classify unseen data. A consistent set of methodologies were applied in our machine learning process, including a "bag-of-words (BOW)" approach, "prior polarity", and "information gain" (Fig. 1).

In the "BOW", the total body of words analyzed (known as the corpora) is represented as an unordered collection of words [9]. For this analysis, unigrams (single elements or words) and bigrams (two adjacent elements in a string of tokens, a 2-word phrase) were used as the basic units of analysis. Higher n-grams (longer phrases) could have been used, but the constraints were computer power and processing time. We also included our classification of certain words in the machine learning approach, known as "prior polarity". The 850 most common single words and the 850 most common 2-word phrases were extracted from the complete set of comments in corpora. The "Information gain" technique was used to limit the number of uni-gram and bi-gram to 1300. Then reduce the size of the BOW by identifying words with the lowest certainty of belonging to a given class, and then removing them—an approach to feature selection. This process improved the computation time and demonstrates the words with highest predictive accuracy [11]. Table 3 shows Top 10 n-grams.

A model or classifier is constructed to predict categorical labels. Most decision-making models are usually based upon classification methods. These techniques also called classifiers enable the categorization of data (or entities) into pre-defined classes. The use of classification algorithms involves a training set consisting of pre-classified examples. Several algorithms used for classification, such as Naïve Bayes (NB), Random forest (RF), J.48, Lazy.IBK, Support Vector Machine (SVM), etc. For each method, the accuracy, precision, recall, the F measure, the Receiver Operating Characteristic (ROC) (graphical approach for displaying the tradeoff between true positive rate (TP) and false positive rate (FP) of a classifier), and the time taken to complete the task were calculated. To reduce computing processing time of the classification, we limited the words in the learning process to the top 100 words by frequency. All text was converted to lower case, and we removed all punctuation. Typographical errors and misspellings were not corrected.

$$Accuracy = \frac{TP + TN}{N} \tag{1}$$

$$Precesion = \frac{TP}{TP + FP} \tag{2}$$

$$Recall = \frac{TP}{TP + FN} \tag{3}$$

$$F - Measure = \frac{2 \times Precesion \times Recall}{Precesion + Recall} \tag{4}$$

FN, TN is False Negative, True Negative and N is the number of classified instances.

Table 1. A number of reviews and doctors by specialty areas.

	Specialty	Reviews	Reviews %	Doctors	Doctors %	Rev/Doc
1	Cardiologist	531	9.55	80	18.96	6.63
	Oncologist	704	12.66	21	4.98	33.52
	Neurologist	1141	20.53	130	30.80	8.78
	Orthopedics	577	10.38	34	8.06	16.97
	Pulmonologist	1349	24.27	84	19.91	16.06
	ENT	553	9.95	27	6.40	20.48
	Endocrinologist	319	5.74	25	5.92	12.76
	Nephrologist	386	6.94	21	4.98	18.38
2	Cardiologist	263	9.02	125	16.49	2.10
	Oncologist	277	9.50	98	12.93	2.83
	Neurologist	220	7.54	96	12.66	2.30
	Orthopedics	833	28.57	69	9.10	12.07
	Pulmonologist	268	9.19	97	12.80	2.76
	ENT	400	13.72	117	15.44	3.42
	Endocrinologist	308	10.56	100	13.19	3.08
	Nephrologist	347	11.90	56	7.39	6.20

RateMDs = 1, Healthgrades = 2

Table 2. Descriptive statistics of reviews length

RateMDs				Healthgrades		
Specialty	Average	Median	Max.len	Average	Median	Max.len
Cardiologist	57.3(3.1)	39(3)	575(20)	35.6(3.8)	39(4)	76(12)
Oncologist	66.4(2.6)	48(2)	890(20)	42.3(5.1)	48(5)	63(19)
Neurologist	77.1(3.3)	57(3)	758(23)	40.9(4.9)	48(5)	64(13)
Orthopedics	79.3(2.8)	63(2)	803(18)	46.7(4.4)	41(4)	106(18)
Pulmonologist	60.5(2.6)	44(2)	474(13)	39.2(4.6)	44.5(4.5)	63(17)
ENT	77.2(3.6)	56(3)	871(34)	36.3(4.2)	36(4)	1074(28)
Endocrinologist	68.4(2.3)	55(2)	485(9)	39.3(4.6)	46(4.5)	63(11)
Nephrologist	66.1(2.7)	46(2)	460(14)	27.1(2.9)	20(2)	108(16)

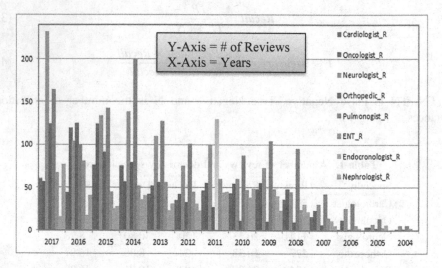

Fig. 2. Total number of reviews by specialty over time on RateMDs

3.2   Topic Modeling

Topic modeling is a refined text-mining technique used for our research work, i.e., understanding the U.S. health consumers by identifying topics on the RateMDs and Healthgrades platforms. Topic modeling is a statistical method to uncover abstract topics from a collection of documents. The Topic name is abstracted and summarized by researchers based on the most frequently appearing keywords in a review because computer algorithms can only detect the pattern of which keywords cluster statistically but cannot summarize what topic those keywords represent. Also, online reviews usually consist of a mixture of different topics [2]. Topic modeling can statistically capture those topics by using different algorithms. We used ONMF method for topic modeling to analyze the U.S. health consumers' reviews about their physicians by using the following method.

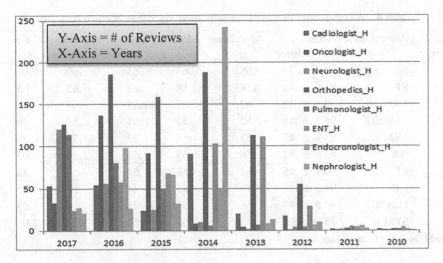

Fig. 3. Total number of reviews by specialty over time on Healthgrades

Table 3. The top 10 uni-gram or bi-gram phrases by information gain

Rate MDs		Healthgrades	
1. Wait	6. Fantastic	1. Rude and	6. Grateful
2. Am happy	7. Competent	2. Best	7. Expert
3. Helpful	8. Rude with	3. Worst	8. Professional
4. Wonderful	9. Pain in	4. Highly recommend	9. Listens
5. Pleasant	10. Impressed with	5. Appointment	10. Caring

In vector space model, a corpus of reviews is represented by an $m \times n$ matrix X, where m is the vocabulary size, and n is the number of documents. A common assumption of topic modeling is that a latent topic can be represented as a distribution over the words. Then, a topic is a vector w in Rm, and an $m \times k$ topic-word matrix W can be obtained by vertically combining k topics. With W, a document can be seen as a distribution over the k topics, which can be represented as a $k \times 1$ vector h. Since using limited topics (usually $k << n$) to precisely fit all documents is impossible, it is common to use WH to approximate the document matrix. H is the topic document matrix, where each column contains the topic distribution of a document. Good W and H could ensure that the difference between WH and the original document matrix X is small. In the case of text streams, the documents arrive continuously. The document matrix X consists of document matrices from different time slots. In time slot t, suppose the current $m \times n$ document matrix is Xt, then the NMF methods detect topics as follows: Given a topic number k, it tries to find an $m \times k$ topic-word matrix Wt and $k \times n$ topic-document matrixes Ht, which satisfy the following function:

$$argmin Wc, Hc \|Xt - WtHt\|2 \qquad st. Wt, Ht \geq 0$$

Table 4. A comparison of various classification algorithms for two data sets.

Plat form	Algorithms	Accuracy (%) ± Error	Precision	Recall	F-Measure	ROC-Curve	Time (s)
1	NB	73.4 ± .37	.65	.65	.65	.69	.08
	RF	92.6 ± .46	.58	.58	.62	.62	1.5
	J.48	83.5 ± .42	.62	.62	.62	.64	.35
	Lazy.IBK	96.7 ± .48	.52	.52	.51	.52	.10
	SVM	93.6 ± .47	.53	.53	.53	.53	.20
2	NB	83.6 ± .42	.66	.63	.61	.59	.03
	RF	90.9 ± .45	.61	.58	.54	.61	.35
	J.48	94.3 ± .47	.76	.55	.44	.53	.03
	Lazy.IBK	93.8 ± .47	.56	.53	.48	.54	.03
	SVM	75 ± .38	.63	.63	.62	.63	.03

RateMDs = 1, Healthgrades = 2

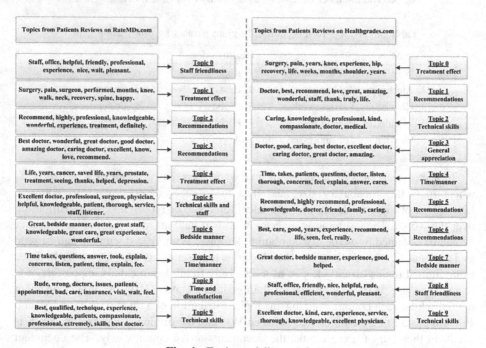

Fig. 4. Topic modeling results

In this study, we need to do some preprocessing before directly applying ONMF method. Our parameters contain n_samples = 5560 for RateMDs and 2916 for Health grades, n_features = 1000, n_topics = 10, n_top_words = 20. We first employ a term frequency-inverse document frequency vectorizer (TfidfVectorizer) with max_df = 0.95, min_df = 2. Then we remove nonsense words, such as stop words in English (e.g., of, I, we, in, is, of, the), and many highly frequent words (e.g., doctor, physician, hospital). Then we applied n_gram tokenizer algorithm to extract meaningful tokens. The extracted tokens may have various lengths from one to a possibly very large number. Each token is considered an atomic entity, meaning that all characters in each token will not be separated for further processing. In step 2, we fit the ONMF algorithm model with n_samples and n_features. Finally, we run scikit-learn facilities to find the top ten topics, each consist of twenty words. To remove redundancy and make topics more informative we apply stemming and lemmatizer algorithm that results in ten topics with ten words with the highest probability in that topic.

We list the topic modeling results of the two platforms' patients' reviews side by side. Based on our text mining python program, we abstracted 10 topics each from RateMDs and Healthgrades patients reviews. Our text mining program assigns the index number to each topic, and it has no particular meaning. The boxes connected by arrows to a topic, we show the top ten keywords for each topic on these platforms. The theme of each topic under the topic index is summarized in Fig. 4.

The results show that both RateMDs and Healthgrades have topics related to staff friendliness, medical/surgery, recommendation, treatment effect, technical skills and staff, bedside manner, time/manner, time/dissatisfaction, and technical skills, as well as appreciation. We also see that the physician reviews on these two websites contain different topics, which may reflect the differences in evaluation of healthcare systems. First, RateMDs patients talked more about physician recommendation to other patients, physician bedside manners and technical skills. Healthgrades patients talked more about recommendations (3/10 topics). Second, in the reviews about technical skills, RateMDs patients mainly focused on physician knowledge and experience, while Healthgrades patients mentioned care and kindness in the technical skills reviews.

4 Discussion and Results

In this section, we discuss the similarity and the difference of the physician reviews between the RateMDs and Healthgrades, particularly on the health system and health service side. Study results identify that sentiment analysis of online physician reviews on these two platforms is possible with a reasonable degree of accuracy and that it is possible to identify salient aspects of reviews and topics discussed in these reviews. These results suggest a potential mechanism to make use of the massive amounts of text on the internet in which people describe their care, and that further exploration of the information contained within the free-text comments may be an important avenue for understanding patient experience, to complement traditional approaches.

From the descriptive statistics in Tables 1 and 2, on RateMDs we can see that pulmonologists have a higher percentage of reviews while oncologists have highest reviews per doctor. On the other hand, orthopedics have the highest percentage of reviews and reviews per doctor on Healthgrades. Orthopedics doctors also have a highest average length of reviews on both platforms. On RateMDs neurologists have received the highest number of reviews in 2017, while nephrologists received a higher number of reviews in 2014 on Healthgrades. On RateMDs, pulmonologists have highest while endocrinologists have the lowest number of reviews. While on

Healthgrades orthopedics have highest and neurologists have lowest review volume. This variation reflects the unbalance in both the quality and the volume of services among both platforms. Figures 2 and 3 shows the distribution of the review volume from 2004–17.

Sentiment analysis via a machine learning approach is only as good as the learning set that is used to inform it. In applications of sentiment analysis to e-health perspective, researchers have had to train the system themselves by reviewing unstructured feedback and ascribing characteristics to them, to allow the algorithm to learn. We used two online physician reviews datasets based on different risk specialties.

A comparative analysis of various machine learning classification algorithms has been made using two datasets taken from RateMDs and Healthgrades. Various performance measures for both the datasets are shown in Table 4. In the analysis, six different measures were used for comparing various classification algorithms. All the measures played a significant role in making any classification decision. It can be noted that on RateMDs, NB classification algorithm while on Healthgrades all classification algorithms except RF took minimum time to classify data. On RateMDs, NB while on Healthgrades, SVM gives less accuracy, i.e., accurately classified instances are comparatively smaller in number. RF, Lazy.IBK and SVM have quite a good accuracy with a little increase in time used for classification on RateMDs. RF, J.48, and Lazy.IBK yielded maximum accuracy, but in RF algorithm, the time taken to build classification model is much higher than other classifiers, or we can say maximum in all the classifiers in most of the cases on Healthgrades. The classification time in RF is more as compared to other best classifiers on both platforms. In RateMDs platform, the Recall and Precision are generally low due to unbalanced sample. Rest of the models also lies in between the best and worst ones.

We also found some common and distinct topics among the different specialty areas on these two platforms. We can see that the most common topics across eight specialty areas are the "Technical skills, bedside manner, and recommendations" (Fig. 4). The goal of these platforms is to help the U.S. patients to find good doctors or good specialists for their health problems. Our findings also reveal that some topics are quite common across two platforms, for example, "technical skills" and "bedside manner". This is not only because they focus on patient care, but also that the platforms elicit such kinds of reviews. Both physician rating platforms ask reviewers to give rating scores based on these two dimensions before writing text reviews. "Recommendations" and "staff friendliness" are another two common topics across specialty areas. All other topics were found only once across both platforms, e.g. "general surgery results appreciation" is seen more on Healthgrades than RateMDs. For the RateMDs, we found that U.S patients talked about "appointment, waiting time and insurance," while Healthgrades patients focused more on "appreciation and care". We also found that many reviewers on both platforms in the U.S. recommended doctors explicitly if they were satisfied with their experiences [3]. This indicates, they consciously realize that other patients may read their posts later. Finally, both platforms patients specifically discussed "treatment effect" under all the specialties.

5 Implications, Limitations, and Conclusions

This paper is the first attempt to compare online doctor reviews across two platforms concerning different disease risk specialties; based on text mining and the online NMF topic modeling. Results do show that patient reviews can assist health care organizations and providers to understand patients' need at this big-data age.

A solution to the challenge of "big data" is to find automated methods for analyzing unstructured feedback, which is a potentially rich source of learning. In this respect, health care is no different to many other industries although it has perhaps been slower than other sectors to recognize its importance. As our confidence in techniques of data mining and sentiment analysis grow, information of this sort could be routinely collected, processed, and interpreted by health-care providers and regulators to monitor performance. Moreover, information could also be taken from many other online sources. As in current study of cross-platform analysis, the information could be crawled and then processed into timely and relevant data, to be a valuable tool for health-care service quality improvement and patients search for competent physicians.

In assessing physicians' reviews, we find that there are common topics that both platforms patients care about, such as technical skills, bedside manner, and treatment effect. Those topics are all related to patient personal experience, which is the core component of healthcare service anywhere. Understanding the voice of patients on these topics can help healthcare providers and healthcare administrators to improve the development of a patient-centered care system. Now that patient-centered care is a stated goal for many organizations and healthcare providers in the U.S., patients' direct experiences and subjective opinions are very important [3].

Our findings provide evidence that online doctor reviews represent a vibrant and ever-growing online asset that reflect the reality of the healthcare, thus, on one hand; it could help providers to understand patients' needs and improve the quality of care. Alternatively, patients can leverage this public online asset to select the physician that would provide the best service for their health problems. In sum, online doctor reviews are a win-win resource for both physicians and patients, on both platforms.

There are several limitations in this study. Online comments left without solicitation on a website are likely to have a natural selection bias towards examples of both good and bad care. It is expected that these online reviews are contributed more by those in particular demographic groups including younger and more affluent people [11]. Further, there are certain aspects of health consumer reviews that are very hard for sentiment analysis to process. Mockery, cynicism, and comedy, frequently adopted by English speakers' patients when talking about their care, cannot be easily detected using this process. It is important the use of prior polarity to improve the results and mitigate some colloquial phrasing, but difficulties were understanding those that depend on context. For example, phrases that cropped up repeatedly, such as "smelled urine" or "like an angel", could be easily characterized as negative or positive. The meaning of other frequently used phrases, however, was hard to establish without an understanding of their context. The best example of this was the phrase a "glass of juice". It was referred to in many different comments in these data, but without knowing the context, is it impossible to allocate it a direct sentiment. "They didn't even offer me a glass of juice" is very different to "The nurse even offers me a glass of juice". Our current algorithm could not yet make use of references to a glass of juice or similar phrases like a cup of coffee that would be clear and obvious looked at by eye on a case-by-case basis. Future attempts to improve NLP ability for patient experience would have to develop the capacity to interpret this level of context-specific and idiomatic content accurately. We appreciate that in this research, we are not using the most state-of-the-art machine learning algorithms used in tourism and restaurant industries [17, 18], but hope that further work might be able to adopt this. Second, in our topic modeling algorithm computational cost is typically high due to ONMF, but the software about these methods is quite new, and there's no doubt that these will be improved in future. Third, we looked at only two regions of the country with a sample of comments and the results may not be generalizable. Future research can investigate the thousands of comments sample from other regions and deception phenomenon.

Acknowledgments. This research is supported by the National Natural Science Foundation, People's Republic of China (No.71531013, 71401047, 71729001).

References

1. Greaves, F., et al.: Associations between internet-based patient ratings and conventional surveys of patient experience in the English NHS: an observational study. BMJ Qual. Saf. **21**, 600 (2012)
2. Hao, H., Zhang, K.: The voice of chinese health consumers: a text mining approach to web-based physician reviews. J. Med. Internet Res. **18**, e108 (2016)
3. Hao, H., Zhang, K., Wang, W., Gao, G.: A tale of two countries: International comparison of online doctor reviews between China and the United States. Int. J. Med. Inform. **99**, 37–44 (2017)
4. Wallace, B.C., Paul, M.J., Sarkar, U., Trikalinos, T.A., Dredze, M.: A large-scale quantitative analysis of latent factors and sentiment in online doctor reviews. J. Am. Med. Inform. Assoc. **21**, 1098–1103 (2014)
5. Kadry, B., Chu, F.L., Kadry, B., Gammas, D., Macario, A.: Analysis of 4999 online physician ratings indicates that most patients give physicians a favorable rating. J. Med. Internet Res. **13**, e95 (2011)
6. Emmert, M., Meier, F., Pisch, F., Sander, U.: Physician choice making and characteristics associated with using physician-rating websites: cross-sectional study. J. Med. Internet Res. **15**, e187 (2013)
7. Xiang, Z., Du, Q., Ma, Y., Fan, W.: A comparative analysis of major online review platforms: Implications for social media analytics in hospitality and tourism. Tour. Manag. **58**, 51–65 (2017)
8. Liu, Y., Bi, J.-W., Fan, Z.-P.: Ranking products through online reviews: a method based on sentiment analysis technique and intuitionistic fuzzy set theory. Inf. Fusion **36**, 149–161 (2017)
9. Giatsoglou, M., Vozalis, M.G., Diamantaras, K., Vakali, A., Sarigiannidis, G., Chatzisavvas, K.C.: Sentiment analysis leveraging emotions and word embeddings. Expert Syst. Appl. **69**, 214–224 (2017)

10. Alemi, F., Torii, M., Clementz, L., Aron, D.C.: Feasibility of real-time satisfaction surveys through automated analysis of patients' unstructured comments and sentiments. Qual. Manag. Health Care **21**, 9–19 (2012)
11. Greaves, F., Ramirez-Cano, D., Millett, C., Darzi, A., Donaldson, L.: Use of sentiment analysis for capturing patient experience from free-text comments posted online. J. Med. Internet Res. **15**, e239 (2013)
12. Tu, D., Chen, L., Lv, M., Shi, H., Chen, G.: Hierarchical online NMF for detecting and tracking topic hierarchies in a text stream. Pattern Recogn. **76**, 203–214 (2018)
13. Klein, C., Clutton, P., Polito, V.: Topic modeling reveals distinct interests within an online conspiracy forum. Front. Psychol. **9**, 189 (2018)
14. Gao, G.G., McCullough, S.J., Agarwal, R., Jha, K.A.: A changing landscape of physician quality reporting: analysis of patients? Online ratings of their physicians over a 5-year period. J. Med. Internet Res. **14**, e38 (2012)
15. Jack, R.A., Burn, M.B., McCulloch, P.C., Liberman, S.R., Varner, K.E., Harris, J.D.: Does experience matter? A meta-analysis of physician rating websites of orthopaedic surgeons. Musculoskelet. Surg. **102**, 63–71 (2018)
16. Alemi, F., Torii, M., Clementz, L., Aron, D.C.: Feasibility of real-time satisfaction surveys through automated analysis of patients' unstructured comments and sentiments. Qual. Manag. Health Care **21**, 9–19 (2012)
17. Guo, Y., Barnes, S.J., Jia, Q.: Mining meaning from online ratings and reviews: tourist satisfaction analysis using latent dirichlet allocation. Tourism Manag. **59**, 467–483 (2017)
18. García-Pablos, A., Cuadros, M., Rigau, G.: W2VLDA: almost unsupervised system for aspect based sentiment analysis. Expert Syst. Appl. **91**, 127–137 (2018)

What Affects Patients' Online Decisions: An Empirical Study of Online Appointment Service Based on Text Mining

Guanjun Liu, Lusha Zhou, and Jiang Wu[✉]

School of Information Management,
Center for E-commerce Research and Development,
Wuhan University, Wuhan 430072, Hubei, China
jiangw@whu.edu.cn

Abstract. The emergence of online health communities enables patients' comments on doctors to express their opinion on service and also make it possible for patients seeking doctors' information before seeing doctor. Making appointment online and then go to see a doctor offline on schedule become popular in China due to its convenience. Both econometric estimations and text mining are used to explore the factors that influence patients' selection of doctors in OAS. The results show that online satisfaction does affect patients to choose doctor, although offline attributes, such as doctor's title and the tier level of hospital, are also considered. We find that overall satisfaction and review volume both have positive impacts on patients' online decisions. As for the specific dimensions of satisfactions extracted from reviews, the service attitude, technical level, explanation clarity, and doctor ethics also positively affect the number of OAS. The moderating effect between doctor's online recommendation and title is negative, as patients care more about doctor's online reviews when she has a low title and vice versa. In addition, the results reveal that patients with high-risk disease are more sensitive to doctor's review volume. Our findings can help doctors design their strategy of online appointment service, and also help online health communities refine their review system so that patients can express their attitudes more specifically.

Keywords: Online health community · Patient satisfaction
Online appointment service · Text mining · Sentiment analysis

1 Introduction

With the explosive growth of internet information resources, more and more patients begin to find health information online. It is universally acknowledged that online information resources are of varying quality, but the emergence and development of online health communities (OHC) solved this problem. People start to rely on OHC to search information, case in point, about 72% American internet users go to OHC for health information [1]. According to iResearch, online health applications (including mobile apps and websites) have more than 2 billion visits monthly in China [2].

Online health community provides a platform on which doctors can better serve and help patients. For example, by participating in online communities, patients can consult

H. Chen et al. (Eds.): ICSH 2018, LNCS 10983, pp. 204–210, 2018.
https://doi.org/10.1007/978-3-030-03649-2_20

doctors directly about health problems by telephone and just cost a little. Besides, online appointment service (OAS) is an easy access to patients who require more consultation and treatment [3, 4]. OHC benefits both doctors and patients in that doctors can make full use of their spare times, while patients can find more health information, suggestion and emotional support that help them recover more effectively [5].

However, most of the existing literatures only investigated online service of OHC, in which patients seek answers from each other (patient to patient OHC), or in which doctors provide service to patients (patient to doctor OHC). Little study has been done about OAS where patients make appointment online and take treatments in hospital, and patients can use both online reviews and offline reputation to choose their desired doctors. Our study attempts to fill this research gap.

This paper makes contributions to OHC research by reconciling an important problem: whether online patients' satisfaction and offline attributes affect patients' decision of choosing doctors in OAS. Our data were collected from one of the largest OHC in the world, where there are more than 170,000 doctors from different Chinese famous hospitals. In our study, we used text mining to find more detailed dimensions of patients' satisfaction and calculated the score of specific topics based on emotion dictionaries. Both doctor's online reputation and offline reputation are tested in this paper. What's more, we measured the moderate effect of disease risk on patients' satisfaction and review volume.

2 Research Hypotheses

Existing literatures rarely study reviews' effect on patients' choosing doctors, which is an emerging area of consideration. We divide patients' satisfaction into overall satisfaction and specified satisfaction to test their effects on doctor's appointment. We also test for the moderating effect of disease risk on satisfaction's influence on doctor's appointment, and the interaction between doctor's position rank and online recommendation on patients' choosing doctor behavior online.

In an OAS, there are many factors that affect patients to select a doctor, such as hospital tier level [6], doctor's title [7], patients' satisfaction [8], online reviews, disease risk, and website recommendation. Therefore, we have the following hypotheses:

H1a: The number of doctor's OAS is positively correlated with her title.
H1b: The number of doctor's OAS is positively correlated with the tier lever of her hospital.
H2: The number of doctor's OAS is positively correlated with the patients' overall satisfaction.
H3: The number of doctor's OAS is positively correlated with the volume of reviews.
H4a: The number of doctor's OAS is positively correlated with the score of doctor's service attitude.
H4b: The number of doctor's OAS is positively correlated with the score of doctor's technical level.

H4c: The number of doctor's OAS is positively correlated with the score of doctor's clarity for explanation.

H4d: The number of doctor's OAS is positively correlated with the score of doctor's ethics.

H4e: The number of doctor's OAS is positively correlated with the score of service process.

H4f: The number of doctor's OAS is positively correlated with the score of hospital infrastructure.

H5a: The effect of patients' overall satisfaction on the number of OAS can be moderated by disease risk, and patients with risker disease attach more importance on patients' overall satisfaction.

H5b: The effect of review volume on the number of OAS can be moderated by disease risk, and patients with risker disease attach more importance on the volume of reviews.

H6: The title and recommendation score can negatively moderate each other's effects on number of OAS.

3 Data and Methods

3.1 Data Collection

To test our research hypotheses, we collect data once a week from one of the largest online medical platforms, "Good Doctor Online (http://www.haodf.com/)". It is a data set of 3,191 doctors, from July 7, 2017 to August 27, 2017, and includes 23,722 records after deleting the records with some information missing. For each doctor in our data set, we collected her personal information, hospital information, satisfaction information and patients' reviews. This data set also consists of 10 specific kinds of diseases, with 5 high-risk diseases and 5 low-risk diseases according to the mortality and relevant data for major diseases from the China Health Statistics Yearbook 2016. According to the yearbook and other's studies [9], we choose 5 kinds of lethal diseases as high-risk disease (leukemia, lung cancer, cirrhosis, coronary heart disease and diabetes) and 5 kinds of non-lethal diseases as low-risk disease (hypertension, rheumatoid arthritis, gastritis, depression and menoxenia).

3.2 Measures for Reviews Topics and Sentiments

There are a vast number of reviews in OAS platform. They vary in topic, sentiment and volume. For this study, we collected and downloaded more than 79,800 patients' reviews about 3,191 focal doctors. Further, we analyzed the topics and sentiments of patients' reviews by Latent Dirichlet Allocation (LDA) and sentiment lexicons and used the sentiment score as the patients' satisfaction of focal doctor. In the process of topic identification, there are fifty themes and can be divided into three categories: patient, doctor and hospital. By summing up all themes, we selected the most often discussed topics: Service, Technical, Explanation, Ethics, Process and Infrastructure. Then we calculated the sentiment score of each topic identified in each review based on

Hownet sentiment lexicon and obtained the satisfaction scores of each doctor in six different topics.

3.3 Model Specification

Our empirical variables are shown in Table 1. The dependent variable *NumOAS* is defined as the number of OAS received by the focal doctor in a week, which refers to how many patients choose to use this OHC to make appointments with the doctor for services. The independent variables include doctor's idle time (*IdleTime*), doctor's title (*Title*), the tier level of her hospital (*Level*), the number of reviews given by the patients (*ReviewNum*), the overall satisfaction on the platform (Satisfaction), the score of satisfaction's specific dimensions (Service, Technical, Explanation, Ethics, Process, Infrastructure). We control the number of people in the province where the doctor works (Population), the virtual gifts patients gave to doctors (*Gifts*), the recommendation score given by the website (*Recommend*), the number of years that a doctor registered on website (*Year*), the number of articles which a doctor has published on her homepages (*Article*), as well as patients' disease risk (*Risky*).

The correlation analysis indicates that the correlation coefficients between each pair of independent and control variables. We can find that the four dimensions of doctors' satisfaction obtained by text mining are highly correlated (service attitude, technical level, explanation clarity and ethics), so we build regression models separately when testing their impacts. To test our hypotheses, we formulate the following empirical models, as shown in Eqs. (1), (2), (3) and (4).

$$
\begin{aligned}
NumOAS_t = {} & IdleTime_t + Title_{t-1} + Level_{t-1} + \ln(ReviewNum)_{t-1} \\
& + Satisfaction_{t-1} + Recommend_{t-1} + Service_{t-1} \\
& + Process_{t-1} + Infrastructure_{t-1} + Year_{t-1} + Risky_{t-1} \\
& + \ln(Gift)_{t-1} + \ln(Population)_{t-1} + \ln(Article)_{t-1} \\
& + TimeDummy_i + DiseaseDummy_i + Constant + \varepsilon
\end{aligned}
\tag{1}
$$

$$
\begin{aligned}
NumOAS_t = {} & IdleTime_t + Title_{t-1} + Level_{t-1} + \ln(ReviewNum)_{t-1} \\
& + Satisfaction_{t-1} + Recommend_{t-1} + Technical_{t-1} \\
& + Process_{t-1} + Infrastructure_{t-1} + Year_{t-1} + Risky_{t-1} \\
& + \ln(Gift)_{t-1} + \ln(Population)_{t-1} + \ln(Article)_{t-1} \\
& + TimeDummy_i + DiseaseDummy_i + Constant + \varepsilon
\end{aligned}
\tag{2}
$$

$$
\begin{aligned}
NumOAS_t = {} & IdleTime_t + Title_{t-1} + Level_{t-1} + \ln(ReviewNum)_{t-1} \\
& + Satisfaction_{t-1} + Recommend_{t-1} + Explanation_{t-1} \\
& + Process_{t-1} + Infrastructure_{t-1} + Year_{t-1} + Risky_{t-1} \\
& + \ln(Gift)_{t-1} + \ln(Population)_{t-1} + \ln(Article)_{t-1} \\
& + TimeDummy_i + DiseaseDummy_i + Constant + \varepsilon
\end{aligned}
\tag{3}
$$

$$
\begin{aligned}
NumOAS_t = {} & IdleTime_t + Title_{t-1} + Level_{t-1} + ln(ReviewNum)_{t-1} \\
& + Satisfaction_{t-1} + Recommend_{t-1} + Ethics_{t-1} + Process_{t-1} \\
& + Infrastructure_{t-1} + Year_{t-1} + Risky_{t-1} + ln(Gift)_{t-1} \\
& + ln(Population)_{t-1} + ln(Article)_{t-1} + TimeDummy_i \\
& + DiseaseDummy_i + Constant + \varepsilon
\end{aligned} \tag{4}
$$

4 Results

We estimated our models using negative binomial regression and all our empirical models were done by STATA. The empirical results in Table 1 contain the interaction effect of doctor's title and website recommendation and the moderate effects of disease

Table 1. Regression results

	Model 1	Model 2	Model 3	Model 4
IdleTime	0.035***	0.034***	0.035***	0.034***
Title	1.916***	1.909***	1.927***	1.934***
Level	0.443***	0.441***	0.439***	0.444***
ln(ReviewNum)	0.357***	0.357***	0.356***	0.356***
Risky	−0.068	−0.061	−0.059	−0.057
Satisfaction	0.729***	0.715***	0.719***	0.719***
Recommend	2.072***	2.066***	2.086***	2.090***
Service	0.105*			
Technical		0.154**		
Explanation			0.125**	
Ethics				0.117*
Process	−0.013	−0.022	−0.014	−0.020
Infrastructure	0.007	−0.004	−0.002	−0.012
Title × Recommend	−0.383***	−0.381***	−0.386***	−0.387***
Risky × ReviewNum	0.088**	0.087**	0.085**	0.084**
Risky × Satisfaction	−0.220	−0.215	−0.227	−0.227
Year	−0.049***	−0.049***	−0.048***	−0.049***
ln(Gift)	0.039*	0.041*	0.037	0.040*
ln(Population)	−0.064**	−0.066**	−0.063**	−0.064**
ln(Article)	−0.004	−0.005	−0.005	−0.004
Constant	−10.493***	−10.447***	−10.506***	−10.549***
Time dummy	√	√	√	√
Disease dummy	√	√	√	√
Log likelihood	−31047.2	−31044	−31043.6	−31043.6
Wald chi2	2111.09	2118.16	2118.19	2113.91
Prob > chi2				
Observations	23,722	23,722	23,722	23,722
Number of x_id	3,191	3,191	3,191	3,191

***$p < 0.01$, **$p < 0.05$, *$p < 0.1$

risk on the number of reviews and overall satisfaction. Hypotheses H4a–H4d were tested respectively in the four models.

It is shown that all the variables have significant influences on the number of OAS received by the focal doctor except for medical process ($p > 0.1$), hospital infrastructure ($p > 0.1$) and the moderate effect of disease risk on overall satisfaction ($p > 0.1$). Therefore, we should reject H4e, H4f and H5a. The results show that the doctors with a high score of overall satisfaction ($p < 0.01$) and a large review volume ($p < 0.01$) are more popular among patients. Furthermore, the doctor's title ($p < 0.01$) and hospital's tier level ($p < 0.01$) have positive effect on OAS. As for the effect of detailed dimensions for satisfaction, the results reveal that service attitude ($\beta = 0.105$, $p < 0.1$), technical level ($\beta = 0.154$, $p < 0.05$), explanation clarity ($\beta = 0.125$, $p < 0.05$), and doctor ethics ($\beta = 0.117$, $p < 0.1$) positively affect the OAS. Therefore, H1a, H1b, H2, H3, H4a–H4d and H5b are all supported.

The results show that the interaction effect between doctor's title and website recommendation score is significantly negative ($p < 0.01$). It indicates that although the doctor's title is inferior, a high website recommendation still can bring a higher OAS to her. This provides doctors an opportunity to get more OAS by raising the recommendation score, for example, participating in the various online activities can increase word of mouth in patients. Besides, the disease risk can moderate the effect of review volume on OAS ($p < 0.05$), indicating that patients with risky diseases are more sensitive to the number of reviews for doctor.

In summary, this paper investigates factors that influence patients' selection of doctors in OAS. Except for H4e, H4f and H5a, all the other hypotheses are supported.

5 Conclusions

This paper investigates what affect patients to select doctors in online booking service in hospitals (OAS). The main finding is online satisfaction such as overall satisfaction, service attitude, technical level, explanation clarity and medical ethics do affect patients choose doctor positively, although offline attributes such as doctor's title and the tier level of her hospital are also considered. Furthermore, the results indicate that review volume has positive effect on the number of OAS and patients with high-risk diseases are more sensitive to that. Therefore, doctors should encourage their patients to comment on the website and attach more importance to their attitude and expression when serving online and offline. Our findings also help OAS platform to refine their system design. Because of the moderate effect of recommendation, the system need to encourage doctors with low professional title or without title to pay more attention to online services in order to get good online reviews, which can attract more patients to make appointments. In the future, we will take the doctor's online consultation services into account and model it to explore the supply and demand in OAS.

References

1. Pew Research Center. http://www.pewresearch.org/fact-tank/2014/01/15/the-social-life-of-health-information/
2. iResearch Center. http://www.iresearch.com.cn/Detail/report?id=2551&isfree=0
3. Wu, H., Lu, N.J.: Online written consultation, telephone consultation and offline appointment: an examination of the channel effect in online health communities. Int. J. Med. Inform. **107**, 107–119 (2017)
4. Zhang, M.M., Zhang, C.X., Sun, Q.W., Cai, Q.C., Yang, H., Zhang, Y.J.: Questionnaire survey about use of an online appointment booking system in one large tertiary public hospital outpatient service center in China. BMC Med. Inform. Decis. Making **14**, 49 (2014)
5. Mey, Y.S., Sankaranarayanan, S.: Near Field Communication based Patient Appointment (2013)
6. Liu, X.X., Guo, X.T., Wu, H., Wu, T.S.: The impact of individual and organizational reputation on physicians' appointments online. Int. J. Electron. Commer. **20**, 551–577 (2016)
7. Hall, J.A., Dornan, M.C.: What patients like about their medical-care and how often they are asked – a meta-analysis of the satisfaction literature. Soc. Sci. Med. **27**, 935–939 (1988)
8. Kersnik, J.: Determinants of customer satisfaction with the health care system, with the possibility to choose a personal physician and with a family doctor in a transition country. Health Policy **57**, 155–164 (2001)
9. Yang, H., Guo, X., Wu, T.: Exploring the influence of the online physician service delivery process on patient satisfaction. Decis. Support Syst. **78**, 113–121 (2015)

Bayesian Network Retrieval Discrimination Criteria Model Based on Unbalanced Information

Man Xu[1] , Dan Gan[2] , Jiang Shen[2(✉)] , and Bang An[2]

[1] Business School, Nankai University, Tianjin 300071, China
[2] College of Management and Economics, Tianjin University,
Tianjin 300072, China
motoshen@163.com

Abstract. Unbalanced sample data are usually ignored in the process of case matching, but these data also lead to misclassification during case matching. To solve this problem, a discrimination criteria model based on the Bayesian network and corresponding algorithm is proposed in our paper. The Bayesian network cost sensitivity learning in this model uses the minimization theorem of loss function. We also introduce a ROC curve to evaluate the performance of the retrieval model and verify the validity of the model by using diagnostic data for clinical heart disease. Our results indicate that this method can effectively eliminate the cost sensitivity of imbalanced datasets and improve the accuracy of the retrieval results.

Keywords: Case matching · Bayesian network · Unbalanced data
Cost-sensitivity

1 Introduction

Datasets are often incomplete due to the absence of a sample, and an imbalance in the number of positive and negative samples causes the overall sample to be unbalanced [1]. Data incompleteness refers to a lack of sample data. Data imbalance is a result of having both positive and negative samples in the overall distribution. Both data incompleteness and imbalance have nonstructural characteristics; their processing methods are complex, and there is no uniform processing method.

At present, research on non-equilibrium data mainly focuses on the algorithm and data layers [2]. The algorithm layer processing method modifies the algorithm according to data set bias so that the case matching plane tends to have a small number of categories, thereby improving the recognition rate of those categories. Data layer processing is data re-sampling, including undersampling and oversampling. Undersampling removes some of the samples and is likely to cause information loss; oversampling increases the number of samples so that the original data can be retained and also makes it easy to marginalize the sample. Incompleteness or imbalance in the data leads to a decrease in the recognition rate of a rare dataset, which is important in

© Springer Nature Switzerland AG 2018
H. Chen et al. (Eds.): ICSH 2018, LNCS 10983, pp. 211–223, 2018.
https://doi.org/10.1007/978-3-030-03649-2_21

increasing the accuracy and specificity of the search results [3] and is the main factor for the efficiency of case matching [4].

Jing et al. proposed a robust weighted online extreme learning machine algorithm that has a cost-sensitive learning theory to solve the problem of dynamic data imbalance [5]. Feng et al. [6] used rough set and fuzzy set methods to obtain uncertain and incomplete system information in a complex system. Leung et al. [7] also used the rough set theory to obtain information from non-complete information systems and proposed similar concepts to exploit useful information in incomplete retrieval. Rajput et al. [8] used the improved Bayesian network to address incomplete data that resulted in redundancy problems and reduced retrieval efficiency. Uramoto [9] used data mining to explore the association of information between cases to ensure the effective handling of incomplete information, and Fernández et al. [10] used fuzzy logic to obtain information based on rule retrieval from unbalanced data, but the method resulted in misclassification and loss. The existing case matching mechanism cannot provide an effective method for resolving misclassifications of unbalanced data sets.

The discrimination criterion is the most common selection criterion in Bayesian networks. It measures the model structure according to the classification performance of a classifier. Classification accuracy is an important basis for evaluating the Bayesian network retrieval model, so the criterion based on minimizing the error classification rate is used for Bayesian network retrieval. The criterion based on minimizing the error classification rate assumes that all categories of misclassification losses are the same; however, the losses caused by different categories of misclassifications are not necessarily the same, and the classification model that satisfies the minimization of false classification criteria is not necessarily able to satisfy the minimization that error classification loss requires. For example, for medical samples categorized by patient health, in which only 1% of patients are represented, a 99% classification accuracy can be obtained, but this model cannot diagnose the patient, so it is useless [11]. Unbalanced data lead to misdiagnoses and false negatives within the case matching classification, and these two types of misclassifications produce different losses. In this study, cost-sensitive learning in different categories of misclassification is considered, and the classification is chosen based on the minimization of misclassification criteria, which resolves the problem of the misclassification of the loss of inconsistency.

In summary, existing research on data retrieval regarding the randomness, polymorphisms and ambiguity of data is discussed, but incomplete and non-equilibrium data are usually regarded as abnormal values and are ignored, thus affecting the efficiency of case matching. This paper examines the problems of misdiagnoses and false negatives that occur in case matching classification caused by unbalanced data and constructs a Bayesian networks retrieval discriminate criterion model based on this unbalanced data. The cost function minimization theorem is used to make the Bayesian networks more cost-sensitive, and a retrieval algorithm for the minimum misclassification loss is proposed. Finally, we evaluate the comprehensive performance of the proposed case matching model for both the misclassification rate and sensitivity using the AUC [12].

2 Knowledge Representations

2.1 State Space Representation

Using state-space to represent the data set, suppose that the finite set of random variables in the matrix is $U, U = \{X, C\}$. Using a function to represent $F, X \to C$, $X = \{X_1, X_2, \cdots, X_n\}$, x_i is the value of property i X_i, C is the class variable, $C = \{C_1, C_2, \cdots, C_n\}$, c_j is value of the j class c_j, and $x = (x_1, \cdots, x_n)^T \in X \subset R^n$. A map for the class $c_j \in \{-1, 1\}, j = 1, 2$, can be represented as:

$$F(x) = \text{sgn}[f(x)] \tag{1}$$

Function $f : X \to R$, when $x \geq 0$, $\text{sgn}(x) = 1$, if not, $\text{sgn}(x) = -1$

2.2 Bayesian Network Constructions

Use the probability distribution $\Pr(x)$ to describe the stochastic process of case matching for eigenvector x and use the random sample variable C, in which $\Pr(c_j)$ is used to describe the classifier, then the prior probability of c_j is $\Pr(c_j)$.

$$\Pr(c_j) = \frac{\{N_i | C(x_i) = c_j, i = 1, 2, \ldots, N_i\}}{N} \tag{2}$$

N_i is the number of samples in the sub dataset and N is the number of samples.

The property variable is distributed according to the constraint conditional probability to form Bayesian network B. To define the conditional probability of U:

$$\Pr(X_1, X_2, \cdots, X_n) = \prod_{i=1}^{n} \Pr[X_i | P_a(X_i)]$$

For retrieval case $x = (x_1, \cdots, x_n)$, the prior classification probability of class c_j is $\Pr(c_j)$. After Bayesian network retrieval, we obtain the posterior classification probability distribution $\Pr(c_j | x_1, \cdots, x_n)$. In the Bayesian retrieval model,

$$\Pr(C = c_j | X = x_i) = \frac{\Pr(C = c_j) \cdot \Pr(X = x_i | C = c_j)}{\Pr(X = x_i)} \tag{3}$$

$\Pr(X = x_i | C = c_j)$ is the conditional probability.

Assuming that α is a regularization factor, according to the chain rule of probability, the Eq. (3) can be represented as

$$\Pr(c_j | x_1, \cdots, x_n) = \alpha \cdot \Pr(c_j) \cdot \prod_{i=1}^{n} \Pr(x_i | x_1, \cdots, x_{i-1}, c_j) \tag{4}$$

and assuming that property X_i is only related to class variable C, then

$$\Pr(c_j|x_1,\cdots,x_n) = \alpha \cdot \Pr(c_j) \cdot \prod_{i=1}^{n} \Pr(x_i|c_j) \tag{5}$$

For the information classification case $x = (x_1,\cdots,x_n)$, we can first classify the training sample set to subset D_j according to the class label using the training sample set to estimate the prior classification probability of each class. Then, the final class is divided according to the Bayesian maximum posterior classification probability. After class selection by the Bayesian classifier, the maximum class of its posterior classification probability $\Pr(c_j|x_1,\cdots,x_n)$ is the final class.

3 The Criterion Based on the Minimal Misclassification Cost

3.1 Misclassification Cost Model

Take the result of Eq. (3) in its short form, s; the threshold of classification reliability is σ,

$$s_j = \begin{cases} 1 & F(x) \le \sigma \\ -1 & F(x) > \sigma \end{cases}, j = 1, 2 \tag{6}$$

It is assumed that $F_0(x) = TP/(TP + FN)$ is the ratio of the predictive result number in the actual positive class sample number. Then, $1 - F_0(x)$ is the misclassification rate.

It is assumed that the specificity of classification is the ratio of the predictive negative class sample result number in the actual negative sample number, $1 - F_1(x) = TN/(TN + FP)$.

Then, $F_1(x)$ is the filtering rate. In the equation, $TP(TN)$ represents the number of positive (negative) samples that are evaluated correctly in the test set. $FN(FP)$ represents the number of positive (negative) samples that are evaluated incorrectly in the test set. Let $F_0(\sigma)$ represent the vertical axis and $F_1(\sigma)$ represent the horizontal axis. The resulting figure is the Receiver Operating Characteristic Curve, ROC. Point $(0, 0)$ on the ROC represents the model where all samples are estimated to be negative, point $(0, 1)$ represents a wrong classification, and point $(1, 0)$ represents a correct classification. The AUC (Area Under the Curve) is used to evaluate the integrated performance of the retrieval model.

$$AUC = \int_0^{+\infty} F_0(F_1^{-1}(s))ds \tag{7}$$

Definition 1: Assume that the eigenvector $x = (x_1,\cdots,x_n)^T \in X \subset R^n$ map on class $c_j \in C = \{-1, 1\}, j = 1, 2$ and considering the effects of the misclassification rate $1 - F_0(\sigma)$ and filtering rate $F_1(\sigma)$, the cost function is named the classification cost, $L(x, c)$. The misclassification cost function is defined as:

$$L(x,c) = L_p(s_i, c_j) = \{|s_i - c_j|^p, p \geq 1\} \tag{8}$$

$$L(x,c) = \begin{cases} 0, & s_j = c_j \\ \lambda_1, & c_1 = 1, s_1 = -1, \lambda_j > 0 \\ \lambda_2, & c_2 = -1, s_2 = 1 \end{cases} \tag{9}$$

λ_1 and λ_2 are misclassification costs. When $\lambda_1 = \lambda_2$, this process is not sensible for the misclassification cost; when the two are not equal, this process is sensible.

3.2 The Average Cost of Misclassification

The next step is to introduce ROC average cost analysis and case matching efficacy and then use the Bayesian maximum posterior probability rule to identify the c_j class of x:$\Pr(c_j|x_1, \cdots, x_n) = \max_{j=1,\cdots,l} \Pr(c_j|x)$, which is the minimal probability rule. Then, the minimum misclassification cost of the Bayesian retrieval cost is $\Pr(c_j|x_1, \cdots, x_n) = \max_{j=1,\cdots,l} \Pr(c_j|x)$.

Assuming that $\Pr(x_i|c_j)$ is the probability when the actual class is c_j, the ROC average function of loss is formed by the distribution probability of the misclassification rate $1 - F_0(x)$ and filtering rate $1 - F_0(x)$. $\Pr_{c_j}$ represents the probability of c_j.

After considering the misclassification cost based on the Bayesian network misclassification minimum error rule, the resulting classification function of the minimal gross risks expectation is:

$$f^* = \arg\min_f E_{X,C}[L_m(x,c)]$$

Through the cost-insensitive sufficient condition of optimization classification, we obtain:

$$f^* = \min_{\Pr_{c_j}} \max_x E_{X,C}\left[\ln \frac{\Pr_{C|X}(c_1|x)\lambda_1}{\Pr_{C|X}(c_2|x)\lambda_2}\right] \tag{10}$$

3.3 Misclassification Cost Minimization

Theory 1: Assuming that $\alpha = \frac{\sum_j \lambda_j}{2}$, $\beta = \frac{1}{2}\ln(\frac{\lambda_2}{\lambda_2})$, and $\Pr_c(x) = \frac{e^{\alpha f(x)+\beta}}{e^{\alpha f(x)+\beta} + e^{-\alpha f(x)-\beta}}$, then $I(\cdot)$ is an indicator function and the function of the misclassification expected loss is

$$E_{X,C}[L(x,c)] = \left[I(c_i = 1)e^{c_i \cdot \lambda_1 f(x)} + I(c_i = -1)e^{-c_i \cdot \lambda_2 f(x)}\right]$$
$$- E_{X,C}\left[s_i \cdot \ln_c(\Pr(x)) + (1 - s_i)\ln(1 - \Pr_c(x))\right] \tag{11}$$

Using the asymmetric symbolic logic transformation of $\Pr_{C_j|X}(1|X)$ results in misclassification cost minimization.

$$f(x) = \frac{1}{\sum_j \lambda_j} \ln \frac{\Pr(c_j = 1|X)\lambda_1}{\Pr(c_j = c^*|X)\lambda_2} \tag{12}$$

Proof: To evaluate the minimum of the classification sensitive function of the exponential loss in the first term in Eq. (12), we need to determine the minimum expected loss function $f(x)$ about x according to the cost sensitive optimality principle:

$$l_e(x) = E_{X|C}\left[(I(c_i = 1)e^{c_i \cdot \lambda_1 f(x)} + I(c_i = -1)e^{-c_i \cdot \lambda_2 f(x)})|X\right]$$
$$= \Pr_{X|C}(1|x)e^{\lambda_1 f(x)} + \Pr_{X|C}(-1|x)e^{\lambda_2 f(x)}.$$

Assuming that the derivative is 0,

$$\frac{\partial l_e(x)}{\partial f(x)} = -\lambda_1 P_{C|X}(1|x)e^{-\lambda_1 f(x)} + \lambda_2 P_{C|X}(-1|x)e^{\lambda_2 f(x)} = 0.$$

We obtain $\frac{\Pr(c_j=1|x)\lambda_1}{\Pr(c_j=c^*|x)\lambda_2} = e^{f(x)\cdot \sum_j \lambda_j}$ and $f(x) = \frac{1}{\sum_j \lambda_j} \ln \frac{\Pr(c_j=1|x)\lambda_1}{\Pr(c_j=c^*|x)\lambda_2}$, where the second derivative is not negative, and then, $f(x)$ is the minimum loss function.

To evaluate the minimum of the classification cost sensitive function of the binomial loss in the second term, we also need to evaluate the minimal expected loss function $f(x)$ about x.

$$l_b(x) = -E_{C|X}\left[((c' \ln(\Pr_c(x)) + (1 - c') \ln(1 - \Pr_c(x))|x\right]$$
$$= -\Pr_{C|X}(1|x)\ln(\Pr_c(x)) - \Pr_{C|X}(0|x)\ln(1 - \Pr_c(x)).$$

$\Pr_c(x)$ is given by the prior probability equation. To evaluate the minimum of $\Pr_c(x)$, we assume the derivative to be 0.

$$\frac{\partial l_b(x)}{\partial \Pr_c(x)} = -\frac{1}{\Pr_c(x)} P_{c|x}(1|x) + \frac{1}{1 - \Pr_c(x)} \Pr_{c|x}(0|x) = 0.$$

It is $\ln \frac{\Pr_c(x)}{1-\Pr_c(x)} = \ln \frac{P_{C|X}(1|x)}{P_{C|X}(0|x)}$. Use conditions α and β to transfer this function into $2(\alpha f(x) + \beta) = \ln \frac{P_{C|X}(1|x)}{P_{C|X}(0|x)}$; it is $f(x) = \frac{1}{\sum_j \lambda_j} \ln \frac{\Pr(c_j=1|X)\lambda_1}{\Pr(c_j=c^*|X)\lambda_2}$.

As $\frac{\partial^2 l_b(x)}{\partial \Pr_c(x)^2} \geq 0$ and $\Pr_\lambda(x)$ is monotonically increasing about the function $f(x)$, it is the minimum value and the proof is complete.

4   Retrieval Strategies and Steps

Let the training sample be $\Gamma = \{(x_i, c_i), i = 1, 2, \cdots, N\}$ and miscategorized losses be λ_1, λ_2; then, the empirical probability of symptom i from the sample is $\Pr(x_i)$.

Retrieval Steps:

Step 1: Knowledge representation and problem identification. Build an undirected graph and let the attribute variables be its joints. The weights of the sides connecting joints x_i and x_j $(i \neq j)$ can be regarded as conditional mutual entropy.

$$I(x_i; x_j | c) = \sum_{x_i, x_j c} \Pr(x_i, x_j, c) \log \left(\frac{\Pr(x_i, x_j | c)}{\Pr(x_i | c) \Pr(x_j | c)} \right) \tag{13}$$

Step 2: Certify the retrieval strategy. Build a span tree of the highest weight according to the root joint searched through $I(x_i; x_j | c)$. Assume that all arcs point outwards from the root joint and consider another arc that connects the variable joint and attribute joint.

Step 3: Perform an iterative search under the state-space representation. According to miscategorized losses λ_1, λ_2 and $f(x)$, verify the M amount of Bayesian retrieval models using the AdaBoost [15] algorithm.

When $m = 1$, repeatedly conduct sampling with replacement under the same possibility of $\Pr_1(i) = 1/N$. The new training set D_1, retrieved by the sampling training set Γ, should be used to build the Bayesian network $B(x, D_1)$ to estimate all of the sample points (x_i, c_i) in Γ. If $B(x, D_1)$ estimates (x_i, y_i) are wrong, let; otherwise, $d_1(i) = 0$. Then, calculate $\psi_1 = \sum_n \Pr_1(i) d_1(i)$, $v_1 = (1 - \psi_1)/\psi_1$ and $\tau_1 = \ln(v_1)$.

When $m = 2, \cdots, M$, calculate $\Pr_m(i) = \Pr_{m-1}(n) \beta_{m-1}^{d_{m-1}(i)} / \sum_n \Pr_{m-1}(i) \beta_{m-1}^{d_{m-1}(i)}$ after updating the sampling possibility of round m. Repeatedly conduct sampling from Γ with replacement under the possibility of $\Pr_m(i)$, and approach a new training set D_m. Next, build the Bayesian network $B(x, D_m)$ by using D_m to estimate all of the sample points (x_i, y_i) in Γ. If $B(x, D_m)$ estimates (x_i, y_i) are wrong, let $d_m(i) = 1$; otherwise, $d_m(i) = 0$. Then, calculate $\psi_m = \sum_n \Pr_m(i) d_m(i)$, $v_m = (1 - \psi_m)/\psi_m$, $\tau_m = \ln(v_m)$.

Calculate $W_m = \tau_m / \sum_m \tau_m$ and combine the M Bayesian networks together to acquire the final retrieval rule function $F(x)$, and let $I(\bullet)$ be an indicator function so

$$F(x) = \arg \max_{c_j \in \{1,2\}} \left\{ \sum_m W_m I(f(x, D_m) = c_j) \right\} \tag{14}$$

Then, the retrieval rule function $F(x)$ is obtained.

Step 4: Output case matching results. Acquire the categorization result s according to the retrieval rule function $F(x)$ and threshold σ. In this way, we can interpret the Bayesian network retrieval results into understandable knowledge.

5   Experiment and Results Analysis

5.1   Number of Clinical Medical Diagnoses

Due to the different conditions of patients and experimental inaccuracies, clinical information can be incomplete and unbalanced. We chose our 303 attribute-vacant test samples from a heart-c dataset of the UCI database. Each sample contains 13 characteristics, described as $\{f_1, f_2, \ldots, f_{13}\}$. Separately, they make up 270×13 and 303×13 datasets. Each test sample has a categorization indicator c, and $c = \{c_1, c_2\}$. When samples from the positive class comprise less than 10% of the total samples, it is called a higher standard unbalanced dataset. After normalization, the sample can be divided into two parts: a 200 sample training set and testing set. Let ϕ be the missing sample value. Samples are shown below in graph 1 (Table 1).

Table 1. Example of the uncertainty information contained in heart-c

Id	Age	Sex	Cp	Trestbps	Chol	Fbs	Exang	Ca	Restecg	Thalach	Oldpeak	Thal	Slope	Disease
211	49	0	2	115	265	0	1	2	0	175	0	2	ϕ	0
212	49	0	3	130	338	1	1	2	1	130	1.5	1	1	1
221	58	0	2	130	213	0	1	1	1	140	0	0	ϕ	1
236	48	0	3	160	329	0	0	0	0	92	ϕ	0	1	0
240	52	0	3	170	ϕ	0	1	3	0	126	1.5	2	1	1
245	54	0	3	140	ϕ	0	1	3	0	118	0	2	ϕ	1
247	55	0	3	140	268	0	0	3	0	128	1.5	1	1	1
249	57	0	3	150	255	0	0	2	0	92	3	0	1	0
240	52	0	3	170	ϕ	0	1	0	0	126	1.5	0	1	1
245	54	0	3	140	ϕ	0	1	1	0	118	0	0	ϕ	1
281	43	0	3	140	288	0	1	2	0	135	2	2	1	1

5.2   Model Validation and Results Analysis

After normalization of the data set, the next step is to determine the uncertain information.

$$\theta_{ijk}^{(t+1)} = \arg\max E\left[p(D|\theta)\Big|D, \theta^{(t)}, S\right] = \frac{f\left(a_i^k, \pi(a_i)^j\right)}{\sum f\left(a_i^k, \pi(a_i)^j\right)} \tag{15}$$

For the 200 samples included in the training set for heart-c, use the Bayesian network to conduct parameter learning to obtain $B = (S, P)$.

Use the CBNF model to match the uncertain information, then obtain B.

$$\theta = M_1(U, T, A, V) = \begin{cases} 1 & v_j^{u_i} = v_{jk}^{u_i}, v_j^t = v_{jk}^t \\ \frac{1 - \theta_{jhk}^t}{(v_j^{u_i} - v_j^t)^2} & v_j^{u_i} = v_{jk}^{u_i}, v_j^t = \phi \\ \frac{1 - \theta_{jhk}^{u_i}}{(v_j^{u_i} - v_j^t)^2} & v_j^{u_i} = \phi, v_j^t = v_{jk}^t \end{cases} \tag{16}$$

$$u_i \in U, t \in T, a_i \in A, v_j \in V$$

The testing set's random value is θ. The possibility of case $v_j^t = \phi$ in the heart-c dataset is described as $v_j^{u_i} = v_{jk}^{u_i}$. For the uncertain sample in the heart-c dataset, the optimized feature set of case t (ID = 240) is $\{f_{13}, f_3, f_{12}, f_{10}, f_8\}$ and consists of the heart beat condition (Thal), chest pain type (Cp), recipient vessel amount (Ca), ST decrease due to exercising (Oldpeak) and peak heart rate (Thalach) (Table 2).

Table 2. Normalized case attribute eigenvalue

Attributes	a_3	a_8	a_{10}	a_{12}	a_{13}
$v_j^{u_i}$	0.3333	1	0	0	0.3333
v_j^t	0.6667	0	ϕ	0.5	0.6667

For u_i in $B = (S, P)$, the value of the parent node set $\pi(a_l)$ is certified as the hth possible value and probability of node set a_j is referred to as $\theta_{jhk}^{u_i}$ and is the kth value.

During the matching process, due to the eigenvalue absence of the target case a_{10}, we need to estimate the results based on its other attributes. From $B = (S, P)$ we can obtain $\pi(a_{10}) = \{a_3, a_8\}$ (Table 3).

Table 3. Attributes of the conditional probability distribution table

Number h	a_3	a_8	$p(a_{10} \mid a_3 a_8)$ 0	1
1	1	0	0.542	0.458
2	1	1	0.336	0.664
3	2	0	0.784	0.216
4	2	1	0.817	0.183
5	3	0	0.098	0.902
6	3	1	0.517	0.483
7	4	0	0.363	0.637
8	4	1	0.715	0.285

The next step is to determine that the parent node set value of attribute a_{10} is $h = 3$, $\{a_3 = 2, a_8 = 0\}$. Then, the a_{10} possibility distribution is shown below in graph 4 (Table 4).

Table 4. The probability distribution of attribute value a_{10} in t

The attribute value of target case	$v_j^{u_i} = 0$	$v_j^{u_i} = 1$
$p(a_{10}\|a_3\ a_8)$	0.784	0.216

Knowing that the attribute value a_{10} of u_3 is $v_j^{u_i}$, and the attribute value a_{10} of t is $v_j^{u_i}$; then, $\theta_{jhk}^{u_i} = \theta = 0.784$.

Similarly, attribute value a_{10}'s probability of u_3 and X_{293} is $\theta_{jhk}^{u_i} = \theta = 0.784$, and attribute value a_{13}'s probability of u_3 and X_{301} is $\theta_{jhk}^{u_i} = \theta = 0.984$. The similarity of t is shown in Table 5, which is calculated by using formula (15),

Table 5. Example of search results for the CBNF method (heart-c dataset)

Case	Discrete eigenvalue normalization					True	Most similar		Results
	a_3	a_9	a_{10}	a_{12}	a_{13}		Case	Similarity	
X_{201}	0.3333	0.5	0.3333	0.3333	0.3333	C_1	X_3	99.73%	C_1
X_{216}	0.6667	0.5	0.3333	0.3333	0.6667	C_1	X_{107}	96.38%	C_1
X_{222}	0	0.5	1	1	0.6667	C_2	X_{251}	96.24%	C_2
X_{247}	0	0	1	0.6667	1	C_1	X_{25}	94.41%	C_1
X_{262}	0.6667	0	1	0.3333	0.6667	C_2	X_{173}	99.53%	C_2
X_{269}	0	0.5	0.3333	1	0.3333	C_1	X_{96}	98.94%	C_1
X_{293}	0.6667	0	ϕ	0.3333	0.3333	C_1	X_{96}	98.94%	C_2
X_{301}	0.3333	0.5	0.3333	1	ϕ	C_1	X_{96}	98.94%	C_1

In the experiment results, X269, X293, and X301 from heart-c data set are uncertain. Their uncertain value can be calculated by formula 14: $\phi = 0.784$.

5.3 Comparison of the Search Efficiency Based on the AUC

In this experiment, we assume that the miscategorization losses of the samples from the same category are the same. The next step is to compare the results acquired by different methods, including the Bayesian network method and others. When λ_1/λ_2 is large, the weight of the positive sample assigned by the Bayesian fusion search is large. We next conduct a categorization test on them because neither λ_1 or λ_2 can be obtained directly. It is known from the constraint that the misclassification loss range is $[-1, 1]$; let $\lambda_1 = 1$ and the range of λ_2 is $[0.1, 0.9]$. If a sample from the case matching is completely correct, then $\lambda_1 = \lambda_2 = 1$. The result of the CBNF model compared with the traditional tree enhancement Bayesian (TBN) is shown in Fig. 1.

When λ_2 increases from 0.1 to 0.9, λ_1/λ_2 becomes less variable. At the same time, the F value, $F_0(x)$ and accuracy are likely to fluctuate to a certain degree and reach an optimal status. $Precison = TP/(TP + FP)$ and $F - measure = 2/(1/F_0(x) + 1/P)$ represent the harmonic mean between precision and sensitivity.

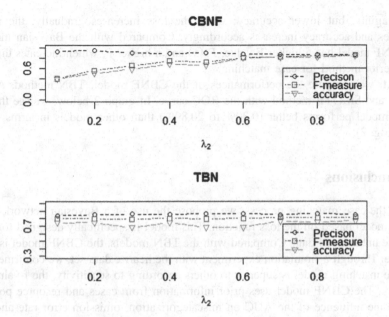

Fig. 1. The results of the cost-sensitive comparison between the CBNF model and TBN method

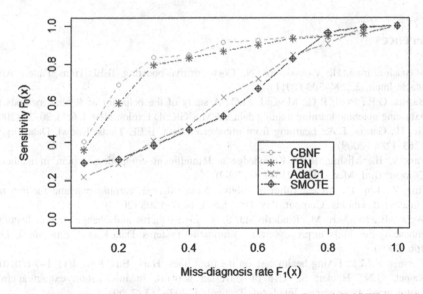

Fig. 2. The ROC curve of the CBNF model and TBN, AdaC1 and SMOTE methods

Graph 4 illustrates that: the agility level is higher than the accuracy level in terms of the CBNF model and Bayesian methods, with the agility line lying above the F value line and accuracy line lying below the F value line; the CBNF model is more sensitive to the miscategorization loss issue. When the cost is high, the CBNF model has a higher agility, but lower accuracy; when the loss increases gradually, the agility decreases and accuracy increases accordingly. Compared with the Bayesian method, the CBNF model has a higher F value, $F_0(x)$ and a higher P, which indicates that it is the superior method for case matching.

Next, we compare the performances of the CBNF model, TBN method, AdaC1 method and SMOTE method with the ROC curve. In graph 2 below, we see that the CBNF model performs better (0.30% to 20.89%) than other models in terms of the AUC (Fig. 2).

6 Conclusions

During the case matching process, we propose the use of a Bayesian network information model based on the loss function. This model is specifically designed for cost-sensitive unbalanced data. Compared with the TBN models, the CBNF model is more accurate. Through a simulation experiment with the heart-c data-set, we confirmed that our case matching model is superior to others according to sensitivity, the f-value and accuracy. The CBNF model uses prior information from cases and resource pools to analyze the influence of the AUC on miscategorization, omission error rate and cost sensitivity. Considering the cost of miscategorization, these results provide a better retrieval strategy.

References

1. Masnadi-Shirazi, H., Vasconcelos, N.: Cost-sensitive boosting. IEEE Trans. Pattern Anal. Mach. Intell. **2**, 294–309 (2011)
2. Batista, G.E., Prati, R.C., Monard, M.C.: A study of the behavior of several methods for balancing machine learning training data. ACM SIGKDD Explor. Newsl. **6**(1), 20–29 (2004)
3. He, H., Garcia, E.A.: Learning from imbalanced data. IEEE Trans. Knowl. Data Eng. **9**, 1263–1284 (2009)
4. Pandey, B., Mishra, R.B.: Knowledge and intelligent computing system in medicine. Comput. Biol. Med. **39**(3), 215–230 (2009)
5. Jing, Z., Lin, F.: An algorithm of robust online extreme learning machine for dynamic imbalanced datasets. Comput. Res. Dev. **52**(7), 1487–1498 (2015)
6. Weber, B., Reichert, M., Rinderle-Ma, S.: Change patterns and change support features–enhancing flexibility in process-aware information systems. Data Knowl. Eng. **66**(3), 438–466 (2008)
7. Bohmer, R.M.J.: Fixing health care on the front lines. Harv. Bus. Rev. **4**(1), 1–7 (2010)
8. Rajput, Q.N., Haider, S.: Use of Bayesian network in information extraction from unstructured data sources. Int. J. Inf. Technol. **4**, 207–213 (2009)
9. Uramoto, N., Matsuzawa, H., et al.: A text-mining system for knowledge discovery from biomedical documents. IBM Syst. J. **43**(3), 516–533 (2010)
10. Heeb, N.V., Bach, C., Am, M.P.F.: On the 2-tuples based genetic tuning performance for fuzzy rule based classification systems in imbalanced data-sets. Inf. Sci. **180**(8), 1268–1291 (2010)
11. Gao, Y.F., Tang, Y.L., Chen, Y.W.: Bayesian networks structure learning based on cost-sensitive criterion. J. Chin. Comput. Syst. **30**(2), 313–316 (2009)

12. Waegeman, W., De Baets, B., Boullart, L.: ROC analysis in ordinal regression learning. Pattern Recognit. Lett. **29**(1), 1–9 (2008)
13. Zhang, X., Li, X., Feng, Y., et al.: The use of ROC and AUC in the validation of objective image fusion evaluation metrics. Signal Process. **115**, 38–48 (2015)
14. Dmochowski, J.P., Sajda, P., et al.: Maximum likelihood in cost-sensitive learning: model specification, approximations, and upper bounds. J. Mach. Learn. Res. **11**(18), 3313–3332 (2010)
15. Dey, D., Sarkar, S., De, P.: A probabilistic decision model for entity matching in heterogeneous Databases. Manag. Sci. **44**(10), 1379–1387 (1998)
16. Asuncion, A., Newman, D.: UCI machine learning repository. University of California, Irvine, School of Information and Computer Sciences (2007). http://www.ics.uci.edu/mlearn/MLRepository.html

Readmission Prediction Using Trajectory-Based Deep Learning Approach

Jiaheng Xie[✉], Bin Zhang, and Daniel Zeng

University of Arizona, Tucson, USA
xiej@email.arizona.edu

Abstract. Hospital readmission refers to the situation where a patient is re-hospitalized with the same primary diagnosis after discharge. It causes $26 billion preventable expense to the U.S. health systems annually and may indicate suboptimal care for patients. Predicting readmission risk is essential to alleviate such financial and medical consequences. Yet such prediction is challenging due to the dynamic and complex nature of the hospitalization trajectory. The state-of-the-art studies apply statistical models with unified parameters for all patients and use static predictors in a period, failing to consider patients' heterogeneous illness trajectories. Our approach – TADEL (Trajectory-BAsed DEep Learning) – addresses the present challenge and captures various illness trajectories. We evaluate TADEL on a unique five-year national Medicare claims dataset, reaching a precision of 0.780, a recall of 0.985, and an F1-score of 0.870. This study contributes to IS literature and methodology by formulating the readmission prediction problem and developing a novel personalized readmission risk prediction framework. This framework provides direct implications for health providers to assess patients' readmission risk and take early interventions to avoid potential negative consequences.

Keywords: Hospital readmission · Predictive analytics · Deep learning
Health IT · Design science

1 Introduction

Hospital readmission is a critical concern in disease management. It is usually defined as the situation where a patient discharged from a hospital is admitted again within 30 days (Axon and Williams 2011). The 30-day readmission leads to an annual cost of $26 billion dollars (Center for Health Information and Analysis 2015) and may indicate suboptimal care for patients, such as fragmented and poorly coordinated care, inappropriate transitions between inpatient and outpatient settings, and even medical errors (Dhalla et al. 2014). Taking interventions to alleviate such consequences demands proactive prediction for patients' readmission risk.

Most prior studies apply statistical methods, such as regression and duration models, to predict patients' readmission risk (Bardhan et al. 2015; Jovanovic et al. 2016). However, significant challenges still exist in those methods, because of the complex nature of patients' illness process. Numerous studies have documented that an

© Springer Nature Switzerland AG 2018
H. Chen et al. (Eds.): ICSH 2018, LNCS 10983, pp. 224–230, 2018.
https://doi.org/10.1007/978-3-030-03649-2_22

illness is not a one-stop outcome. Rather, it contains a dynamic trajectory, such as initial, onset, crisis, acute, stable, unstable, downward, and dying (Corbin and Strauss 1991; Woog 1992). The multi-stage illness trajectory viewpoint poses three major challenges for existing statistical models. First, patients visit hospitals in different phases in the illness trajectory, thus having varied health states and hazard. Regression and duration models aim to estimate the readmission risk at the population level. Such homogeneous models are not capable of capturing patients' heterogeneous health states. Second, as some patients may not experience all the eight phases in the illness trajectory, the hospitalization trajectory should differ for different patients. In addition, patients' time and frequency of hospitalizations and illness phase transitions vary significantly. The current statistical models cannot capture such variance in patients' hospitalization trajectory. Third, a multi-stage illness trajectory requires sequential and dynamic predictors to model the process. Existing studies only use static predictors for each patient (Jovanovic et al. 2016; Radovanovic et al. 2015). Even for studies with panel data, each data entry only contains the predictors for a specified time period. This static feature representation neglects information at different phases of the illness trajectory. To address the abovementioned three challenges, we aim to develop a more fine-grained model to account for patients' illness trajectory.

Recent advances in deep learning, such as long short-term memory (LSTM), show great promise in processing sequential data and remembering long term information (Xie et al. 2017). This unique feature may improve the readmission prediction by incorporating the complete illness trajectory. However, standard LSTMs assume that each health state has a constant contribution to the next health state, ignoring different hospitalization patterns of various patients. During a series of hospitalizations, the time intervals between successive hospitalizations vary from days to months. The potencies of such varied-time hospitalizations should differ. To utilize a dynamic sequential representation and account for patients' heterogeneous health conditions and hospitalization trajectories, we aim to base on an LSTM design while enhancing it by weighting the potencies of different states in the hospitalization trajectory.

This study contributes to healthcare theory by examining the validity of illness trajectory theory in the context of hospital readmission. We also contribute to methodology by developing a novel trajectory-based deep learning approach. The proposed approach also has the potential to tackle any other sequential data with differed potencies in different states, such as online shopping history, crowdfunding investment records, and online course learning process. To IS literature, we formulate the hospital readmission prediction problem and develop a risk predictive approach to improve clinical decision making. This problem together with the proposed approach can be generalized to many other risk assessment context, such as phishing website detection, financial fraud identification, and IT vulnerability assessment.

2 Literature Review

Prior studies developed predictive models to identify patients with high risk of being readmitted within 30 days, so that early interventions can be taken to improve health care for patients and avoid unnecessary cost to the health systems. Most of the existing studies leveraged statistical models, such as regression and duration models, to predict patient's risk of being readmitted in 30 days, with an AUC ranging from 0.6 to 0.8 (Radovanovic et al. 2015; Shadmi et al. 2015). A few studies also applied machine learning models, including SVM and Naïve Bayes (Chen et al. 2015; Yu et al. 2015). To construct the feature set for these models, extant research used static predictors within a study period, such as demographics, augmented medical service uses, and illness severity (Kansagara et al. 2011).

Instead of using a static and homogeneous model, abundant health studies have documented that a patient may experience a series of phases in an illness trajectory (Corbin and Strauss 1991; Woog 1992). Each phase has different level of hazard, resulting in greatly varied risks across patients. Corbin and Strauss (1991) have proposed the illness trajectory theory which details eight phases of an illness trajectory: initial, onset, crisis, acute, stable, unstable, downward, and dying. Various studies successfully leveraged a multi-state approach to model an illness trajectory and outperformed methods without the trajectory. Despite its value in various research applications and its outstanding performance compared to methods without trajectory, the multi-state approach has not been utilized to understand the latent health states during readmission process. Therefore, we are motivated to harness a multi-state design for this study to consider patients' dynamic illness trajectory and heterogeneous hazard.

3 The Proposed Approach

We propose a novel trajectory-based representation to represent the hospitalization trajectory. Let V_t be an array of features for hospitalization at time t. Let N be the number of hospitalizations of a patient in the study time window. We construct a hospitalization trajectory matrix denoted as $[V_1, V_2, \ldots, V_N]$. In the staged trajectory-based deep learning model, each hospitalization will be fed into the model in a stepwise manner.

We design the trajectory-based long short-term memory (LSTM) to process the trajectory-based representation and predict the 30-day readmission risk. An LSTM unit contains a memory cell that stores long term hospitalization information, as shown in Eq. 1. At each time step, this memory cell takes a new hospitalization record $V^{(t)}$ and maintains a portion of prior hospitalization information $h^{(t-1)}$. $tanh(\cdot)$ is the activation function for the memory cell. The operator $\circ$ is element-wise multiplication. W, U, and b are the learnable weight parameters with value between 0 and 1. We further add a decreasing function $\frac{1}{log(e+\Delta_t)}$ to discount the last hidden state, where Δ_t is the time interval between two consecutive hospitalizations, as shown in Eq. 2. The decreasing function could discount the hospitalizations that are far away from the current health state. For instance, a large Δ_t means that the previous hospitalization is far away from the current health state. Thus the decreasing function will be small, indicating a minor impact of the last hospitalization on the next health state. To increase the impact of historical readmission records, we further modify the memory cell by multiplying an indication function $log(e + 1(readmitted))$ to each hospitalization input. When $V^{(t)}$ is a historical readmission record, $1(readmitted)$ returns 1 ($log(e + 1(readmitted)) > 1$), thus amplifying the impact of this record.

$$c^{(t)*} = i^{(t)} \circ \Theta + f^{(t)} \circ c^{(t-1)} \tag{1}$$

$$\Theta = tanh\left(W_u\left(V^{(t)} \times log(e + 1(readmitted)) \right) + U_u\left(h^{(t-1)} \times \frac{1}{log(e + \Delta_t)} \right) + b_u \right) \tag{2}$$

The trajectory-based LSTM unit also contains an input gate $i^{(t)}$, a forget gate $f^{(t)}$, an output gate $o^{(t)}$, and a hidden state $h^{(t)}$. The three gates inherit prior hospitalization information $h^{(t-1)}$ and also receive the current hospitalization record $V^{(t)}$. Similar to the adjustment in the memory cell, we also modify the three gates by discounting the last health state with the function $\frac{1}{log(e + \Delta_t)}$, so that the gates are sensitive to varied time intervals. We also adjust the input $V^{(t)}$ by multiplying the indication function $log(e + 1(readmitted))$ to increase the influence of prior readmission records. Equations 3–6 detail the computation.

$$i^{(t)} = \sigma\left(W_i\left(V^{(t)} \times log(e + 1(readmitted)) \right) + U_i\left(h^{(t-1)} \times \frac{1}{log(e + \Delta_t)} \right) + b_i \right) \tag{3}$$

$$f^{(t)} = \sigma\left(W_f\left(V^{(t)} \times log(e + 1(readmitted)) \right) + U_f\left(h^{(t-1)} \times \frac{1}{log(e + \Delta_t)} \right) + b_f \right) \tag{4}$$

$$o^{(t)} = \sigma\left(W_o\left(V^{(t)} \times log(e + 1(readmitted)) \right) + U_o\left(h^{(t-1)} \times \frac{1}{log(e + \Delta_t)} \right) + b_o \right) \tag{5}$$

$$h^{(t)} = o^{(t)} \circ tanh\left(c^{(t)*} \right) \tag{6}$$

For a patient, the input to the trajectory-based LSTM model is the hospitalization trajectory matrix. The following layer is the trajectory-based LSTM unit to process this matrix recurrently. Finally, a Softmax layer (the following equation) is stacked on top to predict the probability of a patient to be readmitted within 30 days.

4 Empirical Analyses

We utilize patient hospitalization information and health conditions from a five-year national Medicare claims dataset in this study. Based on prior literature (Kansagara et al. 2011; van Walraven et al. 2010), we select four categories of features from the Medicare claims dataset to predict readmission risk. 1. Health status factors (Hammill et al. 2011; Holman et al. 2005). 2. Social determinants of health (Hasan et al. 2010; Silverstein et al. 2008). 3. History of health service utilizations and hospitalizations (Howell et al. 2009; van Walraven et al. 2010). 4. Sociodemographic information (Bottle et al. 2006; Krumholz et al. 2009).

We initially identified 72,709 patients who had at least one 30-day readmission record in 2015 as the readmission group. We then randomly selected another 72,709 patients who had only one hospitalization record (no 30-day readmissions) in 2015 as the control group (non-readmission group). Table 1 shows the model performance. Table 2 shows the significance tests.

Table 1. Model performance

Model	Precision	Recall	F1-score
Naïve Bayes	0.708	0.728	0.718
Logit	0.827	0.703	0.760
SVM	**0.830**	0.687	0.751
HMM	0.522	0.614	0.565
LSTM	0.735	**0.997**	0.846
TADEL[1] (Ours)	0.780	0.985	**0.870**

[1]TADEL: trajectory-based deep learning

Table 2. P-value of T-tests for TADEL against baseline models

Model pair	Precision	Recall	F1-score
TADEL vs Naïve Bayes	<0.001***	<0.001***	<0.001***
TADEL vs Logit	(0.012*)	<0.001***	<0.001***
TADEL vs SVM	(0.009**)	<0.001***	<0.001***
TADEL vs HMM	<0.001***	<0.001***	<0.001***
TADEL vs LSTM	0.015*	(0.055)	0.011*

(.): TADEL < baseline model

Our proposed trajectory-based deep learning (TADEL) outperforms all the baseline models, indicating good design of the trajectory component.

5   Conclusion

Our research objective was to predict patient's 30-day readmission risk while accounting for patient's heterogeneous illness trajectory. We designed a high-performance trajectory-based deep learning framework. The key stakeholders could leverage this framework to take targeted interventions for high-risk patients in order to reduce negative consequences.

References

Axon, R.N., Williams, M.V.: Hospital readmission as an accountability measure. JAMA **305**(5), 504 (2011)

Bardhan, I., Oh, J.H.C., Zheng, Z.E., Kirksey, K.: Predictive analytics for readmission of patients with congestive heart failure. Inf. Syst. Res. **26**(1), 19–39 (2015)

Bottle, A., Aylin, P., Majeed, A.: Identifying patients at high risk of emergency hospital admissions: a logistic regression analysis. J. R. Soc. Med. **99**(8), 406–414 (2006)

Brännström, J., Sönnerborg, A., Svedhem, V., Neogi, U., Marrone, G.: A high rate of HIV-1 acquisition post immigration among migrants in Sweden determined by a CD4 T-cell decline trajectory model. HIV Med. **18**(9), 677–684 (2017)

Center for Health Information and Analysis: Performance of the Massachusetts Health Care System Series: A Focus on Provider Quality (2015)

Chen, R., et al.: Cloud-based predictive modeling system and its application to asthma readmission prediction. In: AMIA Annual Symposium Proceedings. AMIA Symposium vol. 2015, pp. 406–415 (2015)

Coleman, E.A., Min, S.J., Chomiak, A., Kramer, A.M.: Posthospital care transitions: patterns, complications, and risk identification. Health Serv. Res. **39**(5), 1449–1466 (2004)

Corbin, J.M., Strauss, A.: A nursing model for chronic illness management based upon the trajectory framework. Sch. Inq. Nurs. Pract. **5**, 155–1774 (1991)

Dhalla, I.A., et al.: Effect of a postdischarge virtual ward on readmission or death for high-risk patients. JAMA **312**(13), 1305 (2014)

Donnelly, C., McFetridge, L.M., Marshall, A.H., Mitchell, H.J.: A two-stage approach to the joint analysis of longitudinal and survival data utilising the Coxian phase-type distribution. Stat. Methods Med. Res. (2017) https://doi.org/10.1177/0962280217706727

Glance, L.G., et al.: Hospital readmission after noncardiac surgery. JAMA Surg. **149**(5), 439 (2014)

Halfon, P., Eggli, Y., Pêtre-Rohrbach, I., Meylan, D., Marazzi, A., Burnand, B.: Validation of the potentially avoidable hospital readmission rate as a routine indicator of the quality of hospital care. Med. Care **44**(11), 972–981 (2006)

Hammill, B.G., et al.: Incremental value of clinical data beyond claims data in predicting 30-day outcomes after heart failure hospitalization. Circ. Cardiovasc. Qual. Outcomes **4**(1), 60–67 (2011)

Hasan, O., et al.: Hospital readmission in general medicine patients: a prediction model. J. Gen. Intern. Med. **25**(3), 211–219 (2010)

Holman, C.D.J., Preen, D.B., Baynham, N.J., Finn, J.C., Semmens, J.B.: A multipurpose comorbidity scoring system performed better than the Charlson index. J. Clin. Epidemiol. **58** (10), 1006–1014 (2005)

Howell, S., Coory, M., Martin, J., Duckett, S.: Using routine inpatient data to identify patients at risk of hospital readmission. BMC Health Serv. Res. **9**(1), 96 (2009)

Hser, Y.I., Longshore, D., Anglin, M.D.: The life course perspective on drug use. Eval. Rev. **31** (6), 515–547 (2007)

Jovanovic, M., Radovanovic, S., Vukicevic, M., Van Poucke, S., Delibasic, B.: Building interpretable predictive models for pediatric hospital readmission using Tree-Lasso logistic regression. Artif. Intell. Med. **72**, 12–21 (2016)

Kansagara, D., et al.: Risk prediction models for hospital readmission. JAMA **306**(15), 1688 (2011)

Krumholz, H.M., et al.: Patterns of hospital performance in acute myocardial infarction and heart failure 30-day mortality and readmission. Circ. Cardiovasc. Qual. Outcomes **2**(5), 407–413 (2009)

Mishel, M.H.: Reconceptualization of the uncertainty in illness theory. Image J. Nurs. Scholarsh. **22**(4), 256–262 (1990)

Paul, S.S., et al.: Two-year trajectory of fall risk in people with parkinson disease: a latent class analysis. Arch. Phys. Med. Rehabil. **97**(3), 372–379.e1 (2016)

Radovanovic, S., Vukicevic, M., Kovacevic, A., Stiglic, G., Obradovic, Z.: Domain knowledge based hierarchical feature selection for 30-day hospital readmission prediction. In: Holmes, John H., Bellazzi, R., Sacchi, L., Peek, N. (eds.) AIME 2015. LNCS (LNAI), vol. 9105, pp. 96–100. Springer, Cham (2015). https://doi.org/10.1007/978-3-319-19551-3_11

Shadmi, E., Flaks-Manov, N., Hoshen, M., Goldman, O., Bitterman, H., Balicer, R.D.: Predicting 30-day readmissions with preadmission electronic health record data. Med. Care **53**(3), 283–289 (2015)

Silverstein, M.D., Qin, H., Mercer, S.Q., Fong, J., Haydar, Z.: Risk factors for 30-day hospital readmission in patients ≥ 65 years of age. Proc. (Bayl. Univ. Med. Cent.) **21**(4), 363–372 (2008)

Vukicevic, M., Radovanovic, S., Kovacevic, A., Stiglic, G., Obradovic, Z.: Improving hospital readmission prediction using domain knowledge based virtual examples. In: Uden, L., Heričko, M., Ting, I.-H. (eds.) KMO 2015. LNBIP, vol. 224, pp. 695–706. Springer, Cham (2015). https://doi.org/10.1007/978-3-319-21009-4_51

van Walraven, C., et al.: Derivation and validation of an index to predict early death or unplanned readmission after discharge from hospital to the community. CMAJ **182**(6), 551–557 (2010)

Woog, P.: The Chronic Illness Trajectory Framework: The Corbin and Strauss Nursing Model. Springer Publishing Company, New York (1992)

Xie, J., Liu, X., Zeng, D.D.: Mining e-cigarette adverse events in social media using Bi-LSTM recurrent neural network with word embedding representation. J. Am. Med. Inform. Assoc. **25**, 72–80 (2017)

Yu, S., Farooq, F., Esbroeck, A., Fung, G., Anand, V., Krishnapuram, B.: Predicting readmission risk with institution-specific prediction models. Artif. Intell. Med. **65**(2), 89–96 (2015)

ICSH 2018: LSTM based Sentiment Analysis for Patient Experience Narratives in E-survey Tools

Chenxi Xia, Dong Zhao, Jing Wang, Jing Liu, and Jingdong Ma(✉)

School of Medicine and Health Management, Tongji Medical College,
Huazhong University of Science and Technology, 13 Hangkong Road,
Wuhan 430030, Hubei, China
JDMA@hust.edu.cn

Abstract. Background: Analysis of patient experience narratives is helpful to improve care service and to promote patient satisfaction. As more and more E-survey tools went on line, a huge amount of patient comments has become a challenge to analysts. Sentiment analysis is a fully explored machine learning method to classify texts according their sentimental orientation. However, it is seldom applied to the analysis of patient comments, especially in China. Objectives: This paper aims to test the performance of the classical sentiment analysis methods and find an applicable solution of Chinese patient experience narratives analysis. Data: 20,000 patient experience narratives are collected from two hospital's E-survey tools, a mobile patient follow-up system and a WeChat App of patient comments. Methods: Five machine learning methods, Support Vector Machine (SVM), Random Forests (RF), Gradient Boost Decision Tree (GBDT), XGBoost and Long Short-Term Memory (LSTM), are used to explore the sentiment analysis performance of Chinese patient comments. $\chi 2$ statistics is used for feature selection. And Skip-gram model is used for word-embedding. Results: The experiment results showed that LSTM achieved much better performance than SVM did. The F-Measure values of LSTM for positive category and negative category are both 98.87, which is better than other traditional machine learning methods. Conclusion: The result of this paper suggests that LSTM based sentiment analysis is a practical method to exploit the ever-increasing patient experience narratives.

Keywords: Patient experience · Sentiment analysis · Free text
Electronic survey

1 Introduction

With healthcare becoming more patient centered and value driven, patient experiences have drawn increasing interests from multiple stakeholders, highlighting the importance of measuring, reporting, and improving outcomes that are meaningful to patients. Incorporating patient's needs and perspectives are considered as indispensable for quality improvement in healthcare delivery [1, 2]. Recently, the healthcare regulators shifted towards a market-driven approach of turning patient satisfaction surveys into a

© Springer Nature Switzerland AG 2018
H. Chen et al. (Eds.): ICSH 2018, LNCS 10983, pp. 231–239, 2018.
https://doi.org/10.1007/978-3-030-03649-2_23

quality improvement tool for overall organizational performance. Traditionally, patient satisfaction surveys are delivered to patients in various ways, including post, telephone, and face to face. Enabling by information and communication technologies (ICTs), more and more healthcare managers tend to collect the satisfaction information via electronic ways, adopting a variety of E-survey tools such as online websites, mobile apps, social media, or a mixture of these [3–5]. Apart from the advantages in cost and efficiency, E-survey tools are typically useful for collecting the unstructured information such as patient comments, experience sharing or complaints. Thanks to the convenience of electronic survey, healthcare delivery organizations now receive huge volume of information containing patient experience narratives. These patient experience narratives can provide important and additional knowledge to healthcare delivery organizations regarding to safety and quality enhancement. Moreover, analyzing data on negative patient experiences strengthens the ability to detect systematic problems in care delivery system. However, current approaches for handling such narratives heavily rely on manually coding or triaging, which are both time and labor consuming, and eventually result in an underuse of such valuable information source [6, 7].

Progress in natural language processing and machine learning algorithm provides promising alternatives over the manual ways in handling patient experience narratives. With the natural language processing techniques, the patients' free text descriptions of their care could be converted into a social intelligence dataset by analyzing the collected statements for sentiment and reliability, transforming them into an aggregated, quantitative measure of experience for the care delivery organizations. Hereinto, sentiment analysis is a very useful and important research area. Sentiment analysis methods aim to determine the attitude expressed with respect to some theme or the overall contextual polarity of a document. Originating in the field of web mining, the development of sentiment analysis methods often concentrates on processing texts in e-commerce area such as customer reviews [8–10]. In the area of healthcare, sentiment analysis is attracting growing interest. There are literatures that documented using sentiment analysis to mining patient opinion toward health care providers in social media or online physician rating websites [11–13]. These researches have shown the potential of sentiment analysis in handling patient experience narratives. However, most of these studies used the downloaded user generated content as data source, which is poor quality and would lead to unreliable results. Existing sentiment analysis methods developed for processing unstructured text in web media treat the task as a classification problem: a classifier is trained to detect the polarity at sentence or document level. A series of super-vised methods such as naive Bayes, support vector machines (SVM) and maximum entropy classification have been used in sentiment analysis [14]. More recently, neural networks have been shown several advantages over the previous mentioned methods in training high quality classifier. Yet, there in a dearth of relevant researches in processing patient experience narratives [15].

In this study, we used five machine-learning methods, Random Forests (RF), Gradient Boost Decision Tree (GBDT), XGBoost and Long Short-Term Memory (LSTM), to explore the sentiment analysis performance of Chinese patient comments. The results suggest that LSTM based sentiment analysis is a practical method to exploit the ever-increasing patient experience narratives.

2 Related Works

As a hot topic of Nature Language Processing, sentiment analysis, or sentiment Classification, has been studied for many years. Early sentiment classification was often used to identify consumer reviews [16–19]. Today, sentiment classification has emerged in politics, economic, medical [12, 13, 20] and other fields. Ayata [21] used LSTM to predict political orientation through twitter data, and achieved 77.92% accuracy rate. Romanowski A [22] used twitter data for sentiment classification to predict stock price.

2.1 Sentiment Classification Methods

With the continuous development of sentiment classification research, more and more new methods have been proposed, and the performance of sentiment classification is constantly improving. We split the methods of emotional classification into the following two categories.

Sentiment dictionary. based methods classify documents according to manual established sentiment dictionaries and heuristic rules. Hu [23] classifies on-line product reviews with 84.2% accuracy. Ding [24] proposed a holistic lexicon-based approach and reached 91% F-value on customer reviews. A good sentiment dictionary [25–27] is the key component of dictionary-based method and needs to be established in advance. Manual corrections are often needed when the dictionary applied to different domains.

Supervised machine learning is the prevailing solution of sentiment classification in nowadays. Support Vector Machines (SVM), Maximum Entropy (ME), Naive Bayes (NB), and other traditional machine learning methods are fully explored on the topic. Pang [28] used the three methods of NB, ME, and SVM and achieved the highest accuracy of 82.9%. The performance of this approach relies on the quality of feature engineering[6,17,] [29, 30]. However, a good solution often requires cooperation of domain experts for feature extraction. Recently, deep learning methods have gradually been favored by researchers, especially after the word vector method [31] solves the problem of dimensional explosions [32] and semantic gaps. Researchers began to use the Convolution Neural Network (CNN), Recursive Neural Network (ReNN), and Recurrent Neural Network (RNN) to perform sentiment analysis of massive corpus and obtained better performance. Poria [33] used a deep CNN for aspect extraction to obtained better accuracy. Ganin [34] proposed a Domain-Adversarial Neural Networks to analyze Amazon reviews and achieved a significantly better performance than NN and SVM. Chau [35] combined deep learning and sub-tree mining, and achieved 0.14%–6.93% improvements of accuracy over LSTM + GRNN model.

2.2 Sentiment Classification of Patient Experiences Narratives

Elmessiry [14] automatically classified the complaints of 14335 patients with six machine learning methods. Del Arco FMP [36] conducted a sentiment analysis of patient opinions in Spanish. Gillespie [6] established a classification framework for patient complaints. Greaves [12] use sentiment analysis to categorize 6412 online free-text comments, and reached 89% agreement with patient quantitative ratings. Hopper

[13] use sentiment analysis and time-to-next-compliant method to convert patient reviews and help health service providers improve patient satisfaction. ElMessiry [20] use LIWC lexicons and a Naïve Bayes classifier to categorize patients' compliments, and yields 3% greater accuracy over traditional methods.

3   Data

We collected patient experience narratives from two hospital's E-survey tools, a mobile patient follow-up system and a WeChat App of patient comments. The patient narratives of the follow-up system were input and labelled as positive or negative narratives by some hospital employees. The narratives of the WeChat App were input by patients or their family members, and labelled by two medical school students. Then the labelled narratives were cross-checked and rectified to achieve 100% agreement between the two annotators. Finally, we randomly sampled 10,000 narratives, half positive and half negative, from each of the system. At last, we got a corpus of 20,000 patient experience narratives. Tow samples of the patient narratives are listed in Table 1.

Table 1. Samples of the patient experience narratives

Category	Original text
negative	在住院期间医生给病人做了很多检查都没有检查出什么病，所有诊断都只是在怀疑，医生也没有做任何解释。在 10 月 21 号晚上病人突发肚子痛，痛得打滚，当时是廖建恩医生值班，他来给病人看过后没告诉病人家属应该怎么处理和用什么药，以至于病人家属很着急，去问护士，护士也说不知道医生开了什么药。所以病人家属很不满意。
Positive	有一次病人去医生办公室找医生询问病情，不小心看到桌面的病例研讨记录，正好是他的病情，病人觉得能把自己的病交给这样负责的团队很放心。

4   Method

4.1   Word Segmentation

We did word segmentation of each patient narrative with ICTCLAS [37], a commonly used Chinese word segmentation package. Two professional vocabularies, CMeSH [38] (Chinese Medical Subject Headings) and ICD-10 [39] (International Classification of Diseases-10) were used as external vocabularies with ICTCLAS.

4.2   Classification

We classified the patient narratives with five methods, SVM [40], Random Forests (RF) [41], Gradient Boost Decision Tree (GBDT) [42] and XGBoost [43], and Long Short-Term Memory (LSTM) [44].

We classified the patient narratives with SVM, RF, and GBDT in the following 5 steps.

(1) We generated a document-word-matrix at first. Each row of the matrix represented a narrative, and each column represented a word appearing in one of the narratives.
(2) We filtered out the words other than nouns, verbs, adjectives, or adverbs.
(3) We selected the most distinctive words by χ^2 statistics [45–47]. Only the top 5% words of each category were preserved.
(4) The value of each element of the document-word-matrix is calculated by TFIDF [48].
(5) The classifiers were trained and tested.

We classified the patient narratives with LSTM in the following 3 steps.

(1) We did word embedding with Skip-Gram model [31]. The corpus used for word embedding includes Chinese Wikipedia and professional documents of the health domain, e.g., papers and books. After word segmentation and removing non-word characters, the corpus contains about 195 million words. The result of word embedding is a vocabulary of 448820 words. Each word is represented by a vector of 200 elements.
(2) Each word of the patient narratives was mapped to the corresponding vector. Each patient narrative was transformed into a sequence of word vectors. The words or characters with no corresponding entry in the word embedding vocabulary were removed. Finally, each sequence was padded with 0 to the maximum length of all patient narrative sequences.
(3) The LSTM classifiers were trained and tested. The super-parameters of the LSTM model are listed in Table 2.

Table 2. The super-parameters of the LSTM model

Super-parameter	Value
Dimension of hidden state	128
Optimizer	ADAM [49]
Learning rate	0.01
Epoches	100
L2 regularization coefficient for the weights	1e-4
Gradient normalization strategy	ClipElementWiseAbsoluteValue [31] #

For each gradient g, set g = sign(g) max(1.0, |g|). i.e., if a parameter gradient has absolute value greater than 1.0, truncate it.

4.3   Performance Evaluation

We used 5-fold cross validation to test the performance of all classifiers. We split the corpus of 20,000 patient narratives into 5 groups. Each group contains 2,000 positive samples and 2,000 negative samples. Half of the 2000 samples come from the follow-up system, and another half comes from the WeChat app. Each time, one group was used as test samples, and the other 4 groups were used as train samples. The precision, recall, and F1-Measure were calculated for the all classifiers. And finally, the results were averaged.

5   Results

The results of our experiments are shown in Table 3.

Table 3. The performance of sentiment classification

Category	Measure	Classifier				
		LSTM	SVM	RF	GBDT	XGBoost
Negative	Precision	98.75	81.07	97.07	95.98	97.57
	Recall	98.99	100.00	97.80	97.85	98.30
	F1-measure	98.87	89.55	97.43	96.91	97.93
Positive	Precision	98.99	100.00	97.78	97.81	98.29
	Recall	98.74	76.65	97.05	95.90	97.55
	F1-measure	98.87	86.79	97.42	96.84	97.92

6   Discussion

As we can see from the results, The LSTM model is much better than the SVM model, and slightly better than RF, GBDT, and XGBoost. Other papers suggested the same conclusion, although in other languages or in other domains [21, 50, 51]. The better performance of LSTM is underpinned by the following two facts. At first, the input fed into traditional machine learning methods is a document-word-matrix. In other words, the features of each patient narrative are word lemmas. It means that "love" and "like" are totally different two features. However, the input of LSTM is a sequence of vectors. Each vector is generated by word-embedding and is a distributed version of the semantics of the corresponding word. The vectors of synonym or near-synonym are similar to each other. Secondly, the LSTM model is designed to recognize patterns in sequences of data, especially patterns over many time steps, or word distance, e.g., the relationship of a negative word and a praiseful expression.

The Skip-Gram + LSTM framework is a practical solution of sentiment analysis of Chinese patient experience narratives. However, the solution must be supported by two pillars, a high-quality word embedding vocabulary generated from a corpus with enough words, and a train set of enough and balanced or near-balanced examples.

7 Conclusion

The result of this paper suggests that LSTM model combining with Skip-Gram model is a practical solution to of patient experience narratives' sentiment analysis. This solution can help exploit the ever-increasing patient experience narratives, strengthen the ability to detect systematic problems in care delivery system, and promote patient satisfaction.

References

1. Al-Abri, R., Al-Balushi, A.: Patient satisfaction survey as a tool towards quality improvement. Oman Med. J. **29**, 3 (2014)
2. Zgierska, A., Rabago, D., Miller, M.M.: Impact of patient satisfaction ratings on physicians and clinical care. Patient Prefer. Adherence **8**, 437 (2014)
3. Boos, J., et al.: Electronic kiosks for patient satisfaction survey in radiology. Am. J. Roentgenol. **208**, 577–584 (2017)
4. McPeake, J., Bateson, M., O'Neill, A.: Electronic surveys: how to maximise success. Nurse Res. (2014+) **21**, 24 (2014)
5. Repplinger, M.D., et al.: The impact of an emergency department front-end redesign on patient-reported satisfaction survey results. West. J. Emerg. Med. **18**, 1068 (2017)
6. Gillespie, A., Reader, T.W.: The healthcare complaints analysis tool: development and reliability testing of a method for service monitoring and organisational learning. BMJ Qual. Saf. **25**, 937–946 (2016)
7. Reader, T.W., Gillespie, A., Roberts, J.: Patient complaints in healthcare systems: a systematic review and coding taxonomy. BMJ Qual. Saf. **23**, 678–689 (2014)
8. Hamouda, A.E.-D.A., El-taher, F.E.-Z.: Sentiment analyzer for arabic comments system. Int. J. Adv. Comput. Sci. Appl. **4**, 99–103 (2013)
9. Shamshurin, I.: Data representation in machine learning-based sentiment analysis of customer reviews. In: Kuznetsov, S.O., Mandal, D.P., Kundu, M.K., Pal, S.K. (eds.) PReMI 2011. LNCS, vol. 6744, pp. 254–260. Springer, Heidelberg (2011). https://doi.org/10.1007/978-3-642-21786-9_42
10. Zeb, S., Qamar, U., Hussain, F.: Sentiment analysis on user reviews through lexicon and rule-based approach. In: Morishima, A., et al. (eds.) APWeb 2016. LNCS, vol. 9865, pp. 55–63. Springer, Cham (2016). https://doi.org/10.1007/978-3-319-45835-9_5
11. Alemi, F., Torii, M., Clementz, L., Aron, D.C.: Feasibility of real-time satisfaction surveys through automated analysis of patients' unstructured comments and sentiments. Qual. Manag. Healthc. **21**, 9–19 (2012)
12. Greaves, F., Ramirez-Cano, D., Millett, C., Darzi, A., Donaldson, L.: Use of sentiment analysis for capturing patient experience from free-text comments posted online. J. Med. Internet Res. **15**, e239 (2013)
13. Hopper, A.M., Uriyo, M.: Using sentiment analysis to review patient satisfaction data located on the internet. J. Health Organ. Manag. **29**, 221–233 (2015)
14. Elmessiry, A., Cooper, W.O., Catron, T.F., Karrass, J., Zhang, Z., Singh, M.P.: Triaging patient complaints: monte carlo cross-validation of six machine learning classifiers. JMIR Med. Inform. **5**, e19 (2017)

15. Tang, D., Qin, B., Liu, T.: Deep learning for sentiment analysis: successful approaches and future challenges. Wiley Interdiscip. Rev.: Data Min. Knowl. Discov. **5**, 292–303 (2015)

16. Gräbner, D., Zanker, M., Fliedl, G., Fuchs, M.: Classification of customer reviews based on sentiment analysis. na (2012)

17. Zhang, Z., Ye, Q., Zhang, Z., Li, Y.: Sentiment classification of Internet restaurant reviews written in Cantonese. Expert Syst. Appl. **38**, 7674–7682 (2011)

18. Zhang, D., Xu, H., Su, Z., Xu, Y.: Chinese comments sentiment classification based on word2vec and SVMperf. Expert Syst. Appl. **42**, 1857–1863 (2015)

19. Mouthami, K., Devi, K.N., Bhaskaran, V.M.: Sentiment analysis and classification based on textual reviews. In: 2013 international conference on Information communication and embedded systems (ICICES), pp. 271–276. IEEE (2013)

20. ElMessiry, A., Zhang, Z., Cooper, W.O., Catron, T.F., Karrass, J., Singh, M.P.: Leveraging sentiment analysis for classifying patient complaints. In: Proceedings of the 8th ACM International Conference on Bioinformatics, Computational Biology, and Health Informatics - ACM-BCB 2017, pp. 44–51 (2017)

21. Ayata, D., Saraçlar, M., Özgür, A.: Political opinion/sentiment prediction via long short term memory recurrent neural networks on Twitter. In: 2017 25th Signal Processing and Communications Applications Conference (SIU), pp. 1–4. IEEE (2017)

22. Romanowski, A., Skuza, M.: Towards predicting stock price moves with aid of sentiment analysis of Twitter social network data and big data processing environment. In: Pełech-Pilichowski, T., Mach-Król, M., Olszak, C.M. (eds.) Advances in Business ICT: New Ideas from Ongoing Research. SCI, vol. 658, pp. 105–123. Springer, Cham (2017). https://doi.org/10.1007/978-3-319-47208-9_7

23. Hu, M., Liu, B.: Mining and summarizing customer reviews. In: Proceedings of the tenth ACM SIGKDD International Conference on KNOWLEDGE DISCOVERY and Data Mining, pp. 168–177. ACM (2004)

24. Ding, X., Liu, B., Yu, P.S.: A holistic lexicon-based approach to opinion mining. In: Proceedings of the 2008 International Conference on Web Search and Data Mining, pp. 231–240. ACM (2008)

25. Stone, P.J., Dunphy, D.C., Smith, M.S.: The general inquirer: a computer approach to content analysis (1966)

26. Pennebaker, J.W., Francis, M.E., Booth, R.J.: Linguistic inquiry and word count: LIWC 2001. Mahway: Lawrence Erlbaum Assoc. **71**, 2001 (2001)

27. Baccianella, S., Esuli, A., Sebastiani, F.: Sentiwordnet 3.0: an enhanced lexical resource for sentiment analysis and opinion mining. In: LREC, pp. 2200–2204 (2010)

28. Pang, B., Lee, L., Vaithyanathan, S.: Thumbs up?: sentiment classification using machine learning techniques. In: Proceedings of the ACL-02 Conference on Empirical methods in Natural Language Processing-Volume 10, pp. 79–86. Association for Computational Linguistics (2002)

29. Dave, K., Lawrence, S., Pennock, D.M.: Mining the peanut gallery: opinion extraction and semantic classification of product reviews. In: Proceedings of the 12th International Conference on World Wide Web, pp. 519–528. ACM (2003)

30. Mullen, T., Collier, N.: Sentiment analysis using support vector machines with diverse information sources. In: Proceedings of the 2004 Conference on Empirical Methods in Natural Language Processing (2004)

31. Mikolov, T.: Statistical language models based on neural networks. Presentation at Google, Mountain View, 2nd April 2012

32. Bengio, Y., Ducharme, R., Vincent, P., Jauvin, C.: A neural probabilistic language model. J. Mach. Learn. Res. **3**, 1137–1155 (2003)

33. Poria, S., Cambria, E., Gelbukh, A.: Aspect extraction for opinion mining with a deep convolutional neural network. Knowl.-Based Syst. **108**, 42–49 (2016)

34. Ganin, Y., et al.: Domain-adversarial training of neural networks. J. Mach. Learn. Res. **17**, 1–35 (2016)

35. Chau, N.P., Phan, V.A., Le Nguyen, M.: Deep learning and sub-tree mining for document level sentiment classification. In: 2016 Eighth International Conference on Knowledge and Systems Engineering (KSE), pp. 268–273. IEEE (2016)

36. del Arco, F.M.P., Valdivia, M.T.M., Zafra, S.M.J., González, M.D.M., Cámara, E.M.: COPOS: corpus of patient opinions in Spanish. Application of sentiment analysis techniques. Proces. Leng. Nat. **57**, 83–90 (2016)

37. Zhang, H.-P., Yu, H.-K., Xiong, D.-Y., Liu, Q.: HHMM-based Chinese lexical analyzer ICTCLAS. In: Proceedings of the Second SIGHAN Workshop on Chinese Language Processing-Volume 17, pp. 184–187. Association for Computational Linguistics (2003)

38. http://cmesh.imicams.ac.cn/index.action?action=index. Accessed 01 Apr 2018

39. 来斯惟: 基于神经网络的词和文档语义向量表示方法研究. 中国科学院大学 (2016)

40. Cortes, C., Vapnik, V.: Support-vector networks. Mach. Learn. **20**, 273–297 (1995)

41. Liaw, A., Wiener, M.: Classification and regression by randomForest. R News **2**, 18–22 (2002)

42. Friedman, J.H.: Greedy function approximation: a gradient boosting machine. Ann. Stat. **29**, 1189–1232 (2001)

43. Chen, T., Guestrin, C.: Xgboost: A scalable tree boosting system. In: Proceedings of the 22nd ACM SIGKDD International Conference on Knowledge Discovery and Data Mining, pp. 785–794. ACM (2016)

44. Hochreiter, S., Schmidhuber, J.: Long short-term memory. Neural Comput. **9**, 1735–1780 (1997)

45. Galavotti, L., Sebastiani, F., Simi, M.: Experiments on the use of feature selection and negative evidence in automated text categorization. In: Borbinha, J., Baker, T. (eds.) ECDL 2000. LNCS, vol. 1923, pp. 59–68. Springer, Heidelberg (2000). https://doi.org/10.1007/3-540-45268-0_6

46. Caropreso, M.F., Matwin, S., Sebastiani, F.: A learner-independent evaluation of the usefulness of statistical phrases for automated text categorization. In: Text databases and Document Management: Theory and practice, vol. 5478, pp. 78–102 (2001)

47. Sebastiani, F., Sperduti, A., Valdambrini, N.: An improved boosting algorithm and its application to text categorization. In: Proceedings of the Ninth International Conference on Information and Knowledge Management, pp. 78–85. ACM (2000)

48. Salton, G., Buckley, C.: Term-weighting approaches in automatic text retrieval. Inf. Process. Manag. **24**, 513–523 (1988)

49. Kinga, D., Adam, J.B.: A method for stochastic optimization. In: International Conference on Learning Representations (ICLR) (2014)

50. Li, J., Xu, H., He, X., Deng, J., Sun, X.: Tweet modeling with LSTM recurrent neural networks for hashtag recommendation. In: 2016 International Joint Conference on Neural Networks (IJCNN), pp. 1570–1577. IEEE (2016)

51. Uysal, A.K., Murphey, Y.L.: Sentiment classification: feature selection based approaches versus deep learning. In: 2017 IEEE International Conference on Computer and Information Technology (CIT), pp. 23–30. IEEE (2017)

A Deep Learning Based Pipeline for Image Grading of Diabetic Retinopathy

Yu Wang[1(✉)], G. Alan Wang[2], Weiguo Fan[3], and Jiexun Li[4]

[1] Department of Computer Science, Virginia Tech, Blacksburg, USA
vuw316@vt.edu
[2] Department of Business Information Technology,
Virginia Tech, Blacksburg, USA
[3] Department of Accounting and Information Systems, Virginia Tech,
Blacksburg, USA
[4] Department of Decision Sciences, Western Washington, Bellingham, USA

Abstract. Diabetic Retinopathy (DR) is one of the principal sources of blindness due to diabetes mellitus. It can be identified by lesions of the retina, namely, microaneurysms, hemorrhages, and exudates. DR can be effectively prevented or delayed if discovered early enough and well-managed. Prior image processing studies on diabetic retinopathy typically extract features manually but are time-consuming and not accurate. In this research, we propose a research framework using advanced retina image processing, deep learning, and boosting algorithm for high-performance DR grading. First, we preprocess the retina image datasets to highlight signs of DR, then employ a convolutional neural network to extract features of retina images, and finally apply a boosting tree algorithm to make a prediction. Experimental results show that our pipeline has excellent performance when grading diabetic retinopathy score on Kaggle dataset.

Keywords: Retina image · Image grading · Diabetic retinopathy
Early detection · Feature extraction · ConvNN · Deep learning
Boosting tree

1 Introduction

Diabetes mellitus is a chronic, progressive disease caused by inherited or acquired deficiency in production of insulin by the pancreas. According to the WHO (World Health Organization), at the end of 2014, 422 million people in the world had diabetes - a prevalence of 8.5% among the adult population. Many of these deaths (43%) occur under the age of 70 [1]. However, with a balanced diet, proper physical activity, immediate medication and regular screening for complications, diabetes can be treated, and its consequences avoided.

Diabetic retinopathy is a diabetes complication that affects eyes, triggered by high blood sugar level. It is a main cause of loss of vision and occurs as a result of long-term accumulated harm to the small blood vessels in the retina.

H. Chen et al. (Eds.): ICSH 2018, LNCS 10983, pp. 240–248, 2018.
https://doi.org/10.1007/978-3-030-03649-2_24

People can still live well with diabetes if early diagnosis occurs; the longer a person lives with undiagnosed and untreated diabetes, the worse the health outcomes are likely to be. Easy access to automatic diagnostics for diabetes is therefore essential.

Currently, people mainly use handcrafted methods to detect DR. Doctors can detect DR by the signs of lesions associated with the abnormalities in blood vessels caused by diabetes. This method is useful, but it requires many resources. For example, the infrastructure required for handling DR is always short in places where the proportion of diabetes is high, and DR identification is most needed. As the rate of people with diabetes continues to grow, the expertise and equipment needed to alleviate sightless caused by DR will become even more inadequate.

The computer-aided diagnosis has recently become more and more popular. One important motivation is the superior performance of deep learning. In many research areas, like the spotting of lung cancer or brain tumors, deep learning has been used to ascertain the severity from medical images; it has achieved fantastic performance, even competitive with experienced doctors.

The performance of diabetic retinopathy grading task, mainly relies on how well can features be extracted. Recognition considers some very micro details, like microaneurysms, and some larger features, such as exudates, and sometimes their position relative to each other on images of the eye. For ordinary people, those lesions may be hard to detect because of many noises, thus achieving good results in the grading task would be very difficult. Sample image shown in Fig. 1.

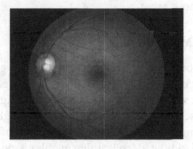

Fig. 1. Sample color retina image from Kaggle (Color figure online)

Deep learning, in many image classification area, achieved state of art performance, especially useful to extract features from images. To this end, we introduce an competitive framework for DR grading. The framework takes retina image as input, go through image preprocessing, 121-layer DenseNet training and features extraction, finally using gradient boosting decision tree to grade DR from features.

We use high-resolution retina image datasets provided by Kaggle as training and evaluation. The retina images are labeled with 5 level in Table 1.

The rest of the paper is organized as follows. Section 2 reviews related work about deep learning in medical image and highlight the research gap. Section 3 describes our proposed research framework. Section 4 presents the experiments and evaluation results. Section 5 discusses the contributions of this study and directions for future work.

Table 1. Diabetic retinopathy (DR) severity scale

DR level	Findings
Grade 0: no apparent retinopathy	No abnormalities
Grade 1: mild non-proliferative diabetic retinopathy	Microaneurysms only
Grade 2: moderate non-proliferative diabetic retinopathy	More than just microaneurysms but less than Severe NPDR
Grade 3: severe non-proliferative diabetic retinopathy	Any of the following: More than 20 intraretinal hemorrhages in each of 4 quadrants Definite venous beading in 2+ quadrants Prominent IRMA in 1+ quadrant
Grade 4: proliferative diabetic retinopathy	One or more of the following: Neovascularization Vitreous/preretinal hemorrhage

2 Related Work

This study aims to use deep learning methods to extract DR features from retinal images, and grade diabetic retinopathy based on severity level. It is related to deep learning in medical image and diabetic retinopathy, so the following sections review some relevant works in those areas.

2.1 Deep Learning in Medical Image

Deep learning, which has been the new research frontier, has gained popularity in many tasks. The main advantage lies on many deep learning algorithms is that networks composed of many layers, which can transform input data (e.g., image) to outputs (e.g., binary value, True or False) while capturing increasingly higher level features. Unlike traditional machine learning methods, in which the creator of the model has to choose and encode features ahead of time, deep learning enables a model to automatically learn features that matter. That is very important because feature engineering typically is the most time-consuming parts of machine learning practice.

Imaging is a cornerstone of medicine. Experts rely heavily on medical image to diagnosis diseases to treat patients. Medical image analysis is a science analyzing medical puzzles and solving medical problems via images, can be used for diagnosis, segmentation, and therapeutic purposes.

Starting from the end of the 1990s, supervised learning techniques, in which labeled training data is used to build model-based systems, were becoming increasingly popular in the medical image area, like active shape models, atlas model and statistical classifiers. Those machine learning or pattern recognition approaches were very popular. That was a big shift from human-designed systems to training data based systems from which features are extracted. Computer-aided systems were able to determine the optimal decision boundary in high dimensional feature space; however, extraction of distinctive features from images still needed to be done by human experts.

The main difference between deep learning methods and traditional machine learning methods is deep learning methods are able to learn discriminative features automatically, rather than choose and encode features ahead of time.

Within the brain image, deep neural networks (DNNs) have been applied for several applications. In [2], the authors introduced a deep learning based manifold learning method to learn the manifold of 3D brain images. They applied a deep generative model that made up of multiple restricted Boltzmann machines (RBMs) [3] on ADNI dataset, which contains 300 T1-weighted MRIs of Alzheimer's disease (AD) and normal subjects. In order to make accelerate computation process, they applied Convolutional RBMs (convRBMs), a form of RBM that uses weight-sharing to reduce the number of trainable weights. Results show that it is much more efficient to train with a resolution of 128 * 128 * 128 in practice and able to extract brain-related disease features by automatically learning low-dimensional manifold of brain volumes. According to Suk et al. [4], they used stacked auto-encoder (SAE) to discover latent representations from the original biological features, even nonlinear latent features can be found in SAE. They also applied another method: a combination of sparse regression models with deep neural network (as introduced by [5]) on ADNI dataset.

Within chest image, many deep learning based applications were applied in detection, classification of nodules as well. As introduced in [6], the authors built an X-ray image retrieval system by experimenting on binary features, textures features, and deep learning (CNN) features. Best results are achieved by using deep learning features in a classification scheme. According to Wang et al. [7], they proposed using deep feature fusion from the non-medical training and hand-crafted features to reduce the false positive results in lung nodules detection task. Compared to previous methods, their method achieved better results in sensitivity and specificity (69.3% and 96.2%) at 1.19 false positive per image on JSRT (Japanese Society of Radiological Technology) database [8].

2.2 Diabetic Retinopathy Grading

In the 1990s, detecting DR was a very time-consuming and manual process that requires a trained clinician to examine and evaluate digital color fundus photographs of the retina. Although some papers, like Klein et al. [9], proposed methods to detect DR, those were mainly focus on tools, like ophthalmoscopy, non-mydriatic camera, and standard fundus camera, not on methodology.

Recent years, with the improvement in medical image quality and quantity, also with the development of deep learning and computational scale, many works in retina related area achieved good performance, all use simple CNNs for color fundus imaging analysis. In 2016, Fu et al. [10, 11] applied a multi-scale and multi-level CNN with a side out-put layer to learn a rich hierarchical representation, and utilized a Conditional Random Field (CRF) to model the long-range interactions between pixels, then combined CNN with CRF layer into an integrated deep network called DeepVessel to segment the blood vessel. In 2015, Kaggle hold a diabetic retinopathy detection competition, they provided around 35,000 color fundus retina images for training, and around 53,000 for testing. The top teams, like Graham [12], all used end-to-end CNN models and achieved a good performance.

Our framework is very robust and able to fit various input because we use large amount of retina image dataset (around 35 thousand), which contains retina images taken from almost all the different conditions (like different cameras), different race of people, to train the model and evaluate the performance.

3   Research Framework

Figure 2 shows our overall research framework for grading diabetic retinopathy. There are three major components: data preprocessing, deep learning based feature extraction and gradient boosting decision tree. In the following sections we will describe the individual components of the framework in more details.

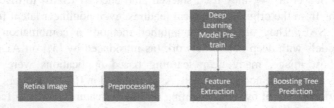

Fig. 2. Research framework for grading diabetic retinopathy

3.1   Data Preprocessing

For diabetic retinopathy grading task, we download the Kaggle Diabetic Retinopathy dataset, which contains 35 thousand retina images and labels. The proportion of this dataset is shown in Table 2. Because DR grading task more relevant to how well we can find lesions of retina, we extract green channel of each image in which lesions are more sensitive and storage can be reduced by 2/3, also, training step in deep learning can be accelerated. Then we apply morphological closing operation and contrast enhancement technique in order to make detection of retina lesions easier. Also, in order to make image suitable for deep learning to train, we transforme image shape to 512 * 512. The original image and image after preprocessing shown in Fig. 3 by the order of a, b.

Table 2. Proportion of Kaggle dataset

Grade level	No. of images
0	25810
1	2443
2	5292
3	873
4	708

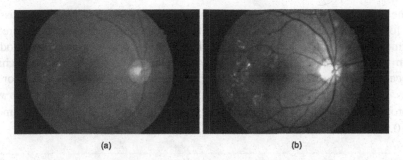

(a)   (b)

Fig. 3. Original image (a) and image after preprocessing (b)

3.2 Feature Extraction

Many current image classification or object detection task apply convolutional neural network to extract features and followed by fully connected layer to make prediction due to superior performance [13–16]. Inspired by [15], we use 121-layer DenseNet architecture as the core component to pre-train the dataset, this network and its prediction performance also been used as our baseline method. In order to alleviate problem caused by highly imbalanced data, we resample the loss weights of data, make them equally in quantity for each level. Besides, we also apply various augmentation methods, like cropping, flipping, and shearing. For our approach, build upon DenseNet, we use it to extract features of retina image first, then apply 50 random augmentations to get 50 outputs from last second fully connected layer (size of 50 * 1024). And finally the mean vector and standard deviation vector are extracted and concatenated as features of that image (size of 2 * 1024).

3.3 Boosting Tree as Prediction

Gradient boosting trees have advantages over neural network when training examples are not large enough, which may lead to overfitting in neural network, and features are well extracted, which tree algorithms can always make good decision on it. In our experiment, we use LightGBM package in Python as tool to train a model based on extracted features. Light Gradient Boosting Machine (LightGBM) is a fast, distributed, high performance gradient boosting framework based on decision tree algorithms. In order to alleviate the local optimal problem, we also apply random search for hyperparameter tuning, we choose top model from 7 random search results.

4 Experiment Results

In this study, we conduct our experiments on Kaggle diabetic retinopathy dataset by performing image grading task. We randomly choose 20% data from each class and combined as testing data, and rest of dataset as training data, that can make sure the distribution of the five classes in the two data sets are equal. Table 3 shows the classification results of our proposed deep learning based hybrid method and the baseline DenseNet based DR score prediction method. This dataset has five classes of label, for each of these classes we calculate the precision, recall and F1 score. The experiment results show that for most of the DR classes, our proposed method outperform than baseline method, especially for levels 1, 2 and 4, our method achieved significantly higher score which is difficult to classify using baseline method or even experts. We also calculate the quadratic kappa score for both of these methods where the proposed method $(k^2 = 0.84)$ outperforms the baseline DenseNet method $(k^2 = 0.79)$.

Method	Kappa score
DenseNet-only	0.70
Our pipeline	**0.84**

Table 3. Experimental Results of DenseNet based method and proposed Deep Learning based method

DR level	Precision		Recall		F1 Score	
	DenseNet	Our method	DenseNet	Our method	DenseNet	Our method
0	0.88	**0.92**	0.99	0.96	0.93	0.94
1	0.56	**0.70**	0.23	**0.31**	0.32	**0.43**
2	0.08	**0.64**	0.17	**0.54**	0.10	**0.58**
3	0.35	**0.67**	0.33	**0.54**	0.34	**0.60**
4	0.43	**0.69**	0.50	**0.60**	0.46	**0.63**

From the results, we can conclude that our deep learning based hybrid model trained on retina images gives a competitive performance on grading DR. This indicates our integrated workflow is robust and can help people to detect DR in real life.

5 Conclusions and Future Research

In this study, we developed an integrated pipeline to automatically grade diabetic retinopathy. We combined image data preprocessing method, convolutional neural network architecture - DenseNet as feature extraction method, and gradient boosting decision tree approach.

The main contributions of our research is that we first apply the state-of-the-art ConvNN based approach for retina image as feature extractor rather than directly make prediction on that. The initial results from our relatively un-optimized approach are quite promising, our approach significantly improved DR grading performance compared with baseline methods by a large margin. Additional optimization will likely result in even better performance. Our proposed framework is highly efficient and effective to grade DR.

Our ongoing works include transforming original image to better extract features of DR; establishing better architecture based on DenseNet; using more advanced machine learning algorithm predict the DR score based on extracted features.

References

1. World Health Organization: Global report on diabetes (2016)
2. Brosch T., Tam R., The Alzheimer's Disease Neuroimaging Initiative: Manifold learning of brain MRIs by deep learning. In: Mori, K., Sakuma, I., Sato, Y., Barillot, C., Navab, N. (eds.) Medical Image Computing and Computer-Assisted Intervention – MICCAI 2013. MICCAI 2013. LNCS, vol 8150. Springer, Heidelberg (2013). https://doi.org/10.1007/978-3-642-40763-5_78
3. Hinton, G.E., Osindero, S., Teh, Y.-W.: A fast learning algorithm for deep belief nets. Neural Comput. 18(7), 1527–1554 (2006)
4. Suk, H.-I., Lee, S.-W., Shen, D., The Alzheimer's Disease Neuroimaging Initiative et al.: Latent feature representation with stacked auto-encoder for AD/MCI diagnosis. Brain Struct. Funct. 220(2), 841–859 (2015)
5. Suk, H.-I., Shen, D.: Deep ensemble sparse regression network for Alzheimer's disease diagnosis. In: Wang, L., Adeli, E., Wang, Q., Shi, Y., Suk, H.-I. (eds.) MLMI 2016. LNCS, vol. 10019, pp. 113–121. Springer, Cham (2016). https://doi.org/10.1007/978-3-319-47157-0_14
6. Anavi, Y., Kogan, I., Gelbart, E., Geva, O., Greenspan, H.: A comparative study for chest radiograph image retrieval using binary texture and deep learning classification. In: 2015 37th Annual International Conference of the IEEE Engineering in Medicine and Biology Society (EMBC), pp. 2940–2943. IEEE (2015)
7. Wang, C., Elazab, A., Wu, J., Hu, Q.: Lung nodule classification using deep feature fusion in chest radiography. Comput. Med. Imaging Graph. 57, 10–18 (2017)
8. Shiraishi, J., et al.: Development of a digital image database for chest radiographs with and without a lung nodule: receiver operating characteristic analysis of radiologists' detection of pulmonary nodules. Am. J. Roentgenol. 174(1), 71–74 (2000)
9. Klein, R., Klein, B.E., Neider, M.W., Hubbard, L.D., Meuer, S.M., Brothers, R.J.: Diabetic retinopathy as detected using ophthalmoscopy, a nonmyciriatic camera and a standard fundus camera. Ophthalmology 92(4), 485–491 (1985)
10. Fu, H., Xu, Y., Lin, S., Kee Wong, D.W., Liu, J.: DeepVessel: retinal vessel segmentation via deep learning and conditional random field. In: Ourselin, S., Joskowicz, L., Sabuncu, M. R., Unal, G., Wells, W. (eds.) MICCAI 2016. LNCS, vol. 9901, pp. 132–139. Springer, Cham (2016). https://doi.org/10.1007/978-3-319-46723-8_16
11. Fu, H., Xu, Y., Wong, D.W.K., Liu, J.: Retinal vessel segmentation via deep learning network and fully-connected conditional random fields. In: 2016 IEEE 13th International Symposium on Biomedical Imaging (ISBI), pp. 698–701. IEEE (2016)
12. Graham, B.: Kaggle diabetic retinopathy detection competition report. University of Warwick (2015)
13. LeCun, Y., Bottou, L., Bengio, Y., Haffner, P.: Gradient-based learning applied to document recognition. Proc. IEEE 86(11), 2278–2324 (1998)
14. Krizhevsky, A., Sutskever, I., Hinton, G.E.: ImageNet classification with deep convolutional neural networks. In: Advances in Neural Information Processing Systems, pp. 1097–1105 (2012)

15. Huang, G., Liu, Z., Weinberger, K. Q., van der Maaten, L.: Densely connected convolutional networks. In: Proceedings of the IEEE Conference on Computer Vision and Pattern Recognition, vol. 1, p. 3 (2017)
16. He, K., Zhang, X., Ren, S., Sun, J.: Deep residual learning for image recognition. In: Proceedings of the IEEE Conference on Computer Vision and Pattern Recognition, pp. 770–778 (2016)

A Deep Learning-Based Method for Sleep Stage Classification Using Physiological Signal

Guanjie Huang[1], Chao-Hsien Chu[1(✉)], and Xiaodan Wu[2]

[1] Pennsylvania State University, University Park, PA 16802, USA
chu@ist.psu.edu
[2] Hebei University of Technology, Tianjin 300130, People's Republic of China

Abstract. A huge number of people suffers from different types of sleep disorders, such as insomnia, narcolepsy, and apnea. A correct classification of their sleep stage is a prerequisite and essential step to effectively diagnose and treat their sleep disorders. Sleep stages are often scored by experts through manually inspecting the patients' polysomnography which are usually needed to be collected in hospitals. It is very laborious for experts and discommodious for patients to go through the process. Accordingly, current studies focused on automatically identifying the sleep stages and nearly all of them need to use hand-crafted features to achieve a decent performance. However, the extraction and selection of these features are time-consuming and require domain knowledge. In this study, we adopt and present a deep learning approach for automatic sleep stage classification using physiological signal. Convolutional Neural Network (CNN) and Long Short-Term Memory (LSTM) of popular deep learning models are employed to automatically learn features from raw physiological signals and identify the sleep stages. Our experiments shown that the proposed deep learning-based method has better performance than previous work. Hence, it can be a promising tool for patients and doctors to monitor the sleep condition and diagnose the sleep disorder timely.

Keywords: Sleep stage classification · Deep learning · Physiological signal
Sleep disorders · Feature extraction

1 Introduction

Sleep, an indispensable physiological activity in our daily life, plays a critical role in keeping people's physical and mental health. An orderly sleep can help people remain vigorous in their daily works. However, a huge number of people suffer from different types of sleep disorders, such as insomnia, narcolepsy, and apnea, etc., which can seriously harm human health. The International Classification of Sleep Disorders (ICSD) has identified over 80 different sleep disorders with associated treatments [3]. A correct classification of the patients' sleep stage is a prerequisite and essential step to effectively diagnose and treat sleep disorders [6, 26, 39]. Because sleep-stage abnormality is correlated with the symptoms of sleep disorders, for instances, obstructive sleep apnea (OSA) decreases the temporal stability of non-rapid eye movement (NREM) and rapid eye movement (REM) sleep bouts [5]. Most obstructive sleep

H. Chen et al. (Eds.): ICSH 2018, LNCS 10983, pp. 249–260, 2018.
https://doi.org/10.1007/978-3-030-03649-2_25

apnea-hypopnea syndrome (OSAHS) are associated with decreased stage N3 sleep [4]. The study by [27] also claimed that the larger ratios of REM/N3 and N1/Wake are related to obstructive sleep apnea (OSA). Thus, sleep stage classification has attracted increased interest for research.

Sleep scoring, proposed by Rechtschaffen and Kales (R&K), is a gold standard used to classify sleep stage and diagnose sleep disorders. The method divided sleep into five stages: REM, and NREM stages 1, 2, 3, and 4 [18]. However, in practice, the rules are often difficult or impossible to follow and deviations are common. It also has some limitations, for instances, low temporal resolution, ignorance of spatial information, insufficient number of stages, low correspondence between electrophysiological activity and stages, and ignorance of other physiological parameters such as autonomous nervous system activity and body motility [17]. The American Academy of Sleep Medicine (AASM) updated and expanded R&K scheme to AASM scoring manuals [33]. According to AASM, the sleep consists of four distinctive stages: stage R sleep, stage N1, N2, and N3, where R corresponds to REM stage, N1 is analogs to stage 1, N2 is similar to stage 2, and N3 can be considered as stages 3 and 4. N1 is a transition stage between wakefulness and sleep, which usually take 1 to 5 min [31]. N2 follows N1 and usually acts as a "baseline" of sleep. N3 can be considered as "deep sleep" which is the most restorative stage of sleep. Stage REM is characterized by the rapid eye movement under eyelids and the occurrence of dream [10].

The standard approach for segmenting the stages is to have the domain experts manually inspect every epochs of the patient's polysomnography (PSG) data based on the R&K rules or AASM. In this study, we use the R&K standard, because the dataset [13] we used for exploration is labeled based on R&K. The PSG data often include electroencephalogram (EEG), electrooculogram (EOG), electromyogram (EMG), electrocardiogram (ECG), respiratory effort signals, blood oxygen saturation, and other measurements [29]. Typically, each epoch is obtained by dividing the entire time series data into epochs of 30 s subsequence. The EEG data from [13] are shown in Fig. 1. We can see that the EEG data in different stages have different patterns. For instances, there is a vertex sharp wave in stage 1 and there are some sawtooth waves in stage R. The expert can score the sleep stages through inspecting these small and big "contexts". The architecture of our model is also inspired by it. However, inspecting epoch by epoch is time-consuming and sometimes involves personal subjective judgment. Hence, an automatic sleep stage classification would be a promising and valuable approach. There are four challenges for automatic sleep stage classification:

Challenge 1: Feature Extraction and Selection. Many studies have been done for automatic sleep stages classification, nearly all of them (e.g., [15, 16, 21, 24, 34, 36]) classified the stages using hand-crafted features. These appropriate features are picked carefully and computed manually based on the expert's domain knowledge. However, these processes are highly labor-intensive and time-consuming [37]. We even need to consider the interaction between features. What's worse, these hand-crafted features might be sub-optimal [22].

Challenge 2: Temporal Information. The classification of sleep stages follows a sequential order [2, 9]. That is, the classification depends on not only the information of current data, but also on the information from the past and the future [33]. However,

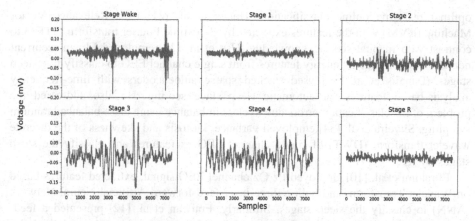

Fig. 1. The samples of 30 s EEG epochs in different sleep stages (sample rate is 250 Hz).

most of the studies (e.g., [16, 21, 24]) only consider the current epoch and did not take advantage of the temporal information from others.

Challenge 3: Patient Impact and Resistance. Though many previous studies (e.g., [7, 10, 11]) achieved good performance in sleep stage classification using multiple physiological data. In the real world, wearing too many sensors during sleep is obtrusive and uncomfortable, which may affect the sleep quality.

Challenge 4: Unlabeled Sleep Data. Currently, the amount of labeled sleep data is limited and thereby it is an obstacle for developing the method for classifying the sleep stages. In fact, there is a huge number of sleep data which is unlabeled. Much of meaningful information are contained in these unlabeled data.

In this study, we focus on tackling the first three challenges. We adopt a newer approach, deep learning, to automatically learn the useful feature representation and integrated it with classification step. The convolutional neural networks (CNN), a popular neural network model, is used to automatically learn the appropriate features with backpropagation. In order to consider the temporal information from the past and the future, the Bidirectional Recurrent Neural Networks (RNN) is adopted to build the classifier. In addition, single EEG is chosen as the biomarker for sleep stage classification, because it is more comfortable compared with PSG recording which needs multiple sensors. We compare its results with other's method [30] for benchmark.

2 Related Works

Many researchers have attempted to classify the sleep stages using extracted features of the physiological data automatically. Radha et al. [28] compared the performance of six different EEG signals using various signal processing feature sets including spectral-domain, time-domain and nonlinear features as data source, and used Random Forest (RF) and Support Vector Machine (SVM) to classify the sleep stages. Their results showed that the RF with spectral linear features of frontal EEG signal achieve the optimal real-time online classification. Huang et al. [21] used Relevance Vector Machine (RVM) with the features extracted by short-time Fourier transform (STFT) to contrast with manual scoring knowledge. Hsu et al. [20] employed Elman recurrent neural classifier with six energy features from single channel EEG to classify five sleep stages. Tsinalis et al. [36] used stacked sparse autoencoders with time-frequency analysis-based features for automatic sleep stage scoring. He also addressed the problem of misclassification errors due to class imbalance using class-balanced random sampling. Silveira et al. [34] employed variance, kurtosis and skewness of the discrete wavelet transform (DWT) of single channel EEG as features and classify the sleep stages by RF.

Ebrahimi et al. [10] employed Pz-Oz channel EEG signal, extracted features based on Wavelet Transform, and built a three-layer feed-forward Artificial Neural Network (ANN) to classify the sleep stages. Similarly, Fraiwan et al. [12] presented a feed-forward ANN based on the techniques of time-frequency analysis, which includes Wigner–Ville distribution (WVD), Hilbert–Hough spectrum (HHS) and continuous wavelet transform (CWT) for automatic sleep stage classification in neonates. Lajnef et al. [24] extracted a wide range of time and frequency-domain features of EEG, EOG and EMG. And a standard sequential forward selection (SFS) was used to select an optimal feature subset in order to facilitate their method of Dendrogram-SVM (DSVM) to classify the sleep stages. Likewise, Chapotot and Becq [7] extracted a variety of features from EEG and EMG, such as Shannon entropy and relative power of a sub-band signal, and selected the effective ones using SFS algorithm. A three-layer feed-forward ANN was then adopted to classify the stages using the selected feature set. Sen et al. [33] conducted a comparative study on EEG-based sleep stage classification in terms of feature selection and classification algorithms. Their results showed that the RF with 12 features, which are selected from 41 features by Fisher score, achieved the best classification rate. Besides using EEG, some studies also employed ECG to identify the sleep stages. Yilmaz et al. [38] demonstrated that sleep stages classification using features of RR-interval of single-lead ECG is feasible. Fonseca et al. [11] selected 80 features from a set of 142 features from ECG and respiratory (RIP) according to SFS-based feature selection, and used a linear discriminant classifier to identify the sleep stages.

These studies all relied on a domain knowledge to design or extract appropriate features. It is quite challengeable as we described in the previous section. Moreover, due to the intricacy of various physiological data, the size of the feature space can become huge so that a feature selection step is always indispensable. Recently, a few studies started to explore the automatic feature learning for sleep stage classification using deep learning. The strength of deep learning methods is end-to-end learning, i.e., feature extraction, feature selection and classification are integrated into a single algorithm using only the raw data as input [36]. Tsinalis et al. [36] used CNNs to learn task-specific filters for sleep stage classification without any prior domain knowledge. Supratak et al. [35] proposed a DeepSleepNet for automatic sleep stage scoring based on raw single-channel EEG. DeepSleepNet consists of two cascaded parts: representation learning and sequence residual learning. Representation learning including two CNNs can extract time-invariant features from raw EEG. Sequence residual learning contains two layers of Bidirectional-Long Short-term Memory (Bidirectional-LSTM) and a shortcut connection, and aims at learning transition rules among sleep stages. These deep-learning related studies are still in exploration stage.

3 Methodology

The objectives of our study are two-fold: (1) to save the efforts of computing the hand-crafted features and (2) to find a suitable method that use less number of signals to increase usability. The proposed method following a deep learning approach which integrates the data preprocessing, the feature extraction, feature selection, and classification into a single end-to-end algorithm. It takes the raw data as input rather than hand-crafted features, and consists of two main modules as shown in Fig. 2. The architecture of proposed deep learning model. the *time-invariant feature* learning and *temporal feature* learning.

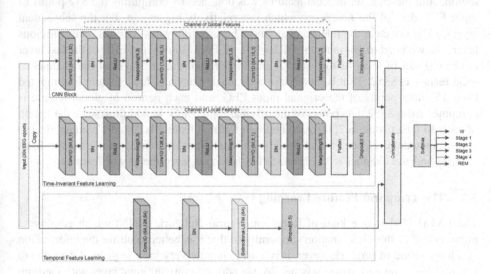

Fig. 2. The architecture of proposed deep learning model.

3.1 The Time-Invariant Feature Learning

The time-invariant feature learning module is made up of multiple Convolutional Neural Network (CNN) blocks. There are two channels in the module of time-invariant feature learning. Each channel of the time-invariant feature learning is mainly composed of three similar CNN blocks. One channel with smaller size of feature maps is designed for capturing the "small contexts" of the signal which are considered as *local features*. Another channel with larger size of feature maps is used to capture the "big contexts" of the signal which we refer them as *global features*.

The CNN block consists of four cascading layers: convolution layer, batch normalization layer, activation layer and pooling layer. After the CNN blocks, one flatten layer and one dropout layer are used. The motivation for constructing such architecture is that the examination of physiological data for sleep stage classification is usually determined in terms of two aspects: the narrow and sharp waves, and the larger trends of the slow change. The smaller feature maps can be used to recognize the narrow and sharp waves which can be considered as local features, such as the occurrence of vertex sharp waves in stage N1. And the larger receptive fields are used to learn the larger context of waves which also can be considered as global features, such as the occurrence of slow waves in stage N3 and N4.

In order to explain how these two channels work, it is important to know the receptive field (RF) and the effective receptive field (ERF). RF represents the area of previous layer which is directly connected to a current layer's neuron [25]. ERF denotes the area of the original input data which is indirectly connected to a current layer's neuron. Both RF and ERF can be affected by the convolutional layer and the pooling layer. Then we can easily see that the channel of local features was obtained by computing the 8 points of input EEG data of in the first layer, which is a very small region. And the channel of local features was obtained by computing the 512 points of input EEG data of the first layer, which is a relatively big region. For the subsequent layers, RF is not clear to understand anymore because it always depends on its previous layer. So, we need to compute the ERF of them. For instance, the ERF of the last layer of the channel of local feature is 157, and the ERF of the last layer of the channel of local feature is 8352. That is, in the last layer, each neuron of local feature is computed from 157 data points of the original input EEG, and each neuron of global feature is computed from 8352 data points of the original input EEG. In addition, since the length of each 30 s EEG data is 7500, each neuron of global feature is actually computed from entire input data. Hence, the channel with small receptive field can learn the local features and the channel with big receptive field can learn the global features.

3.2   The Temporal Feature Learning

The LSTM [19] is one kind of Recurrent Neural Network (RNN) which employs a memory cell to store information temporally so that it is better to utilize the information in a long period of time. However, it is hard to handle very long sequential data due to the gradient issue and memory issue. So, we adopt a convolutional layer with medium size of feature maps to extract a shorter representation of the input data and a batch normalization layer to maintain the stability as shown in Fig. 2.

Figure 3 shows a single cell of LSTM. It contains an input gate i, an output gate o, a forget gate f and a memory cell. The input gate controls which new input feeds into the cell, the forget gate decides which information stored in the cell, and the output gate determines which information is used to compute the output. These gates are connected with each other, and some of the connection are recurrent. Bidirectional LSTM [32] is an extended version of LSTM. It contains two LSTMs, a forward one and a backward one. And hence, it has capability to exploit information from the past and the future.

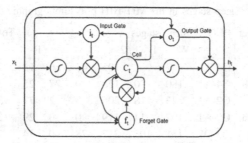

Fig. 3. Long short-term memory cell.

4 Experiment and Results

4.1 Dataset Used

We use the data sets from the MIT-BIH polysomnographic database [13] to examine the relative performance of our proposed model. The database contains over 80 h' worth of four-, six-, and seven-channel polysomnographic recordings during sleep, with sampling rate 250 Hz. Sleep stages were annotated at 30-s intervals based on the R&K rules. It has seven stages: Stages 1, 2, 3, 4, REM, W and MT, where the first five stages are introduced in Sect. 1, W denotes the wake stage, and MT represents the movement time. MT is not presented because it no longer affects the scoring of sleep stages according to AASM. There are 18 subjects in total. Among them, 17 subjects are male, aged from 32 to 56, with weights ranging from 89 to 152 kg. The last one is also male but his age and weight were unknown. The details of the dataset are summarized in Table 1. The numbers in the table denotes the amount of the 30-s EEG epochs. We can easily see that the class distributions of sleep stages are imbalanced. So, we need to balance the dataset in order to learn unbiased features. And the strategy to handle imbalance data will be described in the next section.

4.2 Experiment Setup

In order to leverage the temporal information and improve the efficiency of the training process of the model, the dataset is split up as shown in Fig. 4. Though we have 18 subjects in the dataset, we only utilized 5 of them, i.e., slp01a, slp01b, slp32, slp37 and slp41 in the first experiment. There are two reasons to do so: (1) these data are collected by the same position of sensor, i.e. C4-A1; (2) our benchmark study [30] only picked these subjects and thereby it is easy for us to compare the performance. In Fig. 4, EEG records are divided into epochs of 30 s according to the R&K manual and the annotation of the dataset. Every 32 epochs of EEG record are put in one big chunk following the sequential order of the original data. So the total data can be divided into 2717 epochs and these epochs can be divided into 87 chunks. And then 10-fold cross validation is applied. The reason of using the cross-validation is that, if we split data into training, validation, testing sets, the training set may be too small to learn effective and generalized features.

Table 1. Sleep stages in the MIT-BIH polysomnographic database

Subject	EEG	Sleep stages						Total
		W	1	2	3	4	R	
slp01a	C4-A1	7	1	105	47	66	13	239
slp01b	C4-A1	180	0	128	0	27	25	360
slp02a	O2-A1	43	18	206	5	2	77	351
slp02b	O2-A1	107	14	119	0	0	29	269
slp03	C3-O1	151	105	312	78	0	74	720
slp04	C3-O1	162	60	442	33	0	23	720
slp14	C3-O1	321	188	126	30	12	36	713
slp16	C3-O1	316	108	181	22	2	65	694
slp32	C4-A1	394	27	159	43	17	0	640
slp37	C4-A1	75	21	591	0	0	11	698
slp41	C4-A1	229	230	218	13	0	90	780
slp45	C3-O1	119	54	399	51	52	81	756
slp48	C3-O1	213	241	272	2	0	31	759
slp59	C3-O1	140	105	98	50	30	35	458
slp60	C3-O1	286	344	49	0	0	31	710
slp61	C3-O1	124	88	326	103	0	79	720
slp66	C3-O1	175	143	116	5	0	0	439
slp67x	C3-O1	72	41	40	1	0	0	154
Total		3114	1789	3889	486	212	700	10180

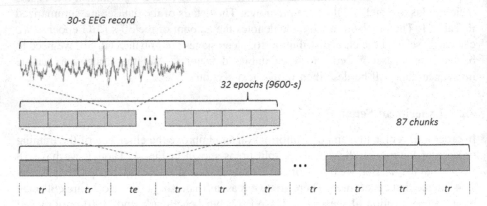

Fig. 4. The illustration of the assembly of the training and testing sets.

All models were implemented using Keras [8] with the TensorFlow [1] backend. They are trained with Adam optimization [23] with learning rate 0.00001, $\beta_1 = 0.9$, $\beta_2 = 0.999$, and $\in = 10^{-7}$, where β_1 and β_2 are used for decaying and $\in$ is used to prevent any division by zero. The reason of using Adam optimizer is that it is robust to the choice of hyper-parameters to some extent [14] and it usually works very well empirically. In addition, in order to prevent the model from overfitting into the noise, the L2 regularization is applied in the first convolutional layer of every channel according to the study by [35]. The categorical cross entropy is adopted as the loss function for the task of classifying the sleep stages.

Since the classes of the dataset are imbalance, a class weight (a.k.a., misclassification cost) scheme was used to fix this issue. Through using the class weight, the minority classes become more important. Specifically, its errors would cost more than those of the other classes. In addition, we have also tried random oversampling of the minority class and random down-sampling of the majority class to balance the dataset separately. However, the oversampling would cause overfitting problem on the data of minority class. And the down-sampling might lose information so that the model cannot correctly learn the features of the majority class.

4.3 Results and Discussion

The computational results of 10-fold cross-validation are summarized in Table 2, which compares our results and the results from [30], which utilized hand-crafted features, in terms of recall (a.k.a., True Positive Rate (TPR)), precision (a.k.a., Positive Predictive Value (PPV)) and F1 score. As shown in Table 2, we can see that if EEG signals are used to predict the sleep stages our proposed method, which uses deep learning method (CNN & LSTM), performed better than [30], which used Hidden Markov Model with hand-crafted features. Though they have carefully designed to extract and select the features, it might be suboptimal due to the difficulty of feature extraction. We used deep learning model to automatically learn the most effective features and use them to classify the stages. So, we considered the deep learning learned a better set of features than [30] in this scenario.

Table 2. Comparison of performance (%) between the proposed method with [30].

		[30]			Proposed method			Method with pretrain		
		TPR	PPV	F1	TPR	PPV	F1	TPR	PPV	F1
Sleep stages	W	80.99	**92.13**	**86.20**	81.24	81.16	81.42	**86.44**	83.24	84.81
	1	**54.55**	**38.24**	**44.96**	51.63	37.71	43.59	51.30	38.11	43.73
	2	32.79	65.79	43.76	65.45	**87.72**	74.96	**69.27**	84.38	**76.09**
	3	44.23	21.70	29.11	**52.43**	28.88	37.24	51.45	**37.60**	**43.44**
	4	**80.95**	**55.74**	**66.02**	74.82	49.08	55.49	65.06	55.67	60.00
	R	70.31	34.09	45.92	**74.82**	46.02	56.98	70.50	**60.49**	65.12
Avg.		60.14	51.28	52.27	64.90	58.28	54.22	**65.67**	**59.91**	**62.20**

Overall, in terms of average results, the proposed method with pretrain performed the best, followed by the proposed method. Specifically, all evaluation metrics of Stages 2, 3, and R are better than the benchmark model. The performance of the classification of Stage W is comparable. The classification of Stages 1 and 4 are less accurate than the benchmark model. We consider the model makes sensible mistakes here.

As shown in Fig. 5, most of the misclassification of Stage 4 are estimated as Stage 3. Stage 3 is defined by 20%–50% of the epoch consists of high voltage (>75 µV), low frequency (<2 Hz) activity, and Stage 4 is low frequency (<2 Hz) activity where more than 50% of the epoch consists of high voltage (>75 µV) according to R&F. That is, they are indistinguishable to each other. Hence, AASM proposed to merge them in to one stage.

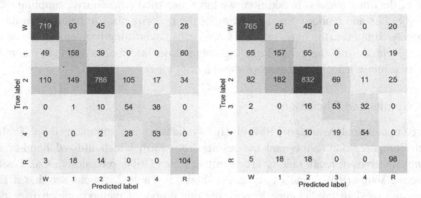

Fig. 5. The confusion matrix - the proposed method (left) and the method with pretrain (right).

However, since the data are limited, the effective features is difficult to be learned. Pretraining on similar data is one approach to overcome this issue. Hence, we pretrain the model on the remaining 13 records of MIT-BIH polysomnographic database [13] before we apply 10-fold cross-validation. The results of the proposed model with pretraining are also shown in Table 2. We can see that the recalls of Wake and Stage 2 are getting better while the others are getting worse. These can be considered as a reasonable change in its performance and there are two sensible reasons: (1) the amount of the pretraining dataset is still relatively small which cannot offer a thorough knowledge of sleep stages, and (2) there is a bias of the data of Stages 1, 3, and 4 between the training/testing dataset and pretraining dataset. In terms of the overall performance, the pretraining helps improve the method.

5   Conclusion and Future Work

In this paper, we propose a deep learning model for automatic sleep stage classification based on raw single-channel EEG without any hand-crafted features. Besides better performance, it also can save a lot of time and efforts of designing, computing and selecting the features manually. We employed CNN to learn the time-invariant features and used Bidirectional-LSTM to learn the temporal information from the past and the future. On the other side, the proposed method only needs one single EEG sensor data rather than using complete PSG recording which requires bunches of sensors. Accordingly, it can also improve the patient experience to some extent.

For future work, we plan to modify and deploy our method on some easily-collected data so that the sleep stages identification will not be so obtrusive any more.

Patient can monitor their sleep condition more easily and comfortably. Furthermore, tackling the unlabeled sleep data is also promising. Because current labeled data are limited and deep learning model usually prefer a huge amount of data to achieve a decent performance. We also plan to compare our results with results obtained from other deep learning models such as [35, 36] as they are not using the same data sets and takes time to compute using our data set.

References

1. Abadi, M., et al.: TensorFlow: a system for large-scale machine learning. In: OSDI, pp. 265–283 (2016)
2. Ancoli-Israel, S., et al.: The AASM manual for the scoring of sleep and associated events: rules, terminology and technical specifications. American Academy of Sleep Medicine, Westchester (2007)
3. American Sleep Disorders Association, et al.: The international classification of sleep disorders: diagnostic and coding manual. American Sleep Disorders Association (1990)
4. Basunia, M., et al.: Relationship of symptoms with sleep-stage abnormalities in obstructive sleep apnea-hypopnea syndrome. J. Community Hosp. Intern. Med. Perspect. 6(4), 32170 (2016)
5. Bianchi, M.T., et al.: Obstructive sleep apnea alters sleep stage transition dynamics. PLoS One 5(6), e11356 (2010)
6. Carskadon, M.A., Rechtschaffen, A.: Monitoring and staging human sleep. Princ. Pract. Sleep Med. 3, 1197–1215 (2000)
7. Chapotot, F., Becq, G.: Automated sleep–wake staging combining robust feature extraction, artificial neural network classification, and flexible decision rules. Int. J. Adapt. Control. Signal Process. 24(5), 409–423 (2010)
8. Chollet, F., et al.: Keras (2015)
9. Dong, H., et al.: Mixed neural network approach for temporal sleep stage classification. IEEE Trans. Neural Syst. Rehabil. Eng. 26(2), 324–333 (2018)
10. Ebrahimi, F., et al.: Automatic sleep stage classification based on EEG signals by using neural networks and wavelet packet coefficients. In: 2008 30th Annual International Conference of the IEEE Engineering in Medicine and Biology Society, EMBS 2008, pp. 1151–1154 (2008)
11. Fonseca, P., et al.: Sleep stage classification with ECG and respiratory effort. Physiol. Meas. 36(10), 2027 (2015)
12. Fraiwan, L., et al.: Time frequency analysis for automated sleep stage identification in fullterm and preterm neonates. J. Med. Syst. 35(4), 693–702 (2011)
13. Goldberger, A.L., et al.: Physiobank, physiotoolkit, and physionet. Circulation 101(23), e215–e220 (2000)
14. Goodfellow, I., et al.: Deep learning. In: ICML2013 Tutor, pp. 1–800 (2011)
15. Güneş, S., et al.: Efficient sleep stage recognition system based on EEG signal using k-means clustering based feature weighting. Expert Syst. Appl. 37(12), 7922–7928 (2010)
16. Hassan, A.R., et al.: Automatic classification of sleep stages from single-channel electroencephalogram, pp. 1–6, November 2015
17. Himanen, S.-L., Hasan, J.: Limitations of rechtschaffen and kales. Sleep Med. Rev. 4(2), 149–167 (2000)

18. Hobson, J.A.: A Manual of Standardized Terminology, Techniques and Scoring System for Sleep Stages of Human Subjects. In: Rechtschaffen, A., Kales, A. (eds.) 58 p. Public Health Service, US Government Printing Office, Washington, DC (1968)). (Electroencephalogr. Clin. Neurophysiol. **26**(6), 644 (1969))

19. Hochreiter, S., Schmidhuber, J.: Long short-term memory. Neural Comput. **9**(8), 1735–1780 (1997)

20. Hsu, Y.-L., et al.: Automatic sleep stage recurrent neural classifier using energy features of EEG signals. Neurocomputing **104**, 105–114 (2013)

21. Huang, C.-S., et al.: Knowledge-based identification of sleep stages based on two forehead electroencephalogram channels. Front. Neurosci. **8**, 263 (2014)

22. Humphrey, E.J., et al.: Feature learning and deep architectures: new directions for music informatics. J. Intell. Inf. Syst. **41**(3), 461–481 (2013)

23. Kingma, D.P., Ba, J.: Adam: a method for stochastic optimization. arXiv Prepr. arXiv:1412. 6980 (2014)

24. Lajnef, T., et al.: Learning machines and sleeping brains: automatic sleep stage classification using decision-tree multi-class support vector machines. J. Neurosci. Methods **250**, 94–105 (2015)

25. Le, H., Borji, A.: What are the receptive, effective receptive, and projective fields of neurons in convolutional neural networks? arXiv Prepr. arXiv:1705.07049(2017)

26. Li, X., et al.: Hyclasss: a hybrid classifier for automatic sleep stage scoring. IEEE J. Biomed. Health Inform. **22**(2), 375–385 (2018)

27. Ng, A.K., Guan, C.: Impact of obstructive sleep apnea on sleep-wake stage ratio. In: 2012 Annual International Conference of the IEEE Engineering in Medicine and Biology Society (EMBC), pp. 4660–4663 (2012)

28. Radha, M., et al.: Comparison of feature and classifier algorithms for online automatic sleep staging based on a single EEG signal. In: 2014 36th Annual International Conference of the IEEE Engineering in Medicine and Biology Society (EMBC), pp. 1876–1880 (2014)

29. Roebuck, A., et al.: A review of signals used in sleep analysis. Physiol. Meas. **35**(1), R1 (2013)

30. Rossow, A.B., et al.: Automatic sleep staging using a single-channel EEG modeling by Kalman filter and HMM. In: Biosignals and Biorobotics Conference (BRC), 2011 ISSNIP, pp. 1–6 (2011)

31. Sanei, S., Chambers, J.A.: EEG Signal Processing. Wiley, Hoboken (2013)

32. Schuster, M., Paliwal, K.K.: Bidirectional recurrent neural networks. IEEE Trans. Signal Process. **45**(11), 2673–2681 (1997)

33. Şen, B., et al.: A comparative study on classification of sleep stage based on EEG signals using feature selection and classification algorithms. J. Med. Syst. **38**(3), 18 (2014)

34. da Silveira, T.L., et al.: Single-channel EEG sleep stage classification based on a streamlined set of statistical features in wavelet domain. Med. Biol. Eng. Comput. **19**, 19 (2016)

35. Supratak, A., et al.: DeepSleepNet: A model for automatic sleep stage scoring based on raw single-channel EEG. IEEE Trans. Neural Syst. Rehabil. Eng. **25**(11), 1998–2008 (2017)

36. Tsinalis, O., et al.: Automatic sleep stage scoring with single-channel EEG using convolutional neural networks. arXiv Prepr. arXiv:1610.01683 (2016)

37. Wang, K., et al.: Research on healthy anomaly detection model based on deep learning from multiple time-series physiological signals. Sci. Program. **2016**, 9 (2016)

38. Yilmaz, B., et al.: Sleep stage and obstructive apneaic epoch classification using single-lead ECG. Biomed. Eng. Online **9**(1), 39 (2010)

39. Zhang, X., et al.: Sleep stage classification based on multi-level feature learning and recurrent neural networks via wearable device. arXiv Prepr. arXiv:1711.00629 (2017)

Chronic Disease Management

Visualizing Knowledge Evolution of Emerging Information Technologies in Chronic Diseases Research

Dongxiao Gu[1], Kang Li[1], Xiaoyu Wang[2(✉)], and Changyong Liang[1]

[1] The School of Management, Hefei University of Technology,
193 Tunxi Road, Hefei 230009, Anhui, China
[2] The 1st Affiliated Hospital, Anhui University of Traditional Chinese Medicine,
117 Meishan Road, Hefei 230031, Anhui, China
329789400@qq.com

Abstract. To provide knowledge support and reference for scholars in technologies and data-driven chronic disease research, investigated knowledge base, research hotspots, development status and concluded future research directions in chronic disease research driven by emerging technologies. We conducted a bibliometric analysis based on 4820 literature data collected from the Web of Science core collection during 2000–2017. The time distribution, space distribution, literature co-citation were analyzed and visualized, the dynamic process of research hotspots in this research filed was revealed, and future development trends were discussed.

Keywords: Emerging technologies · Chronic diseases · Bibliometric analysis Technologies and data-driven

1 Introduction

Chronic diseases, also known as chronic non-communicable diseases, has the characteristics of complex etiology, concealed onset, longer duration, and difficulty in healing. Common chronic diseases include diabetes, hypertension, cardiovascular and cerebrovascular diseases, coronary heart disease, osteoporosis, and etc. [1]. The chronic diseases issue has also attracted the attention of governments of all countries worldwide. They have issued a series of policy documents to actively promote chronic diseases' prevention and management [2]. China, for example, in 2012, China's State Council proposed an initiative to "establish chronic disease prevention and control systems covering urban and rural areas", which is the first comprehensive chronic disease prevention plan at the national level. On February 14, 2017, the General Office of the State Council of the People's Republic of China issued the "2017–2025 Medium and Long-Term Plan for Prevention and Treatment of Chronic Diseases in China". On October 18, 2017, Xi Jinping, the president of the People's Republic of China, pointed out in the report of the 19th CPC National Congress that it is necessary to implement a healthy China strategy and provide a full range of health services for broad masses of people in China.

H. Chen et al. (Eds.): ICSH 2018, LNCS 10983, pp. 263–273, 2018.
https://doi.org/10.1007/978-3-030-03649-2_26

At present, a series of emerging information technologies represented by big data, cloud computing, the Internet of Things, and artificial intelligence are triggering a new wave of industrial revolution worldwide. The literatures associated with emerging information technologies in chronic diseases have also mushroomed. Lv et al. [3] used co-word analysis and cluster analysis and studied chronic disease self-management. Lu [4] used bibliometrics and conduct statistical analysis from the aspects of chronological distribution, geographical distribution, authors, source journals, and fund types, and revealed research status and hot topics in the field of chronic disease management in China during 2005–2014. Taifang et al. [5] reviewed relevant literatures related to elderly chronic diseases in the elderly between 1983–2016, and analyzed the development status and trends of elderly chronic diseases research worldwide. Rajpal, Kumar and Agarwal [6] used data mining methods and studied "hot" and "cold" spots in this research field, and the results show that research on obesity is emerging in the field. Kong, Mou and Hu [7] used unsupervised machine learning methods for the analysis of gene expression profiling, and identified important genes and related pathways of microarray gene expression data of Alzheimer's disease. Khan and Choudhury et al. [8] used bibliometric metadata to analyze longitudinal trends of global obesity research and collaboration. Lledo, Diez and Bertomeu-Motos et al. [9] Compared and visualized two-dimensional and three-dimensional tasks of robot-assisted neurological rehabilitation based on virtual reality in post-stroke patients. Yang, Chen and Ma et al. [10] used microarray datasets to identify the pathogenesis of heart failure caused by different etiologies. Gu and Li et al. [11] used bibliometrics and tracked the knowledge evolution of healthcare big data research.

Generally, lots of research achievements in the field of chronic diseases research driven by emerging information technologies have been achieved. However there are still some issues deserving to be addressed and resolved. No study driven by scientific evidence instead of subjective belief overview the current status and future direction under consideration of entire emerging information technologies in chronic diseases. Meanwhile, existing researches are basically addressing the application of a specific emerging technology in a certain type of chronic disease, rather than from the scope of all kinds of chronic disease. A lack of a comprehensive understanding of emerging information technologies in chronic diseases has disturbed an appropriate allocation of research resources into this area which causes inefficient researches to a great extent.

To fill in this research gap, based on literature data consisting of 4820 articles from web of science database published during 2000 to 2017, this study provides a visual analysis for the development status, hotspots, and trend of emerging information technologies' applications in cancer research field. This study visualized and unveiled the dynamic knowledge structure of emerging information technologies application in chronic diseases research, which will be helpful to understand current state-of-art developments and discuss future research directions of this research filed for scholars in e-health and medical informatics. This study provides scholars in medical information management field with panoramic knowledge support for their better understanding current research status, hotspots and trends in the future.

2 Methodology

2.1 Data Source

We collected data on articles published in core international journals between January 1st, 2000 and December 31, 2017 from the Web of Science (SCI-EXPANDED, SSCI, A&HCI, CPCI-S, CPCI-SSH, ESCI, CCR-EXPANDED and IC included) for our literature analysis. The search strategy we used is TS = (big data OR cloud computing OR Internet of things OR artificial intelligence OR #) AND TS = (hypertension OR coronary disease * OR hyperlipidemia OR diabet * OR ##), and the literature type: (Article), in which the symbol "#" represents twenty other words related to emerging technologies, and the symbol "##" represents twenty eight other words associated with chronic diseases. We connected these words with "OR", we eventually obtained 4820 journal articles. (The retrieval time is January 24, 2018).

2.2 Toolkits

HistCite, CiteSpace, and *Excel* were used to complete our study. *CiteSpace* is a freely available Java application, it is often used to visualize and analyze the status quo and future trends in scientific literatures [12]. It has advantage on finding key points in the development of a field, especially turning point and key point of knowledge [13]. *CiteSpace* was used to obtain author's cooperation network, agency cooperation network, literature co-citations, and research hotspots.

3 Knowledge Map of Time-and-Space Analysis

3.1 Time Distribution Map

We analyzed the number of scientific literature between 2000–2017, and obtained the trend of the increasing number of articles published every year. As shown in Fig. 1, the volume of published articles is generally increasing. The curve of 2000–2014 was relatively flat, basically in line with the exponential growth trend, but that of 2014–2017, the curve growth is very rapid, with a linear upward trend, much higher than index prediction curve. It shows that there will be more and more research results in this research field, and the future research on this field will also continue to maintain a large research hotspot.

We also analyzed investigators' input in this research field. As shown in Fig. 2, the trend of this curves is almost the same with that in Fig. 1. This shows that the size of the author's investment also is increasing steadily.

3.2 Space Distribution Map

Author Distribution
We used *CiteSpace* and generated authors cooperation network map, as shown in Fig. 3, and Top 20 authors were shown in this figure. The author with the most

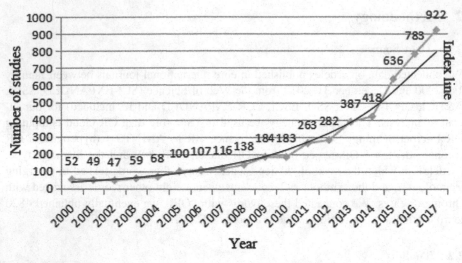

Fig. 1. Annual number of published articles.

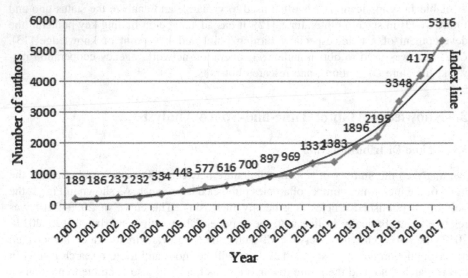

Fig. 2. Annual number of authors.

publication is Acharya UR. He has a total of 44 articles published. In this study, 4820 articles are completed by a total of 20488 authors, of whom 3489 published 2 or more articles. The number of network nodes is 737, the figure of connections between nodes is 752, and the density of the network is 0.0028. The connections between high-yielding authors are not dense enough, which indicates that the cooperation among high-yield authors is not dense. Table 1 lists Top 20 authors and the number of articles published.

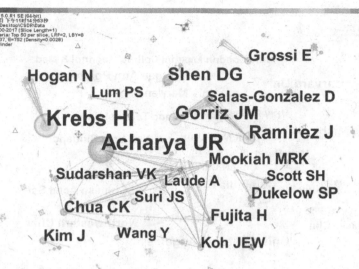

CiteSpace, v. 5.0 R1 SE (64-bit)
2018年1月24日 下午11时14分53秒
C:\Users\Lee\Desktop\CSDR\Data
Timespan: 2000-2017 (Slice Length=1)
Selection Criteria: Top 50 per slice, LRF=2, LBY=8
Network: N=737, E=752 (Density=0.0028)
Pruning: Pathfinder

Fig. 3. Author collaboration network.

Table 1. Authors and the number of articles published (TOP 20).

Author	No. of published articles	Author	No. of published articles
Acharya UR	44	Salas-Gonzalez D	12
Krebs HI	40	Dukelow SP	12
Ramirez J	21	Mookiah MRK	12
Gorriz JM	21	Koh JEW	11
Shen DG	19	Suri JS	11
Hogan N	15	Sudarshan VK	11
Grossi E	13	Scott SH	10
Chua CK	13	Laude A	10
Fujita H	13	Wang Y	10
Kim J	13	Lum PS	10

Institutional Distribution

Then we analyzed the institutions of scientific literature by generating institutional cooperation network map, as shown in Fig. 4. Table 2 shows the Top 10 institutions in the number of published articles. Among them, the Top 2 organizations that published the largest number of articles are Massachusetts Institute of Technology (MIT) and Harvard University, with 84 and 83 articles respectively. The numbers of articles published by the top 20 institutions are 39 or more. It shows that the research in this field has received extensive attention from various authoritative academic research institutions in the world.

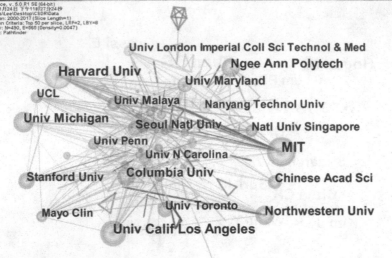

Fig. 4. Institutional collaboration networks.

Table 2. Institutions and the number of articles published (TOP 10).

Institution	No. of published articles	LCS	GCS
MIT	84	396	2952
Harvard University	83	152	3719
University of California, Los Angeles	75	108	1557
University Michigan	63	48	679
University Maryland	58	160	1314
Northwestern University	57	165	1429
Columbia University	55	40	578
Ngee Ann Polytechnic	55	215	916
Stanford University	51	150	1732
Seoul National University	49	28	447

In the *Histcite* system, the frequency of citations is divided into Local Citation Score (LCS) and Global Citation Score (GCS). The LCS refers to the frequency of citations of an article in the current database, and the GCS refers to the frequency of citations of a article in the Web of Science database. According to Table 2, MIT and Harvard University not only published the largest number of articles, but also with the best LCS and GCS. This indicates that the two institutions have great influence in this research field. The University of Michigan ranked 4th with 63 articles, but its LCS and GCS are far less than the University of Maryland and Northwestern University. The influence of the articles published by the University of Michigan is not as big influence as that of those published by the University of Maryland and Northwestern University.

The cooperation between institutions is an important way to enhance the overall research capabilities of institutions, complement the advantages of scientific research resources, as well as share knowledge. And the level of research cooperation between institutions is also one of the indicators reflecting the state of research in a research field. In Fig. 4, the number of network nodes is 490, the number of connections between nodes is 565, and the density of the network is 0.0047, which shows in this research field, the cooperation is extensive and close among different institutions.

4 Literature Co-citation Analysis

We analyzed the co-citations of literatures and generated literature co-citations network map, as shown in Fig. 5. Co-citation network refers to a knowledge network formed when two scientific literatures are cited at the same time by the third or other different literatures [14]. Literature co-citation analysis expresses relationships between literatures through frequency cited by other literatures at the same time. And the higher the reference frequency, the closer the relationship is, and the more similar the academic background of the two literatures is [15].

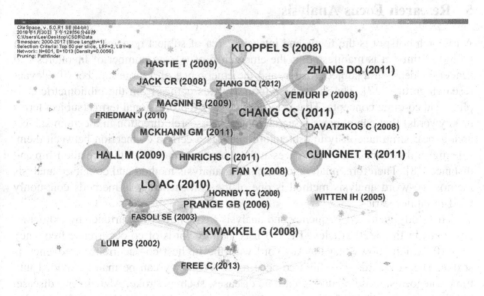

Fig. 5. Article co-citation network. (Color figure online)

Essentially, when certain literatures, journals, or academic groups are repeatedly cited by their counterparts, these knowledge carriers are essentially recognized by the scientific community in which they are located and form a scientific paradigm. This paradigm relationship can be visualized through the analysis of literature co-citation networks [16]. Through the literature co-citation network, the knowledge base of chronic disease research driven by emerging information technologies can be specifically presented.

In Fig. 5, each node represents the referenced literature, the size of the node is proportional to how many times it is cited, the lines between the nodes indicate the co-citation relationship, the thickness of the lines indicates the strength of the co-citation, and the different colors indicate the years in which the literatures are cited. The number of network nodes is 601, the number of connections between nodes is 1013, and the density of the network is 0.0056. In the literature co-citation network, Chang [20] published a literature named LIBSVM: A Library for Support Vector Machines in ACM Transactions on Intelligent Systems and Technology have the most citations (138 times). Chang [20] and Cuingnet [21], Klöppel [22], Jack [23], Ashburner [24] are all connected. And the connection with Ashburner [24] is the thickest, indicating that co-citation relationship between Chang and Ashburner is stronger. It also shows that the scientific literature published by Chang [20] has a strong correlation with that by Ashburner [24], and their subject are similar. Generally the literatures cited in the research field are distributed widely and a completely mature co-citation network system has not formed yet.

5   Research Focus Analysis

A research hotspot is the focus and intensive area of subject research within a certain period of time, it is manifested as the emergence of a large number of literatures and academic ideas on a subject matter, and the emergence of a large number of relevant research groups [17]. The idea of Co-term analysis comes from the bibliometric coupling and co-cited concepts. That is to say, when two professional terms (subject terms or keywords) that can express research topics or research direction in a certain subject area appear simultaneously in a literature, there is a certain connection between them. The higher the number of occurrences at the same time, the closer their relationship and distance [18]. Therefore, relative to the citation analysis method and co-author analysis method, co-word analysis method is one of the content analysis methods commonly used in bibliometrics.

This study analyzed frequency and analysis frequency co-occurrence by extracting keywords in the 4820 articles. Table 3 lists the keywords of co-occurrence frequency Top 10, which shows that the keyword with the highest co-occurrence frequency is stroke. The keywords with high co-occurrence frequency can be mainly divided into three categories, those related to chronic diseases, such as stroke, Alzheimer's disease, obesity, etc., those related to emerging technologies, such as artificial neural networks, support vector machines, machine learning, etc., and those related to research issues to be resolved such as classification, predictions and so on.

The co-word network refers to the objective knowledge network that expresses the structure of the scientific knowledge field constituted by the co-occurrence of keywords, it can be used to depict the knowledge structure of a subject area, and it can be combined with the time series to reveal the evolution of a discipline structure [19]. We analyzed the keywords of literature and generated the keyword co-occurrence network map, as shown in Fig. 6. Each node in this figure represents a keyword, the size of the

Table 3. Keyword frequency (TOP 10).

	Keyword	Frequency	Centrality
1	Stroke	589	0.11
2	Classification	540	0.32
3	Alzheimer's disease	340	0.22
4	Rehabilitation	323	0.28
5	Diagnosis	323	0.13
6	Robotics	318	0.12
7	Artificial neural network	315	0.12
8	Disease	304	0.13
9	Support vector machine	276	0.01
10	Machine learning	275	0.03

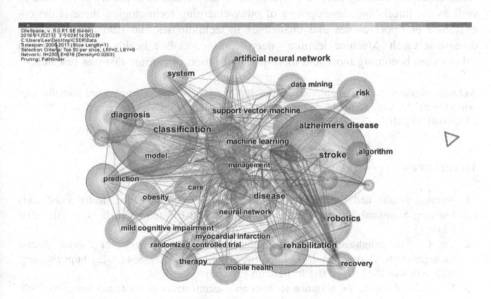

Fig. 6. Keywords co-occurrence network (Color figure online)

node is directly proportional to the frequency of co-occurrence, the connection between nodes represents the co-occurrence relationship between the two keywords in the same literature, and different colors represent the year of the co-occurrence of keywords. The number of network nodes is 250, the number of connections between nodes is 818, and the density of the network is 0.0263. According to this figure, there are strong connections between the keywords, and the entire network is densely connected. It shows that the most of papers published in this research field are multi-topic research.

6 Concluding Remarks and Future Trends

This study analyzed and the time distribution, spatial distribution, literature co-citations, and research hotspots of the research domain knowledge. First of all, regarding the distribution of time, the annual quantity of articles published and the amount of annual authors' input have increased year by year, and the growth rate is rapid in recent years. Secondly, in terms of spatial distribution, the authors' cooperation network density is not high, there is less cooperation among high-yield authors, the cooperation relationship is looser, but the cooperation between institutions is relatively more. Thirdly, the literature co-citation network is not dense enough, and a relatively complete and mature co-citation network system has not yet been formed. Finally, in the keyword co-occurrence network, there are many connections between keywords, and the entire network is densely connected, which indicates that the literatures in this research field are mostly multi-topic research. With the arrival of the era of big data, as well as the flourishing development of other emerging technologies, there is the co-existence of opportunities and challenges in technologies and data–driven chronic disease research. Machine learning, deep learning, mobile health, block chain and robotics are becoming more and more popularly used in chronic diseases research.

Acknowledgements. The dataset collection and analysis of this research were partially supported by the National Natural Science Foundation of China (NSFC) under grant Nos. 71331002, 71301040, 71771075, 71771077, 71573071, and 71601061.

References

1. National Health and Family Planning Commission of PRC: China Health and Family Planning Statistical Yearbook. Peking Union Medical College Press, Beijing (2015). (in Chinese)
2. Lv, L.: The enlightenment of the international theoretical model of chronic disease management to China. Chin. J. Heal. Inform. Manag. **12**(5), 529–534 (2015). https://doi.org/10.3969/j.issn.1672-5166.2015.05.018. (in Chinese)
3. Lv, Y., Li, Z., et al.: Visualization analysis on research status, hotspots and frontiers of self-management of chronic disease. J. Nurs. (China) **20**(7B), 1–5 (2013). https://doi.org/10.3969/j.issn.1008-9969.2013.14.001. (in Chinese)
4. Lu, F.: Literature metrology analysis of chronic disease management research papers. Chin. Nurs. Res. **29**(7C), 2676–2678 (2015). https://doi.org/10.3969/j.issn.1009-6493.2015.21.054. (in Chinese)
5. Taifang, L., Aihua, Z., et al.: Visualization analysis under the international perspective about the chronic disease research of the elderly base on the web of science database. Mod. Prev. Med. **44**(3), 520–524 (2017). (in Chinese)
6. Rajpal, D.K., Kumar, V., Agarwal, P.: Scientific literature mining for drug discovery: a case study on obesity. Drug Dev. Res. **72**(2), 201–208 (2011). https://doi.org/10.1002/ddr.20416
7. Kong, W., Mou, X., Hu, X.: Exploring matrix factorization techniques for significant genes identification of Alzheimer's disease microarray gene expression data. BMC Bioinform. **12**(5), S7 (2011). https://doi.org/10.1186/1471-2105-12-s5-s7

8. Khan, A., Choudhury, N., Uddin, S., Hossain, L., Baur, L.A.: Longitudinal trends in global obesity research and collaboration: a review using bibliometric metadata. Obes. Rev. **17**(4), 377–385 (2016). https://doi.org/10.1111/obr.12372

9. Lledó, L.D., et al.: A comparative analysis of 2D and 3D tasks for virtual reality therapies based on robotic-assisted neurorehabilitation for post-stroke patients. Front. Aging Neurosci. **8**, 205 (2016). https://doi.org/10.3389/fnagi.2016.00205

10. Yang, G., Chen, S., Ma, A., Lu, J., Wang, T.: Identification of the difference in the pathogenesis in heart failure arising from different etiologies using a microarray dataset. Clinics **72**(10), 600–608 (2017). https://doi.org/10.6061/clinics/2017(10)03

11. Gu, D., Li, J., Li, X., Liang, C.: Visualizing the knowledge structure and evolution of big data research in healthcare informatics. Int. J. Med. Inform. **98**, 22–32 (2017). https://doi.org/10.1016/j.ijmedinf.2016.11.006

12. Chen, C.: Searching for intellectual turning points: progressive knowledge domain visualization. Proc. Natl. Acad. Sci. **101**(suppl. 1), 5303–5310 (2004). https://doi.org/10.1073/pnas.0307513100

13. Chen, C.: CiteSpace II: detecting and visualizing emerging trends and transient patterns in scientific literature. J. Assoc. Inf. Sci. Technol. **57**(3), 359–377 (2006). https://doi.org/10.1002/asi.20317

14. Small, H.: Co-citation in the scientific literature: a new measure of the relationship between two documents. J. Assoc. Inf. Sci. Technol. **24**(4), 265–269 (1973). https://doi.org/10.1002/asi.4630240406

15. Xie, P.: Study of international anticancer research trends via co-word and document co-citation visualization analysis. Scientometrics **105**(1), 611–622 (2015). https://doi.org/10.1007/s11192-015-1689-0

16. Lyu, P., Zhang, L.: Scientific knowledge networks in LIS (II): case study on the structure, characteristics and evolution of co-citation networks. J. China Soc. Sci. Tech. Inf. **33**(4), 349–357 (2014). https://doi.org/10.3772/j.issn.10000135.2014.04.002. (in Chinese)

17. Lu, Y., Li, Z., Arthur, D.: Mapping publication status and exploring hotspots in a research field: chronic disease self-management. J. Adv. Nurs. **70**(8), 1837–1844 (2014). https://doi.org/10.1111/jan.12344

18. Zhang, Q., Xu, X.: On discovering the structure map of knowledge management research abroad—integration of a bibliometric analysis and visualization analysis. J. Ind. Eng./Eng. Manag. **22**(4), 30–35 (2008). https://doi.org/10.3969/j.issn.1004-6062.2008. (in Chinese)

19. Leydesdorff, L.: Why words and co-words cannot map the development of the sciences. J. Am. Soc. Inf. Sci. **48**(5), 418–427 (1997)

20. Chang, C.C., Lin, C.J.: LIBSVM: a library for support vector machines. ACM Trans. Intell. Syst. Technol. (TIST) **2**(3), 27 (2011)

21. Cuingnet, R., Gerardin, E., Tessieras, J., et al.: Automatic classification of patients with Alzheimer's disease from structural MRI: a comparison of ten methods using the ADNI database. Neuroimage **56**(2), 766–781 (2011)

22. Klöppel, S., Stonnington, C.M., Chu, C., et al.: Automatic classification of MR scans in Alzheimer's disease. Brain **131**(3), 681–689 (2008)

23. Jack Jr., C.R., Bernstein, M.A., Fox, N.C., et al.: The Alzheimer's disease neuroimaging initiative (ADNI): MRI methods. J. Magn. Reson. Imaging: Off. J. Int. Soc. Magn. Reson. Med. **27**(4), 685–691 (2008)

24. Ashburner, M., Bergman, C.M.: Drosophila melanogaster: a case study of a model genomic sequence and its consequences. Genome Res. **15**(12), 1661–1667 (2005)

Media Message Design via Health Communication Perspective: A Study of Cervical Cancer Prevention

Hua Ran, Shupei Geng[✉], and Di Xiao

The School of Journalism and Communication,
Wuhan University, Wuhan 430072, Hubei, China
284994302@qq.com

Abstract. This paper focuses on the prevention of cervical cancer as a case lestudy, exploring the impact and role of health information on public health and individual health concepts, and further strengthening women's concerns about their own health. Based on 2×2 online random experiment, the experimental materials about cervical cancer are designed with different degree of fear appeals (Low Threat/High Threat Intensity) and different types of information (Narrative/Statistical Evidence). 300 women in appropriate age are the target research participant. The results show that the threat intensity and the type of evidence have impact on the attitude of the participants. The experimentally preset randomized four scenes found a significant difference after the pairwise comparison, and the willingness to prevent of the four scenes present a high trend in the comparison results with the control group. Individuals' perceptions of disease fear and their willingness to prevent cervical cancer are influenced by the intensity of the threat and the type of evidence. For the perception of fear effectiveness, the two types of evidentiary changes in the level of the threat of narrative evidence and the message of the high threat level will significantly affect the fear efficacy score. However, in the measurement of prevention intention, the persuasive effect of narrative evidence under the high threat intensity is significantly higher than that of statistical evidence and vice versa. By measuring the participants' perceptions of fear effectiveness and degree of prevention intention, the media health massage design strategy and the content structure of media health information to maximize the persuasive effect in the limited conditions could be concluded.

Keywords: Health communication · Cervical cancer prevention
Persuasive effect · Fear appeals · Evidence types

1 Introduction

Health issues are closely related to public life. Health information affects public perceptions, attitudes and behaviors. In the context of communication, how the media can effectively transmit health information, construct a cognitive system of health knowledge, and eliminate misunderstandings and conservative concepts are worth being discussed in long-term perspectives. Cervical cancer is the second most common

© Springer Nature Switzerland AG 2018
H. Chen et al. (Eds.): ICSH 2018, LNCS 10983, pp. 274–285, 2018.
https://doi.org/10.1007/978-3-030-03649-2_27

cancer among women in the world. However, this cancer can be clearly identified and preventable at the early stage. Therefore, prevention, inspection and early detection are important principles for the treatment of cervical cancer.

In most cases, women's health issues involve personal privacy, which limits the possibility to public discussion of the disease to some extent. Due to factors such as economic, culture, ideology and value, women are still at a disadvantage in society and family. The stereotypes and misunderstanding of the public on 'sexuality' issues and women's diseases also reflect the imbalance of gender power structure and the inequality of gender status. At present, the general needs of women are neglected and the information related to cervical cancer can not be effectively disseminated, which also directly affects people's involvement in women's health problems. The vicious circle which caused by the lack of information and social prejudice has lead to an incomplete understanding of relevant knowledge of disease and a lack of awareness of women's own protection.

In recent years, there is a close cooperation between medical community and the medical industry. A large number of advanced cervical cancer prevention technologies have been utilized into clinical application. It has been demonstrated that the persistence of two high-risk HPV infections is the most critical factor for cervical cancer. With the HPV vaccine gradually listed in China, the female public has a reliable alternative for cervical cancer screening. However, health information needs to be delivered through the media. In the Chinese market, the public has already developed the habit of acquiring information through various media organizations, including the Internet. Redundant and complicated information will undoubtedly cause confusion and interference to the recipients. Correspondingly, the scientific content also has the opportunity to cultivate female's correct and positive prevention attitude to the cervical cancer. In addition to the increasingly progressive clinical prevention measures, how the media plans to disseminate content and guide the public to choose healthy behaviors is of great significance to improve women's willingness of cervical cancer prevention.

2 Literature Review

2.1 Health Communication and Cervical Cancer Prevention

According to the literature analysis, most of researches are based on nursing, clinical medicine and other fields, and there are just few researches focusing on cervical cancer cognitive construction and basic attitude of individual diseases from the perspective of health transmission. In general, the knowledge of cervical cancer of female is extremely limited, especially in low- and middle-income countries. A qualitative study by Ports (2015) and other scholars on women in Malawi in Africa shows that women's awareness of cervical cancer is at a low level and women's knowledge about cervical cancer is likely to be misunderstood or deviated, such as the risk associated with disease and preventive measures etc. Because of limited conditions, a large numbers of women do not have access to health information. Women in Asia are generally less aware of cervical cancer than in developed regions such as Europe, America and Australia.

At present, HPV vaccine is one of the effective methods to prevent cervical cancer. Most scholars also suggest that individual's attitude to disease cognition, social norms and perception control will affect their willingness to be vaccinated with HPV vaccine (Wong 2014). Dunlop (2010) and other scholars used group experiments and questionnaires to explore the different forms of media information on the public cervical cancer prevention attitude and cognition. They also compared narrative stories with conventional news. Meanwhile the article says that if advertising evokes a strong emotional response from individuals, they are more likely to participate in the discussion of relevant topics. Rogers (2016) used the conversations and scenes that appear in television about HPV to analyze the impact on the public's willingness to vaccinate. He summed up how television content affects the public's willingness to get HPV vaccinated through text rhetoric and scene descriptions. Television provides a scientific and accurate description of the related communication issues and promotes open discussion on sexual health issues, which inspires individuals' willingness to prevent cervical cancer more or less. Lee (2017) analyzed the impact of messaging frameworks and online media channels on the perceived severity of cervical cancer and HPV among young people. Compared with the content framework, the channel of information dissemination has a more significant impact on the individual attitude. Therefore, the author further proposed the design strategy and transmission way of online cervical cancer and HPV information.

2.2 Persuasive Effect

With the further development of information communication technology, people are more dependent on the information transmitted by the mass media to society, and the media will have a deeper impact on individual's concept. Therefore, researches on the persuasive effect of communication have also become the academic and social interest. The theory of persuasion, which have an extensive significance on both academic research and social application, mainly focuses on the influence of discourse and symbols on people, and its core issues involve the psychology of individual and society. In fact, whether in education, election, consumption or voting, the main channels for individuals or groups to use persuasive strategies are communication. Persuasion can influence one's beliefs, attitudes, intentions, motives, and actions (Gass and Seiter 2013). In conclusion, persuasion is the use of means of communication in a specific social environment, so that the audience can meet the expectations of the communicator after receiving the information. Health communication has the connotation of advocating the public to actively choose healthy behavior, and the measurement standard of transmission effect is to test the change and tendency of individual attitude. Thus, it is appropriate to use persuasion theory in health communication research.

Early scholars believe that fear appeal plays a positive role in the change of individual behavior and attitude. With the increase of fear level of information, the persuasion effect is obviously strengthened. In the subsequent study, Janis (1953) suggested that there is a 'inverted U' relationship between fear demands and persuasion effects, which means the moderate intensity of fear demands is the best. In general, low intensity demands cause too little threat and motivation, while high intensity leads to self-defense and rebuttal feelings of information recipients. Different experimental situations bring the different correlation between fear appeal and persuasion effect. Witte's (1992) high-threat fear appeal will trigger two common reactions among the audience: one is fear control, the other is risk control. When the audience believes that recommendations in information that prevent threats from occurring are effective and easy to implement, there is an incentive to control the risks. But if the audience is unable to obtain effective advice, or if they think it is too difficult to reach it, fear control will be taken. Therefore, when the threat presented in the dissemination of information is high, it must be accompanied by highly effective measures, methods and recommendations. This also provides guidance and direction for the design of experimental materials in this text.

The strength of persuasion can be enhanced by constantly proving the point of view in some forms during the process of information presentation. These evidences often appear in different forms and can be divided into two categories: objective statistical evidence and narrative evidence (Perloff 2010). Statistical evidence refers to the use of factual presentation and abstract data to convince the audience, such as the development of related disease data conjecture, indicating that individuals or groups are likely to be affected by health problems. As a matter of fact, statistical evidence includes a quantitative description of events, persons, places, or other phenomena, while narrative evidence includes specific, emotional information (Baesler and Burgoon 1994). For example, describing a special situation in the first person may also affect the receiver in some extent. Narrative evidence is defined as 'the use of case stories or examples to demonstrate that the conclusions provided by the communicator are true' (Preiss 1997). The effect of persuasive communication depends not only on the choice of motivation, but also on the organizational form of opinion information. This paper uses the combination of different types of evidence and different threat degree of information to explore which forms of information can optimize the communication effect through the experimental method, which has certain practical significance.

3 Methods

In this paper, a 2×2 online random experiment is designed by using the experimental method. According to persuasion effect theory, cervical cancer news information with different degree of fear appeal (low threat intensity/high threat intensity) and different information type (narrative evidence/statistical evidence) is designed. The subjects are randomly assigned to any of the four online scenes to answer follow-up questions by reading and understanding the material without being informed of the purpose of the experiment. Simultaneously, the experiment also set up a control group that do not accept any experimental materials. According to the results of the experiment, this paper will explore the difference of women's attitude to cervical cancer prevention and risk perception of disease after receiving different types of health information so that the design strategy and content structure of media health information can be analyzed. The purpose of this paper is to maximize the persuasive effect in the limited framework and conditions. In summary, this paper will mainly explore the following issues:

a. A survey of the attitude and willingness of women toward the prevention of cervical cancer;
b. The influence of different types and threat level of evidence on the cognition and prevention willingness of women towards cervical cancer;
c. Putting forward effective communication strategies for media to disseminate health information.

3.1 Participant Recruitment for Online Experiment

The experiment was conducted in an online questionnaire. Taking Wuhan area as the center, 300 samples were recruited by convenient sampling. The composition of samples shows that the subjects are college students, who are easier to adapt to the experimental arrangements but also have a certain academic background and life base compared with other people in society, including undergraduates, masters and doctors. It is convenient to extract samples because the network of college students' group relations is stable and diverse. According to statistics, the average age of the participants is 24 years old, and most of them have been in or will enter the cervical cancer age group in recent years. In order to keep the cognitive level of the participants in an close interval, the study excluded some students those majoring in psychology and medicine in the process of issuing the questionnaire. After reading materials, the participants need to answer three detailed questions related to the content to test whether they read carefully, so as to ensure the authenticity of the sample and the validity of the data. '1' point for correct answer and '0' point for the wrong answer, the full score of detailed questions is 3. If a participant's score is greater than or equal to 2 points, he is classified as 'valid sample', otherwise 'invalid sample'. Based on the above rules, this experiment eliminated 16 "invalid samples" and then added 16 samples to ensure the total amount is equal to 300.

3.2 Experiment Materials Design

According to the characteristics of independent variables, this study designed four materials of uniform length, content and style based on the regular features of news reports and personal blog pages. Except for the control group, participants in the other four experimental groups will randomly read one of four materials about cervical cancer prevention and answer the following questions. All the four paragraphs are composed of a simple paragraph. The main difference between the statistical and narrative evidence is that the former is objectively described by the third person with authoritative data, while the latter is the subjective and narrative expression of the first person perspective. The low/high threat intensity in the statistical evidence presents the cervical cancer mortality, severity, cervical cancer cure rate and the prevention success rate. In narrative evidence, the intensity of low/high threat is mainly presented by the tone of the patient's self-described and the result of anticancer. Each material refers to a variety of cervical cancer prevention methods, including cervical section screening and HPV vaccination.

3.3   Measures

Two central theoretical constructs were assessed with 5-point Likert scale and scaled such that higher values corresponded with the positive end of the scale: Perceived fear Effectiveness and prevention intention.

Perceived Fear Effectiveness. In Witte's (2000) extended parallel process model, there are five dimensions of fear, perceived-susceptibility, perceived-severity, self-efficacy and response-efficacy. The general questions are: how much did this message make you feel frightened; I am at risk for HPV; I believe that HPV is a severe health problem; I am able to get vaccinated for HPV. According to research themes and materials, this article sets the perception of fear effectiveness as: (i) I think I have a certain risk of contracting the HPV virus; (ii) I think I have a certain risk of developing cervical cancer or precancerous lesions; (iii) I think infection with HPV will have very serious consequences; (iv) I think inoculation of HPV vaccine is effective for cervical cancer prevention; (v) I believe cervical cancer screening is effective for cervical cancer prevention; (vi) If I conduct cervical cancer screening regularly, I feel more confident about my future health status; (vii) If I have been vaccinated with the HPV vaccine, I am more at ease with my future health status.

Prevention Intention. There are three main dimensions for measuring the degree of Prevention intention: the willingness to cervical cancer screening; the willingness to be vaccinated and the willingness to cultivate healthy living habits. Based on previous studies, the following indicators were taken in response to individual prevention intentions (Lee and Cho 2017): (i) I am willing to do cervical cancer screening; (ii) I am willing to be vaccinated to prevent cervical cancer; (iii) I will search the Internet for topics on cervical cancer and HPV in the near future; (iv) I will discuss the topic of cervical cancer and HPV with my family and friends in the near future; (v) I will consciously avoid bad habits.

The experimental assumptions are as follows:

H1: *There is a main effect on the persuasive effects of fear appeal level information on individual's perception of disease risk and prevention intention, and the persuasive effect of high threat level information is higher than that of low threat level;*
H2: *There is a main effect of the type of persuasive evidence on perceiving the individual's perception of disease risk and the willingness to prevent, and the persuasive effect of statistical evidence is superior to narrative evidence;*
H3: *Individuals' perception of disease risk and willingness to prevent cervical cancer are affected by the interaction of threat intensity and the type of evidence.*

3.4   Manipulation Test

In order to test whether the participants successfully accepted the experimental materials, the study conducted preliminary deletions with three material detail questions. If the number of correct answers is less than two (not included), the sample is judged to be invalid. Then the study conducted an independent sample t-test. After receiving the information, participants were significantly higher than the control group in terms of perception of fear effectiveness and prevention intention. *Perceived fear effectiveness:*

M = 24.80, SD = 4.915, t = 4.550, p < 0.01. *Prevention intention:* M = 19.73, SD = 3.627, t = 4.001, p < 0.01. It can be seen that the difference between the experimental group and the control group in the sense of fear effectiveness and the degree of prevention intention is significant, and the experimental group is significantly higher than the control group. Therefore, the intervention of this experimental information material was successful.

4 Results

According to the reliability analysis of the questionnaire, the Kronbach's coefficient of the questionnaire is 0.874; the KMO value of the questionnaire is 0.888 through the Bartle's sphere test. The experimental results are of high statistical significance and can be further analyzed.

For the degree of perception of fear effectiveness, the main effects of the degree of threat and type of evidence are significant, with $F (1,236) = 36.602$, $P < 0.01$; $F (1,236) = 17.504$, $P < 0.01$; the interaction of threat level and evidence type is also significant, with $F (1,236) = 23.776$, $P < 0.01$ (Table 1).

Table 1. Threat level in analysis of variance

Variables	SS	DF	MS	F	P
Threat level (a)	673.350	1	673.350	36.602***	0.000
Evidence types (b)	322.017	1	322.017	17.504***	0.000
a * b	437.400	1	437.400	23.776***	0.000
Error	4341.633	236	18.397		

$^{*} = 0.01 < P \leq 0.05$, $^{**} = 0.001 < P \leq 0.01$, $^{***} = P \leq 0.001$.
The P value indicates significance level.

In-depth analysis of the differences, an independent sample t-test using the degree of threat and type of evidence as independent variables. High threat information is more powerful than low threat information, so that participants can have a higher sense of fear effectiveness, with $t = 5.605$, $P < 0.01$; and narrative evidence information is more likely than statistical evidence to produce after participants receive information panic, with $t = -3.749$, $P < 0.01$.

In order to reveal the interactions in depth, this paper carries out a simple effect test on the degree of threat and type of evidence. The results show that under the condition of statistical evidence information, the simple effect of threat level is not significant, with $F = .689$, $P > 0.1$. However, under the condition of narrative evidence type information, the simple effect of threat level is significant, with $F = 59.689$, $P < 0.01$. At the same time, under the high degree of threat, the perceived level of fear effectiveness of the data-type evidence information and narrative evidence information is significantly different, with $F = 41.040$, $P < 0.01$. In the low-threatening condition, there is no significant difference in the perception of the two types of information evidence by the subjects, $F = .240$, $P > 0.1$. In summary, the two types of proof switching between high and low threat intensity changes and high threat information in the narrative evidence will significantly affect the fear effectiveness score. The other two types of collocations have no significant effect (Fig. 1).

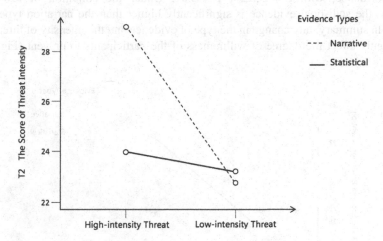

Fig. 1. Plot for the interaction of threat intensity and narrative evidence vs. statistical evidence on the perception of fear effectiveness

For the willingness of disease prevention, the main effect of threat degree is significant, with F (1,236) = 5.061, 0.01 < P < 0.05; the interaction degree of threat degree and evidence type is significant, with F (1,236) = 61.993, P < 0.01 (Table 2).

Table 2. Prevention intention in analysis of variance

Variables	SS	DF	MS	F	P
Threat level (a)	52.267	1	52.267	5.061*	0.025
Evidence types (b)	15.000	1	15.000	1.452	0.229
a * b	640.267	1	640.267	61.993***	0.000
Error	2437.400	236	10.328		

* = 0.01 < P ≤ 0.05, ** = 0.001 < P ≤ 0.01, *** = P ≤ 0.001.
The P value indicates significance level.

In-depth analysis of the differences, an independent sample t-test using the degree of threat and type of evidence as independent variables. In general, the information of the low threat level can improve the willingness of the subjects to prevent cervical cancer more than the high threat level information, with t = −2.006, 0.01 < P < 0.05. In the simple effect analysis of the interactive influence of the two variables of "threat intensity" and "evidence type" on the willingness to prevent, the simple effects of the four scenarios are significant.

In other words, the low-threatening statistical evidence can make the subject more willing to prevent than the statistical evidence with high threat degree, with F = 51.240, P < 0.01. The high-threatening narrative evidence is more likely to motivate the participants' willingness to prevent than the low-threatening narrative evidence, with F = 15.815, P < 0.01. Under high threat intensity, the persuasive effect of narrative evidence on prevention intention is significantly higher than that of statistical evidence, with F = 22.234, P < 0.01. Under the condition of low threat intensity, the statistical evidence is significantly higher than the narration type information. In summary, any change in the type of evidence and the intensity of threats will significantly affect the degree of willingness of the participants to prevent (Fig. 2).

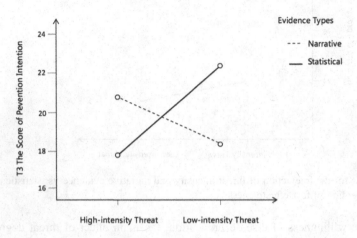

Fig. 2. Plot for the interaction of threat intensity and narrative evidence vs. statistical evidence on prevention intention

5 Discussions and Conclusions

5.1 Implications for Health Messages Design

The media coverage of health information is biased, weak and unprofessional, which leads to the lack of awareness of cervical cancer in public. Therefore, the primary goal of health communication should be improving public health knowledge and popularizing information of cervical cancer prevention. The statistic shows that more than half of the participants will be able to search for the information about cervical cancer in the near future or discuss it with family and friends. It can be said that the health communication content is the main source of non-medical and unprofessional public access to information, and it also has the ability to shape the general health knowledge structure of the society. At present, however, domestic media reports on the spread of various types of cervical cancer, as well as all kinds of social software, have not paid enough attention to cervical cancer-related knowledge. Therefore, the media should disseminate and guide the correct disease-related information and establish a relatively scientific cognitive system for the public, so that the public can avoid deviations in the value judgment of health information to some degree. The media should also exert social responsibilities, strengthen the popularization and penetration of health knowledge, and further highlight the role of health knowledge in the dissemination and education.

According to the experimental results, different types of information have different effect on persuasion effect. The media should accurately grasp the types of information and content structure, select different channels of communication based on their consumers, communication strategies and contents, so as to maximize information efficiency. The media can also strengthen positive psychological interventions for patients or the public and give the public information on the prevention of cervical cancer, thereby avoiding unnecessary panic. The media reports on cervical cancer directly or indirectly highlight the risk factors of the disease, which can positively influence the public's awareness of avoiding the risk of disease. In health communication, moderate fear appeal persuasion can actively guide the public to change unhealthy living habits. The study found that media reports of cervical cancer risk are heavily flooded with emotional persuasion messages. The information enhances the communication effect by evoking the public's 'fear appeal', however, which violates the social responsibilities of the media to guide public opinion and even promote public misbehavior. Therefore, the media should also pay attention to the balance of disease risk and prevention effectiveness in health communication.

At the same time, linear regression analysis is not well presented due to the space limitations. In spite of this, the result shows that the rising of the fear effectiveness score will significantly increase the score of prevention intention. This indicates that there is a greater chance to improve women's prevention intention when enhancing their fear perception, no matter what kind of forms of information they get.

5.2 Contributions

Reviewing the results and literature, most health communication studies are highly specialized which are based on a certain basic knowledge of medical science. Taking the ordinary female public as the research object, this paper provides some clear instructions for the media to design the content and to formulate the dissemination strategy effectively. Theoretically speaking, this paper further analyzes the frame and strategy of media information by using persuasion effect theory, and also tests the practicability of persuasion theory in health communication. It provides a typical case for the study of the measurement of the media communication effect and the way of reporting in the future.

With the renewal of social medical knowledge and the development of diversified information channels, the accumulation of health knowledge and women's cognition of cervical cancer have been significantly improved. However, they still spend less time on addressing the concern of their health. This situation may be closely related to the knowledge and information that people accept via mass media. The study found that woman's health attitude, behavior or belief are partially affected by media report (Watson et al. 2009) and strongly affected by the content of TV and blogs (Daily 2015). Although individual's experience, cultural backgrounds economic status and attitudes can influence their behavior, media is still regarded as one of the channel to bridge the gap between public and health information. This article uses experimental methods to provide a cross-discipline research path combined with psychology for persuasion research in mass communication, which has made breakthroughs and innovations in interdisciplinary research. In conclusion, this article researches the message design strategy of health communication through the cross-section analysis of mass communication and psychology, and also provides a psychological support for the research results of communication.

5.3 Limitations and Future Directions

Above all, in terms of subjects, the study ignored the characteristics of the information receiver – women. The effect of information dissemination depends on the feedback given by receivers. While women's personal health concept, daily life experience, economic status, cultural backgrounds, involvement and other factors all affect their acceptance of health information. At the same time, the process of recruitment is anonymous, which also affects the accuracy of the experimental results to a certain extent. In the next place, from the point of view of communication channels, the study only focuses on the communication effect caused by change or classification of information content, but it doesn't include the potential different effects among various media organizations. Actually, all the parts of the process of communication, such as content, subjects and channels, are worth being focused, which will significantly improve the authority and objectivity of the study. Therefore, future research can not only focus on assessing individual differences, but also consider more specific forms of information—such as the persuasive effect of images of health information. When new combinations of variables are presented in the experiment, the interactive effects of multiple factors t of health communication can be considered.

In terms of experimental operation, the article uses a 2×2 online random experiment. In order to obtain more experimental samples, this paper ignores the space-time difference, so that the control of the experimental environment in this study cannot be unified. Subsequent research will strive to adopt offline experiment to control the experimental conditions and potential variables. Meanwhile, in order to avoid significant individual differences, follow-up research will be based on a specific area or unit to take a random sample of stratification, which is able to ensure that participants' knowledge, economic level and personal perceptions fluctuate in a relatively small range. In summary, future research should increase the effectiveness and maneuverability of the experiment from three aspects: experimental environment, experimental subjects, and material intervention.

Acknowledgment. We thank the women who participated in this research study.

References

Baesler, E.J., Burgoon, J.K.: The temporal effects of story and statistical evidence on belief change. Commun. Res. **21**(5), 582–602 (1994)

Daily, K.: Biased assimilation and need for closure: examining the effects of mixed blogs on vaccine-related beliefs. J. Heal. Commun. **20**(4), 462–471 (2015)

Gass, R.H., Seiter, J.S.: Persuasion, Social Influence, and Compliance Gaining. Pearson/Allyn & Bacon, Boston (2013)

Janis, I.L., Feshbach, S.: Effects of fear-arousing communications. J. Abnorm. Soc. Psychol. **48**(1), 78–92 (1953)

Lee, M.J., Cho, J.: Promoting HPV vaccination online: message design and media choice. Heal. Promot. Pract. **18**(5), 152483991668822 (2017)

Wong, N.C.H.: Predictors of information seeking about the HPV vaccine from parents and doctors among young college women. Commun. Q. **62**(1), 75–96 (2014)

Perloff, R.M.: The Dynamics of Persuasion, 4th edn. Routledge (2010)

Ports, K.A., Reddy, D.M., Rameshbabu, A.: Cervical cancer prevention in Malawi: a qualitative study of women's perspectives. J. Heal. Commun. **20**(1), 97–104 (2015)

Preiss, M.A.R.W.: Comparing the persuasiveness of narrative and statistical evidence using meta-analysis. Commun. Res. Rep. **14**(2), 125–131 (1997)

Rogers, B.: All adventurous women do: HPV, narrative, and HBO's girls. Heal. Commun. **31**(1), 83–90 (2016)

Dunlop, S.M., Kashima, Y., Wakefield, M.: Predictors and consequences of conversations about health promoting media messages. Commun. Monogr. **77**(4), 518–539 (2010)

Watson, M., Shaw, D., Molchanoff, L., McInnes, C.: Challenges: lessons learned and results following the implementation of a human papilloma virus school vaccination program in South Australia. Aust. N. Z. J. Public Heal. **33**, 365–370 (2009)

Witte, K., Allen, M.: A meta-analysis of fear appeals: implications for effective public health campaigns. Heal. Educ. Behav. Off. Publ. Soc. Public Heal. Educ. **27**(5), 591 (2000)

Witte, K.: Putting the fear back into fear appeals: the extended parallel process model. Commun. Monogr. **59**(4), 329–349 (1992)

Information Systems and Institutional Entrepreneurship: How IT Carries Institutional Changes in Chronic Disease Management

Kui Du[1], Yanli Huang[2], Liang Li[3], Xiaolu Luo[4], and Wei Zhang[1(✉)]

[1] University of Massachusetts Boston, Boston, MA 02125, USA
Wei.zhang@umb.edu
[2] Innovation Center, Wuhou Health Bureau, Chengdu 610041, China
[3] University of International, Business and Economics, Beijing 100029, China
[4] Tiaoshanta Health Community Center, Chengdu 610041, China

Abstract. In this working-in-progress paper, we propose a qualitative study of using Information Technologies (IT) to help battle Chromic Disease Management (CDM). Using the institutional entrepreneurship theory, we argue that IT provides the vehicle with which and the context within which healthcare providers can proactively and innovatively improve CDM.

Keywords: Information technologies · Institutional entrepreneurship
Chronic disease management · Patient-Centered Medical Home

1 Introduction

In China, chronic diseases have become the leading threat to public health. From 2003 to 2012, the prevalence of chronic disease doubled from 123.3% to 245.2% (NHFPC 2016). In 2012, chronicle disease mortality nationwide reached 533 out of every 100,000 people, or 86.6% of all deaths (NHFPC 2016); burden of chronic disease accounted for 70% of the total burden of disease (NHFPC 2015). The continuous rise of chronic disease and associated cost – both financial and social – become one of, if not the, leading motivations for China to engage in extensive healthcare reforms and experiments in attempt to curb the trend (World Bank 2016).

In this working-in-progress paper, we propose a qualitative study of one such experiment on chronic disease management (CDM) in the Community Health Centers (CHCs) in Alpha (a pseudo name) district in a metropolitan city in Southwest China. The experiment started in 2015 and attempted to introduce practices based on Patient-Centered Medical Home, a new model for delivering healthcare that originated in the United States (Stange et al. 2010), to chronic disease management in the CHCs. Traditionally in China, chronic disease was treated the same as other diseases: the doctors saw patients when and only when the patients felt ill and the interactions between the patients and doctors ended when patients left the doctors' offices. PCMH, however, emphasizes relationship building between doctors and patients and advocates

H. Chen et al. (Eds.): ICSH 2018, LNCS 10983, pp. 286–291, 2018.
https://doi.org/10.1007/978-3-030-03649-2_28

personalized, comprehensive care instead of care focusing narrowly on disease treatment. The care is delivered in a coordinated way, usually by a team directed by doctors but not just doctors (Stange et al. 2010). In the US implementations, PCMH has demonstrated substantial effectiveness in chronic disease management (Grumbach and Grundy 2010), and drew great interests from the CHCs.

PCMH relies heavily on information technologies such as Electronic Medical Record (EMR). In fact, nearly half of the 166 items of the most popular measure used to assess "medical homeness", the National Committee for Quality Assurance's Physician Practice Connections – Patient-Centered Medical Home tool, are about the use of some IT (Stange et al. 2010). The implementation in the CHCs we study is no different, centering on the adoption of and adaptation to the Electronic Patient Management (EPM) system that aims to support PCMH in the three CHCs. In short, the EPM system essentially embeds the new PCMH practice, thus becoming the focal point of the implementation.

Interestingly but perhaps not surprisingly, the introduction of a new system that embeds a new practice not only engendered great tensions with the previous CDM practice but also ran afoul of government requirements that are of paramount importance in China. While we were amazed by the magnitude of the observed obstacles, we were even more fascinated by how innovatively the obstacles were overcame and subsequently the new practice began to take root in the CHCs, all through the use of the EPM. Viewing the introduction of the PCMH practices as an institutional innovation in CDM, we turn to the theory of institutional entrepreneurship and use it as the theoretical lens through which we can view and understand *how the EPM enables institutional entrepreneurs at CHCs to both establish new CDM practice and gain legitimacy for it.*

2 Institutional Entrepreneurship and Information Systems

Although one of the central claims of institutional theory is that institutions have strong inertia and restrain its constituents from deviating from status quo, gradual and radical changes to institutions, nevertheless, still happen all the time. The constraints imposed by institutional forces, often referred to as the "iron cage" (DiMaggio and Powell 1983), sometimes inhibit innovation and consequently deter technological, economical, and social advancement. A subgroup of institutional theorists then have been long interested in how to effectively reform existing institutions. While sometimes institutions change because of exogenous shocks such as regulatory changes or disruptive innovations, this subgroup of institutional theorists are more focused on endogenous institutional changes and, particularly, how some institutionally embedded agents, either individuals or organizations, can initiate changes to their institutional environments (Garud et al. 2007).

Along this line of academic inquiry, DiMaggio (1988) first coined the term "institutional entrepreneurs," who are actors that initiate changes to transform existing institutions or create new ones. Battilana et al. (2009) further suggested two requirements for change agents to qualify as institutional entrepreneurs: (1) these agents need to initiate divergent changes that could break the existing institutional logic; and (2) these agents need to take active actions, mobilize resources, and intensively participate in implementing these changes. Any theory of institutional entrepreneurship, as Battilana et al. (2009) argue, needs to be a theory of actions, or a theory that depicts the activities through which individual and organizational actors create a vision for divergent change, mobilize allies and leverage resources to pursue the vision, and ultimately reform existing institutions or create new ones. The lack of such theory has been argued as one of the institutional theory's core weaknesses (DiMaggio and Powell 1991).

When studying institutional entrepreneurs' actions, researchers have noticed multiple strategies institutional entrepreneurs often use to pursue institutional changes, such as rhetorical, structural, and cultural strategies (Battilana et al. 2009; Greenwood et al. 2002). These strategies differ in their effectiveness, but overall, even for effective ones, they typically require long time periods and involve intense conflicts among different institutional logics before the new institution can be established. Practitioners are constantly seeking for more effective tools that can induce institutional changes rapidly and more effectively.

Although remaining largely unnoticed, information systems might have the potential to become a new weapon for institutional entrepreneurs to induce institutional changes. Contemporary information systems often have pre-defined business routines and roles embedded in their software codes (Volkoff et al. 2007). The flexibility of information systems customization used to be rather limited, and thus, as Davenport (1998) noted almost two decades ago, *"SAP [an enterprise information system brand] isn't a software package; it's a way of doing business..."* (pp. 125) and *"an enterprise system imposes its own logic on company's strategy, culture, and organization"* (pp. 127). Thus, when institutional entrepreneurs want to introduce new institutional logic, one potential way of doing so is to codify those desired logic in information systems, which consequently become a carrier of institutional logic (Gosain 2004). Then, after system implementation and as the adopting organizations continuously use their information systems, they start to intentionally or unintentionally impose to the users the routines, social structures, and the norms and values embedded in the design of these information systems (Gosain 2004).

At the organization level, scholars have long noticed that organizations often take advantage of implementing a new information system as a window of opportunity to break existing practice and trigger the adoption or development of new ones (Tyre and Orlikowski 1994). At the institutional level, however, we are not yet sure whether institutional entrepreneurs can leverage information systems as a strategic weapon to induce the desired institutional changes. We have a few studies that focus on how institutional entrepreneurs mobilize their resources and make institutional arrangements to facilitate the diffusion of IT innovation (Garud et al. 2002; Wang and Swanson 2007). In these few studies, IT or information systems *per se* are the object of institutional entrepreneurship activities, but not the logic or practice embedded in them. To our knowledge, we have not adequately studied the role of information systems as a carrier of new institutional logic to enable and facilitate institutional entrepreneurship. Moreover, the technological environment has evolved. Advancements in technologies such as cloud computing made IS more flexible and easier to change than before. Thus this paper, at the theoretical level, aims to shed light on the question how institutional entrepreneurs can use today's information systems to induce desired institutional changes.

3 Research Method and Data Collection

We employed the case study method, which fits this study particularly well for three reasons. First, the research on institutional entrepreneurship in the CDM is still a nascent area, and the case study method is a suitable choice for exploratory studies (Edmondson and McManus 2007). Second, we focus on understanding how institutional entrepreneurs used the EPM system to both establish new CDM practice and gain legitimacy for it, and the case study method is ideally suitable for "how" questions as well as exploring the why underlying the observed phenomena (Yin 2009). Third, the focal CDM practice in Alpha district started in 2015 and two of the authors have traced this transformation since January 2016, which continues until today. Under such circumstance, the longitudinal, real-time case study design is especially appropriate (Eisenhardt and Graebner 2007; Yin 2009).

We managed to obtain great access to the research site. Following the principle of triangulation (Yin 2009), we collected data in multiple ways including interviews, field observations, and internal documents from institutional entrepreneurs in both the CHCs and the EPM service provider. In the 16 months since January 2016, two of the authors made six field visits to the CHCs, each averaging four days. During the field trips, in addition to interviewing informers form the CHCs and the EPM service provider, we attended events such knowledge sharing sessions, internal team meetings, and patient education programs at the CHCs. The research team also conducted multiple phone conferences with the informers for the study. So far, we have accumulated more than 50 h of interview and phone conference recordings and a vast collection of documents such as EPM system use manual and training manuals, internal reports on EPM deployment, and internal communications within the CHCs and the EPM service provider and between the CHCs and the EPM service provider.

4 Preliminary Findings and Expected Contributions

Our preliminary data analysis suggested the following:

(1) PCMH is an institutional innovation, and the EPM system is a carrier of the desired PCMH logic (which was also a radical innovation for CDM).
(2) The leadership, doctors, nurses, and staffs at CHCs and the EPM design and deployment team from the service provider acted as institutional entrepreneurs. These entrepreneurs attempted to use the implementation of the EPM system as a trigger to start the institutional changes and as a carrier to implement the changes.
(3) However, at least two tensions emerged. The EPM system contradicted with the practice mandated by the central and local governments (and another IT system enforced by them); it also contradicted with the existing institutional logics embedded in the daily practice of how CHCs had been dealing with chronic disease.

(4) The instructional entrepreneurs made innovative use of the EPM system to solve the tensions. They also made changes to the EMP system to adapt to the local circumstances that hinder the implementation of PCMH.

Currently, we are conducting in-depth data analysis.

With this study, we expect to make both theoretical and practical contributions. Theory-wise, we ultimately hope to establish IS as an effective strategy for institutional entrepreneurship, thus contributing to literature in not only institutional entrepreneurship but also IS usage. Practice-wise, we hope our study help to shed light on how to use IS to usher PCMH into healthcare providers and counter the threat of CDM to public health.

References

Battilana, J., Leca, B., Boxenbaum, E.: How actors change institutions: towards a theory of institutional entrepreneurship. Acad. Manag. Ann. 3(1), 65–107 (2009)

Davenport, T.H.: Putting the enterprise into the enterprise system. Harv. Bus. Rev. 76(4), 121–131 (1998)

DiMaggio, P.J.: Interest and agency in institutional theory. In: Zucker, L. (ed.) Institutional Patterns and Organizations, pp. 3–22. Ballinger, Cambridge (1988)

DiMaggio, P.J., Powell, W.W.: The iron cage revisited - institutional isomorphism and collective rationality in organizational fields. Am. Sociol. Rev. 48(2), 147–160 (1983)

DiMaggio, P.J., Powell, W.W.: Introduction. In: Powell, W.W., DiMaggio, P.J. (eds.) The New Institutionalism in Organizational Analysis, pp. 1–38. The University of Chicago Press, Chicago (1991)

Edmondson, A.C., McManus, S.E.: Methodological fit in management field research. Acad. Manag. Rev. 32(4), 1246–1264 (2007)

Eisenhardt, K.M., Graebner, M.E.: Theory building from cases: opportunities and challenges. Acad. Manag. J. 50(1), 25–32 (2007)

Garud, R., Hardy, C., Maguire, S.: Institutional entrepreneurship as embedded agency: an introduction to the special issue. Organ. Stud. 28(7), 957–969 (2007)

Garud, R., Jain, S., Kumaraswamy, A.: Institutional entrepreneurship in the sponsorship of common technological standards: the case of Sun Microsystems and Java. Acad. Manag. J. 45(1), 196–214 (2002)

Gosain, S.: Enterprise information systems as objects and carriers of institutional forces: the new iron cage? J. Assoc. Inf. Syst. 5(4), 151–182 (2004)

Greenwood, R., Suddaby, R., Hinings, C.R.: Theorizing change: the role of professional associations in the transformation of institutionalized fields. Acad. Manag. J. 45(1), 58–80 (2002)

Grumbach, K., Grundy, P.: Outcomes of implementing patient centered medical home interventions. Patient-Centered Primary Care Collaborative, Washington, DC (2010). http://3ww.pcpcc.net/files/evidence_outcomes_in_pcmh.pdf. Accessed 30 Apr 2017

NHFPC: Chinese disease prevention and control working progresses 2015. National Health and Family Planning Commission of the People's Republic of China (2015). http://www.nhfpc.gov.cn/jkj/s7915v/201504/d5f3f871e02e4d6e912def7ced719353.shtml. Accessed 29 Apr 2017

NHFPC: Nutrition and chronic disease surveillance in Chinese residents 2015 report. National Health and Family Planning Commission of the People's Republic of China. People's Medical Publishing House, Beijing (2016)

Stange, K.C., et al.: Defining and measuring the patient-centered medical home. J. Gen. Intern. Med. **25**(6), 601–612 (2010)

Tyre, M.J., Orlikowski, W.J.: Windows of opportunity - temporal patterns of technological adaptation in organizations. Organ. Sci. **5**(1), 98–118 (1994)

Volkoff, O., Strong, D.M., Elmes, M.B.: Technological embeddedness and organizational change. Organ. Sci. **18**(5), 832–848 (2007)

Wang, P., Swanson, E.B.: Launching professional services automation: institutional entrepreneurship for information technology innovations. Inf. Organ. **17**(2), 59–88 (2007)

World Bank: Deepening health reform in China: building high-quality and value-based service delivery - policy summary. World Bank Group, Washington, D.C (2016). http://documents. worldbank.org/curated/en/800911469159433307/Deepening-health-reform-in-China-building-high-quality-and-value-based-service-delivery-policy-summary. Accessed 29 Apr 2017

Yin, R.K.: Case Study Research: Design and Methods. Sage Inc., Thousand Oaks (2009)

The Development of a Smart Personalized Evidence Based Medicine Diabetes Risk Factor Calculator

Lei Wang[1], Defu He[1], Xiaowei Ni[1], Ruyi Zou[1], Xinlu Yuan[2],
Yujuan Shang[1], Xinping Hu[1], Xingyun Geng[1], Kui Jiang[1],
Jiancheng Dong[1], and Huiqun Wu[1(✉)]

[1] Department of Medical Informatics, Medical School of Nantong University,
Nantong, China
wuhuiqun@ntu.edu.cn
[2] Department of Endocrinology, Affiliated Hospital of Nantong University,
Nantong, China

Abstract. Type 2 diabetes mellitus (T2DM) is a chronic disease affected with complex risk factors and has been regarded as one of the major social burdens due to its high occurrence. In this study, we aim to incorporate the idea of evidence based medicine (EBM) into our diabetes risk factor App development. We acquired and extracted the relative risk of different risk factors from relevant literature by searching academic databases. A total of 19 items of risk factors in our daily lives has been finally selected. To design App graphic interface, a total of three pages were designed to let user answer the questions and show the results of their level or risk to have T2DM. We validated the feasibility of our App in 100 users and the results were promising. Therefore, the personalized EBM diabetes risk factor calculator might be a feasible approach to remind those T2DM risky populations by revealing their potential risk factors, thus making implementation of personalized and prevention medicine achievable at hand.

Keywords: Evidence based medicine · Personalize medicine · Diabetes
Mobile medicine

1 Introduction

Type 2 diabetes mellitus (T2DM) is a chronic disease affected with complex risk factors ranged from genetics to life styles [1–3]. T2DM has been regarded as one of the major problems resulting in social burdens due to its high occurrence. However, many people don't realize their risk level of having such popular disease. Most people might visit clinics only when they had typical symptoms such as weight loss, increased drinking and urinating frequency etc. In some worse conditions, patients come to visit clinicians until serious complications like diabetic retinopathy occurred. Hence, the early detection and prediction are crucial for T2DM management. Although blood glucose test is key to T2DM screening and has been validated as a precise measure to diagnose T2DM, it's still not popular in those T2DM suspects especially when their have unobvious symptoms or signs.

Modern technology, however, is rapidly changing the health care system. Due to fast spread and wide usage of mobile phones, the use of mobile applications has been a

© Springer Nature Switzerland AG 2018
H. Chen et al. (Eds.): ICSH 2018, LNCS 10983, pp. 292–300, 2018.
https://doi.org/10.1007/978-3-030-03649-2_29

promising way to implement such T2DM screening assignments [4]. It has been proved that patient self-management of chronic disease like T2DM is a feasible and resource-saving way [5]. Mobile App tailored T2DM risk calculator is an innovative health technique that has become popular during last decade [6, 7].

Although many Apps have been developed for those T2DM patients to self-manage their disease conditions, the Apps for personalized T2DM prediction are still lacking. One of the reasons for that is due to the insufficient clinical evidence for those App designers. Most diabetes risk calculators are not cautious about the included items to calculate users' diabetes risk, which may stem from medical textbooks, news, and clinical experts' suggestions. These items might be low-quality and lack of accuracy. Evidence based medicine (EBM) is an idea that brings reliable clinical trials' results together and has been recently treated as a robust evidence for clinical practice. For this reason, we aim to incorporate the idea of EBM in our App design and turn such EBM evidence into practicable guidelines. We believe that combination of the robust evidence and widely spread as well as easy accessibility of mobile Apps will undoubtedly make personalized T2DM risk prediction more participatory and achievable.

2 Materials and Methods

The workflow of this study was shown (Fig. 1). In this study, we first searched relevant literature databases to obtain clinical trials. Then we screened the risk factors and finally included 19 risk factors in our App [8–20]. The risk ratio (RR) of these factors

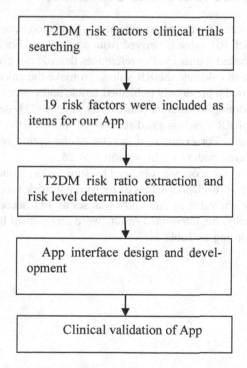

Fig. 1. The workflow of the risk factors selection

were extracted or calculated from the clinical evidence, then, the RRs were converted to different risk points for further summation. Based on these results, App was designed, developed, and validated in clinics.

3 Search Strategy

As an important step in EBM, we acquired the relevant articles by searching relevant academic databases. In this study, we searched PubMed, Embase and Cochrane database and some Chinese domestic academic database such as Wangfang (www. wanfangdata.com.cn), VIP (www.cqvip.com), CNKI (www.cnki.net) for relevant citations until March 2017. While conducting the searches in the database, Medline search terms used were listed as follows: (i) exp diabetes. tw., glucose.tw., hyperglycemia.tw., metabolic syndroms.tw., metabolic disorders.tw.; (ii) risk factors.tw., risks.tw.; (iii) activit*. tw., weight. tw., alcohol. tw., smok*. tw., diet*. tw.; body mass index, fruit. tw., exercise. tw., education. tw.; (iv) and age. tw., gender. tw., sex. tw., sleep. tw., econom*, tw. We combined the terms to generate a subset of citations that address the objective of our research study. We also hand searched the reference lists of relevant articles for eligible studies. We examined the reference lists of all known primary and review articles to identify additional articles not captured by the electronic searches. The detailed search strategy is available from the authors.

4 Relative Risk and Risk Points Conversion

RR is a statistical indicator for the measurement of association between risk factors and clinical outcomes. Each RR value is derived from a reference. For references that give the RR value, we extracted it directly. For references that did not give the RR value, we used the existing data to calculate the RR value. To make the calculation results more interpretable, we referred a previously published article and converted our RRs into the risk points firstly according to different relative risk ranges [21]. As shown in Table 1, the different ranges of RR were assigned to five risk points from 50, 25, 10, 5 and 0 respectively accordingly. For example, if the RR of the option selected by the tester was 2.6, the score corresponding to this option was 25.

Then, the summary risk score was obtained by summation of the risk points of each risk factor. And the final result was achieved by summary risk scores divided a weight value. Herein, the weight value in our study was set as 111 according to our preliminary test results. Finally, the interpreted results were represented by different levels of risk by its range according to Table 2.

Table 1. Relative risk range and risk points calculation

Relative risk (x)	Risk points
0 < x < 0.2; x > 7.0	50
0.2 < x < 0.4; 3.0 < x < 7.0	25
0.4 < x < 0.7; 1.5 < x < 3.0	10
0.7 < x < 0.9; 1.1 < x < 1.5	5
0.9 < x < 1.1	0

Table 2. The different levels of risk ranges and related interpretations

Results	<0	0.01–0.5	0.5 < 0.9	0.9 < 1.1	1.1 < 2.0	2.0 < 5.0	>5.0
Level of risk	Very much below average risk	Much below average risk	Below average risk	About average risk	Above average risk	Much above average risk	Very much above average risk

5 Android App Development

In this experiment, we developed our App based on Java Eclipse SDK installed with Android Development Tools (Version: 23.0.6.1720515). The workflow of our App was designed as follows: when App icon on the Launcher was clicked, the first page with default MainActivity will pop up and a Fragment with its user interface would be loaded. The top ActionBar with back and forward buttons were shown. The questions in need of the user to answer were listed in the fragment, and if the user doesn't complete the essential information, a Toast Notification will pop up until all questions were answered. In this study, an EditText was put at the bottom of the view to input adjusted results, with initial default value as 111. Once the value was set, it could not be changed in the following calculations. As the number of people investigated increased, this value would change a little to obtain more accurate results. The body mass index (BMI) could be automatically achieved and visualized when the height and weight values were input as people completed the first three questions at the first page in our App. In the second page, ListView and BaseAdapter were designed with interval background colors and adaptive list items visualization. The ListView contained RadioGroup of multiple choice question items and TextView of reference at the right bottom corner. ActionBar would be updated if the user drops down for more questions, and if reference icon was clicked, AlertDialog would show the related reference. The user could copy the reference to search more detail information with web browser embedded in their mobile phone.

6 Validation

To validate the accuracy of our software, we included 100 users to install our App. A total of 50 out 100 users are non-diabetic university students, and the other 50 users are clinically diagnosed type 2 diabetes patients from the Department of

Endocrinology, Nantong First People's Hospital. The study protocol was conducted in accordance with the ethical guidelines of the 1995 Declaration of Helsinki, and this study was approved by the Ethics Committee of Nantong First People's Hospital. All users were consented to install the App or to be instructed to use the App, they answered all questions and the test results were recorded for further statistical analysis.

7   Statistical Analysis

Data were analyzed using SPSS 20.0 for Windows software (SPSS, Inc., Chicago, IL). In this experiment, the summary of RRs was expressed as $\bar{\chi} \pm$ SD. Student T test was used to compare the summary of RRs between the normal control groups and diabetic groups. The P value less than 0.05 was treated as statistically significant.

8   Results

8.1   The Visualization of the App Interface for User to Answer Questions

There were three screen pages in our developed App. The first page was shown for the user to input the basic demographic data like age and gender. The second page was shown for the user to select different items of risk factors. For each item, multiple choices of each factor with different RR were listed for selection (Fig. 2).

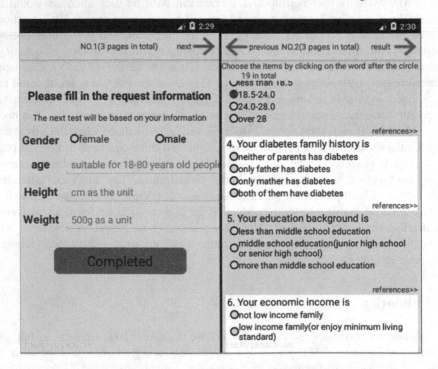

Fig. 2. The screenshot of input page

8.2 Risk Level Calculation and Visualization of the Result

When all questions have been completed, the user could click the result button at the right upper corner to turn to the third page, that is, the result page. The result page in our App demonstrated the results calculated by our algorithm and presented the personalized risk levels to the user. In the result page, all detailed relative risk of the question would show and the final level of risk would indicate the overall level of risk status in different colors, which would range from green to red as the risk level increased (Fig. 3).

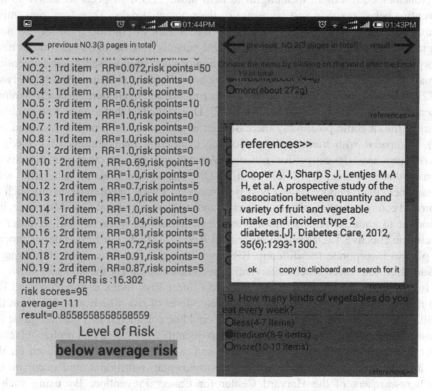

Fig. 3. The screenshot of the result page (Color figure online)

8.3 Validation Results

In this study, the summary of RR values was 20.47 ± 1.60 in the diabetic group, while in the control group was 16.22 ± 1.12 in the normal control group, with statistical significance ($P < 0.05$), indicating the feasibility of our App in diabetes risk calculation.

9 Discussion

Prevention is the best strategy to reduce healthcare costs due to T2DM complications. With regard to the trend of modern health care is shifting to 'participatory', 'prevention', 'prediction', 'personalized' and 'precision', mobile techniques could be a possible way to achieve this shift. Mobile programs involve the use of diabetes prevention and diabetes screening for potential diabetes patients. This new technology enables us to recognize our risk hazards to have diabetes in our daily lives and could help people to recognize their potential risk to get diabetes in a couple of minutes.

Nonetheless, it's more meaningful to help those T2DM suspects to adhere to the preventive behaviors than just be aware of their potential risks. Therefore, preventive behavioral interventions for T2DM patients are in need of consideration for our next program developing. To intervening the T2DM patients' risk factors, some studies have incorporated additional self-regulation techniques such as goal-setting and intention formation into the App. Some programs have been designed to reduce healthcare costs of T2DM patients over time by changing their routines and to encourage their adherence to healthy eating and exercising behavior [22]. Due to the fact that mobile App has been a part of life, it could potentially increase user engagement and promote sustained use [23]. Compared with traditional face-to-face counseling interventions [24], medical practitioners are advocating for self-management and self-directed interventions to address these challenges [25]. Taken T2DM management as an example, self-management interventions have a positive impact on a wide range of behaviors such as improved eating behavior, physical activity, and stress management [26]. Moreover, it's important to encircle self-monitoring and feedback as an integrate part in order to develop an effective T2DM self-management App [27–31]. In our further development, we plan to incorporate the different RR from each risk factor as input and output a personalized self-management intervention recommendation for the user to follow.

In this study, we referred to the Harvard Cancer Risk Index as we converted RR into risk points and further into an interpretable level of risk which was shown on the result page. The Harvard Cancer Risk Index could be considered as a general guide for assessing an individual's risk of cancer and to quantify established and probable factors affecting cancer incidence. The estimates used in this risk index were based on the existing literature and the judgment of environmental, nutritional, and occupational health researchers of the Harvard Center for Cancer Prevention. By using such a categorical approach to risk class indication, the likely disagreement among investigators could be reduced to some extent. Similar methods have been applied in our App development; however, due to the discrepancy between cancer and T2DM, the conversion principles should be verified. Fortunately, we achieved a good performance in our preliminary test on 100 subjects, and we will test on large sample size clinical trials in our further study. Although the preliminary results we have obtained were promising, the App could not be regard as diagnosis software to take replace of clinical personnel. One reason for that was the risk factors included in our App might be limited to different kinds of the population due to the searching limits for language. Another reason was that some other risk factors had not been included due to lack of high-quality evidence, but they might affect the risk level of diabetes at the same way.

Besides these limits, it should be noted that for some elder populations who are not good at high-tech applications like mobile phones, instruction should be given by other volunteers for better use of the App [32].

In summary, we preferred the use of this App as a reminder for those users who very much higher than the average risks of T2DM to visit clinics and have laboratory test or other examinations to get a clear diagnosis.

10 Conclusion

The personalized EBM diabetes risk factor calculator might be a feasible approach to remind those T2DM risky populations by revealing their potential risk factors, thus making implementation of personalized and prevention medicine achievable at hand.

Acknowledgements. This work was supported by the grant from National Key R&D Program of China (2018YFC1314902), National Natural Science Foundation of China (No. 81501559, 81371663), Natural Science Foundation of the Higher Education Institutions of Jiangsu Province (No. 15KJB310015) and Science and Technology Project of Nantong City (MS12015180).

References

1. Sundaram, M., Kavookjian, J., Patrick, J.H.: Health-related quality of life and quality of life in type 2 diabetes: relationships in a cross-sectional study. Patient **2**(2), 121–133 (2009)
2. Stevens, M.J., Feldman, E.L., Greene, D.A.: The etiology of diabetic neuropathy: the combined roles of metabolic and vascular defects. Diabet. Med. **12**(7), 566–579 (1995)
3. Franz, M.J., et al.: Nutrition principles for the management of diabetes and related complications. Diabetes Care **17**(5), 490–518 (1994)
4. Rollo, M.E., et al.: EHealth technologies to support nutrition and physical activity behaviors in diabetes self-management. Diabetes Metab. Syndr. Obes. **9**, 381–390 (2016)
5. Bodenheimer, T., Lorig, K., Holman, H., Grumbach, K.: Patient self-management of chronic disease in primary care. JAMA **288**, 2469–2475 (2002)
6. Jo, S., Park, H.-A.: Development and evaluation of a smartphone application for managing gestational diabetes mellitus. Healthc. Inform. Res. **22**(1), 11–21 (2016)
7. Williams, J.P., Schroeder, D.: Popular glucose tracking apps and use of mHealth by latinos with diabetes: review. JMIR Mhealth Uhealth **3**(3), e84 (2015)
8. LNCS Homepage. http://www.cdc.gov/diabetes/statistics/prev/national/figbysex.htm
9. He, Y., Zeng, Q., Zhao, X.L.: Association of body mass index and waist circumstance with risk of hypertension and diabetes in Chinese adults. Med. J. Chin. PLA. **40**(10), 803–808 (2015)
10. LNCS Homepage. http://www.cdc.gov/diabetes/statistics/prev/national/figbyeducation.html
11. Larrañaga, I., Arteagoitia, J.M., Rodriguez, J.L., Gonzalez, F., Esnaola, S., Piniés, J.A.: Socio-economic inequalities in the prevalence of type 2 diabetes, cardiovascular risk factors and chronic diabetic complications in the Basque Country, Spain. Diabetic Med. **22**(8), 1047–1053 (2005)
12. Carlsson, S., Midthjell, K., Grill, V.: Smoking is associated with an increased risk of type 2 diabetes but a decreased risk of autoimmune diabetes in adults: an 11-year follow-up of incidence of diabetes in the nord-trøndelag study. Diabetologia **47**(11), 1953–1956 (2004)

13. Gao, M., Li, J.J., Wu, Y.T.: Relationship between length of sleep and incidence risk of type 2 diabetes. Chin. J. Endocrinol. Metab. **30**(5), 393–396 (2014)
14. Wang, H., Liu, D.M., Peng, Y.: Physical activity of moderate intensity and risk of type 2 diabetes mellitus. J. Jinggangshan Univ. (Nat. Sci.) (05), 115–120 (2011)
15. Tang, W., Cai, Y., Huang, X.P.: Survey of depression status in patients with type 2 diabetes mellitus and analysis of risk factors. J. Clin. Med. Pract. (2012)
16. Liu, J., Lan, S.Y.: The epidemiology study advances of risk factors of type 2 diabetes. J. Nantong Univ. (Med. Sci.). **26**(03), 230–232 (2006)
17. Shi, Y., Dong, J.Y., Zhang, Z.L.: Meta-analysis on coffee drinking and type 2 diabetes. J. Nantong Univ. (Med. Sci.) (1), 89–94 (2012)
18. Tong, X., Dong, J., Wu, Z.: Dairy consumption and risk of type 2 diabetes mellitus: a meta-analysis of cohort studies. Eur. J. Clin. Nutr. **65**(9), 1027–1031 (2011)
19. Feskens, E.J.M., Sluik, D., Woudenbergh, G.J.V.: Meat consumption, diabetes, and its complications. Curr. Diabetes Rep. **13**(2), 298–306 (2013)
20. Cooper, A.J., Sharp, S.J., Lentjes, M.A.H.: A prospective study of the association between quantity and variety of fruit and vegetable intake and incident type 2 diabetes. Diabetes Care **35**(6), 1293–1300 (2012)
21. Colditz, G.A., et al.: Harvard report on cancer prevention volume 4: Harvard cancer risk index. Cancer Causes Control. **11**(6), 477–488 (2000). Risk Index Working Group, Harvard Center for Cancer Prevention
22. Cradock, K.A., ÓLaighin, G., Finucane, F.M., Gainforth, H.L., Quinlan, L.R., Ginis, K.A.: Behaviour change techniques targeting both diet and physical activity in type 2 diabetes: a systematic review and meta-analysis. Int. J. Behav. Nutr. Phys. Act **14**(1), 18 (2017)
23. Helander, E., Kaipainen, K., Korhonen, I., Wansink, B.: Factors related to sustained use of a free mobile app for dietary self-monitoring with photography and peer feedback: retrospective cohort study. J. Med. Internet Res. **16**(4), e109 (2014)
24. Miller, R.L., Shinn, M.: Learning from communities: overcoming difficulties in dissemination of prevention and promotion efforts. Am. J. Community Psychol. **35**(3–4), 169–183 (2005)
25. Bodenheimer, T., Lorig, K., Holman, H., Grumbach, K.: Patient self-management of chronic disease in primary care. JAMA **288**(19), 2469–2475 (2002)
26. Gillett, M., et al.: Delivering the diabetes education and self management for ongoing and newly diagnosed (DESMOND) programme for people with newly diagnosed type 2 diabetes: cost effectiveness analysis. BMJ **341**, c4093 (2010)
27. Chodosh, J., et al.: Meta-analysis: chronic disease self-management programs for older adults. Ann. Intern. Med. **143**, 427–438 (2005)
28. Catherine, H.Y., et al.: A web-based intervention to support self-management of patients with type 2 diabetes mellitus: effect on self-efficacy, self-care and diabetes distress. BMC Med. Inform. Decis. Mak. **14**, 117 (2014)
29. Alhuwail, D.: Diabetes applications for Arabic speakers: a critical review of available apps for android and iOS operated smartphones. Stud. Health Technol. Inform. **225**, 587–591 (2016)
30. Ahn, Y., Bae, J., Kim, H.S.: The development of a mobile U-Health program and evaluation for self-diet management for diabetic patients. Nutr. Res. Pract. **10**(3), 342–351 (2016)
31. Ried-Larsen, M., et al.: Implementation of interval walking training in patients with type 2 diabetes in Denmark: rationale, design, and baseline characteristics. Clin. Epidemiol. **8**, 201–209 (2016)
32. Scheibe, M., Reichelt, J., Bellmann, M., Kirch, W.: Acceptance factors of mobile apps for diabetes by patients aged 50 or older: a qualitative study. Med. 2.0. **4**(1), e1 (2015)

A Descriptive Tomographic Content Analysis Method in Chronic Disease Knowledge Network: An Application to Hypertension

Liqin Zhou[ID], Lu An[✉][ID], Zhichao Ba[ID], and Zhiyuan Li[ID]

Center for the Studies of Information Resources, Wuhan University,
Wuhan 430072, China
anlu97@163.com

Abstract. Exploring the hierarchical structure and internal correlation of chronic disease knowledge network is of great significance to distinguish conceptual terms and core directions of chronic disease area. This paper proposed a descriptive Tomographic Content Analysis method to analyze the cross-section of chronic disease knowledge network. K-core values and clustering coefficients were applied to divide the network into layers. Then vectors for each layer were constructed to calculate their cosine similarities to compare their correlation and differences. Finally, network stratification results were compared with the community modules obtained by the traditional social network analysis from a quantitative perspective. To illustrate the method, a number of 26,717 articles related to hypertension in the PubMed database were taken as examples to construct the chronic disease knowledge network. Results show that the chronic disease knowledge network can be divided into the basic layer, the middle layer and the detailed layer. The basic layer can be used to divide the main research directions of chronic diseases. The detailed layer can be used to characterize the specific research and reveal the microscopic forms of the network. The middle layer can be used to explore the network intersection and evolution paths. Compared with the traditional social network analysis method, our proposed method can obtain more in-depth and detailed hierarchical structures and internal correlations of chronic disease knowledge networks.

Keywords: Knowledge network · Tomographic content analysis
Hierarchical structure · Chronic disease · Hypertension

1 Introduction

With the aging population, the rapid development of urbanization and industrialization, and the impact of unhealthy lifestyles, chronic diseases (such as heart disease, cardiovascular disease, cancer and diabetes and so on) of our residents are becoming increasingly severe. Currently, more than 300 million people are diagnosed with chronic disease, and the number is increased at an annual rate of 8.9%. What's more, the disease burden caused by chronic disease accounts for 70% of the total disease burden. It severely occupied medical resources and caused a heavy burden on families, society, and countries [1]. Therefore, more and more scholars have begun to devote

© Springer Nature Switzerland AG 2018
H. Chen et al. (Eds.): ICSH 2018, LNCS 10983, pp. 301–312, 2018.
https://doi.org/10.1007/978-3-030-03649-2_30

themselves to the study of chronic diseases. Chronic disease knowledge network refers to a complex network, which was formed by the social relationships among knowledge nodes in the field of chronic diseases. They can communicate, transfer, and share knowledge resources with each other. Exploring the chronic disease knowledge network can facilitate mining potential knowledge of chronic diseases, identifying research frontier and detecting hot trends of chronic diseases.

Existing literature usually constructed citation or co-occurring networks based on authors, institutions, journals, keywords and subject terms to explore knowledge networks, and used social network analysis methods to visualize their network structures [2]. However, these studies only focused on the overall characteristics of knowledge networks (such as small-world, scale-free features and so on), and lacked of in-depth analysis of their internal structures and microscopic forms [3]. As the hierarchical structure of complex networks had validated [4], exploring the hierarchical structure have became an effective way to further improve knowledge networks. Carmi et al. [5] decomposed the Internet layer by layer based on the k-core value, and classified the network by some parameters, such as the number of nodes at each layer, the maximum connectivity subgraph, and the average distance. Then Hu and Chen [6] decomposed networks with k-core values, and fused them with clustering coefficients and summarized the overall networks. These studies all laid foundation for further exploring the domain knowledge distribution and network correlations.

The main purpose of this paper is to introduce a descriptive Tomographic Content Analysis method to analyze the cross-section of chronic disease knowledge network. The network is decomposed into topological layers by K-core values and clustering coefficients. The position of knowledge entities in each layer are analyzed from a quantitative perspective. Finally, the hierarchical structure and internal correlation are compared with the community modules obtained by traditional social network analysis method. To illustrate the process of the method, a number of 26,717 articles related to Hypertension in PubMed database are taken as an example to construct the chronic disease knowledge network. The proposed method can also be applied to other disciplines or various knowledge networks, such as citation networks, co-authored networks, institutional cooperation networks and so on.

2   Related Research

The hierarchical structure of a complex network is the basic reason for its characteristics of scale-free, Point-degree power-law distribution, modularization, and high-efficiency connectivity [7]. In order to reveal the hierarchical structure of the network, Sales-Pardo et al. [8] adopted the unsupervised box model to construct a hierarchy tree to infer the hierarchical structure of complex networks based on the affinity of nodes. Another more common method is to divide the hierarchical structure of networks based on the k-core value of nodes. Hu and Chen [6] divided the knowledge network into different layers according to the k-core value of nodes, and introduced the three-dimensional closure as basic analysis unit to describe the peer-level aggregation, knowledge fusion, and differentiation of micro-association structures. These studies are helpful for exploring the internal structure and the microscopic forms of knowledge networks. However, research on the internal correlation among various layers of knowledge network is still rare, and there is no unified specification.

Then Teng et al. [9] utilized the correlation frequency as a threshold to extract the hierarchical structure of keyword network and tag network, and verified its scale-free and small-world effects. Lee et al. [10] classified three different bibliometric content networks related to Parkinson's disease according to different query knowledge entities, and took a slice-and-dice approach to analyzing the characteristics and correlations of the networks. But they cannot calculate the internal correlation among layers from a quantitative perspective.

3   Tomographic Content Analysis Method

This paper proposed a descriptive Tomographic Content Analysis method to analyze the cross-section of the network. The network is decomposed into topological layers by the k-core values and network parameters. The positions of knowledge entities in each layer are analyzed in a two-dimensional plane. In order to compare the correlations and differences among various network layers, we defined the position and meaning of nodes in each cross section. At the same time, each node is iteratively merged as a community through a community detection algorithm [11], and the clustering of nodes are regarded as modules. Finally, a metric is introduced to compare the similarities between layers or modules.

3.1   Network Hierarchical Division Based on K-Core Value

The K-core value is one of the most commonly used parameters in complex network analysis. It can be used to reveal the core level of network nodes. As the scale of network grows, K-core value will not change as dramatically as the node degree, but gradually becomes stable [12]. Therefore, K-core is usually used to divide network hierarchical structures, as shown in Fig. 1 [13].

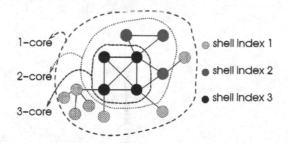

Fig. 1. A simple example of k-core based network layer

The k-core value of nodes can be defined as: the node is connected to at least k nodes with degrees no less than k [14]. The method of obtaining k-core value is to iteratively eliminate nodes whose degree is less than k in total network, so as to obtain stable sub-networks [15]. The basic idea is as follows. In order to be a core node in the network, it must not only reach a certain degree, but also have a certain number of neighboring nodes that are at least as important as itself.

This study refers to the ideal of "first divide and then rejoin" approach [5, 6]. First, the subject terms' co-occurring network are divided into multiple sub-layers by k-core values. Then the sub-layers are merged into several large layers to analyze the detailed forms and associations of various network levels according to the clustering coefficient.

3.2 Hierarchical Structure Analysis

In order to compare the correlations and differences among various network layers, we defined the position and meaning of nodes in each cross section. At the same time, each node was iteratively merged as a community through a community detection algorithm [11] until no new community appears, and the clusters of nodes were regarded as modules. Finally, a metric was introduced to compare the similarities among layers and modules.

To identify the position of knowledge entities, networks were decomposed into topological layers. Each layer was composed by degree centrality and betweenness centrality in a two-dimensional plane, as shown in Fig. 2. Degree centrality refers to the local importance between nodes and their adjacent nodes, while betweenness centrality refers to the global importance between nodes and their non-adjacent nodes. The position of the node on each layer represents its local importance with other nodes and global importance in a particular topic. Each layer can be divided into four quadrants. The HH quadrant represents nodes with a high degree centrality and betweenness centrality, and corresponds to entities that are influential in locally and globally. The HL quadrant represents nodes with high degree centrality and low betweenness centrality, and corresponds to locally influential entities; The LH quadrant represents nodes with low degree centrality and high betweenness centrality, and corresponds to globally influential entities. The LL quadrant indicates that the degree centrality and betweenness centrality are low, and corresponds to entities that are not important in locally and globally.

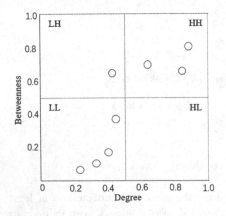

Fig. 2. The position of nodes in each layer

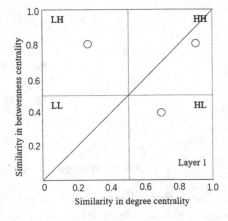

Fig. 3. Similarities among layers or modules

For each layer and each module, the degrees centrality vector and betweenness centrality vector were established. Calculating the cosine similarity for each pair, we can obtain the similarities in degree centrality and betweenness centrality. Similarity values can be used to determine the positions of the x-axis and the y-axis, as shown in Fig. 3. Similar to Fig. 2, Fig. 3 also can be divided into four quadrants: HH, HL, LH, LL. The distance to each node represents the total similarity among two layers or two modules. When all nodes are mapped on the diagonal, it means that knowledge entities in the two layers or two modules have a linear relationship. If the distribution of nodes is inclined to the x-axis, it means that entities from different layers or modules have similar local roles. If the distribution of nodes is inclined to the y-axis, it means that entities from different layers or modules have similar global roles.

The process of Tomographic Content Analysis method is as follow: (1) Construct the subject terms co-occurring network; (2) Divide nodes into different layers based on K-core values and clustering coefficients; (3) Clustering nodes into different modules by traditional social network analysis method; (4) Calculate the degree centrality and betweenness centrality of nodes in each layer or module, and show them in the coordinate; (5) Establishing degree centrality vector and betweenness centrality vector for each layer or module; (6) Calculate the cosine similarity among layers and modules, and mapping them to two-dimensional coordinates for analysis.

4   Results Analysis and Discussion

4.1   Data Collection and Preprocessing

Hypertension is the most common chronic disease and the most important risk factor for cardiovascular diseases. In this study, we used the retrieval strategy of "Hypertension [MeSH Terms] AND ("2000/1/1" [PDat]: "2017/5/1")", and obtained 99,252 articles related to hypertension between 2000 and 2017. To maintain the bibliographic articles both containing abstracts and full texts, we finally obtained 26,717 articles.

Then data was then imported into the Bibliographic Items Co-occurrence Matrix Builder [16]. Through extracting and counting the fields (such as journals, authors, and subject terms), we found that the 26,717 articles were distributed over 1701 journals, involving 171,637 authors and 9,978 subject terms. In order to determine the high-frequency MeSH subject terms, we used the high-low-frequency word boundary formula proposed by Yang [17] to determine the frequency threshold value. Then the subject terms co-occurring matrix was constructed in BICOMB based on the frequency threshold, and then it was imported into Ucinet and converted to an adjacency matrix.

4.2   Hierarchical Division of the Chronic Disease Knowledge Network

The processed original adjacency matrix was imported into NetDraw, and the K-cores option in the analysis menu was chosen to calculate the K-core value of nodes. In order to reduce the complexity of the graph, only Top-100 nodes with the highest occurrence frequency were selected for analysis. Then a total of 19 different K-core values were obtained, with the largest K-core value being 31 and the smallest being 12. The 19 k-shells can be considered as different sub-networks, and their clustering coefficients are calculated, as shown in Table 1.

Table 1. Clustering coefficients for each K-shell

K-shell	Clustering coefficients	K-shell	Clustering coefficients
31	1093.86	20	1
30	1	19	218.944
29	100.67	18	1
27	1	17	1
26	1	16	1
25	1	15	1
24	123.67	14	1
23	1	13	264.67
22	1	12	1
21	1		

According to the clustering coefficients of each K-shell, it can be seen that there are some adjacent layers in 19 sub-layers with similar characteristics and different characteristics. Therefore, according to the size of the clustering coefficient, adjacent layers with similar characteristics can be merged into one large layer, and the sub-layers with different characteristics can be used as the boundary for distinguishing large layers. The subject terms co-occurring network of chronic disease in this paper can be divided into three layers from inside and outside, as shown in Fig. 4.

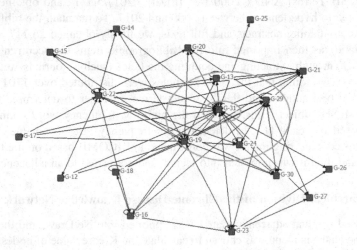

Fig. 4. Hierarchical division of the chronic disease knowledge network based on K-core

The first layer was composed of nodes with a K-core value of 31, because its clustering coefficient is the largest, up to 1093.86; the second layer was composed of nodes with K-core values of 29, 24, 19, and 13, because their clustering coefficients are similar. The third layer was composed of nodes with K-core values of 30, 27, 26, 25, 23, 22, 21, 20, 18, 17, 16, 15, 14, 12. Because the clustering coefficients of these layers are 1. The layered network was shown in Fig. 5.

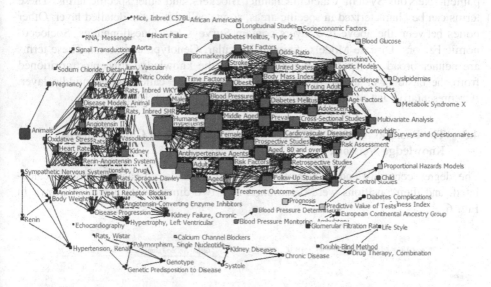

Fig. 5. The layered network of subject terms (Color figure online)

In Fig. 5, the size of the nodes is represented by the node degree, and the color of the nodes are distinguished by K-core values. The first layer contains 37 nodes, the second layer contains 33 nodes, and the third layer contains 30 nodes.

Table 2. A representative list of 10 nodes in each layer

Layer	Number of nodes	MeSH terms
Basic layer	37	Humans, Aged, Risk Factors, Antihypertensive Agents, Cardiovascular Diseases, Treatment Outcome, Prospective Studies, Body Mass Index, Risk Assessment, Multivariate Analysis...
Middle layer	33	Surveys and Questionnaires, Metabolic Syndrome X, Socioeconomic Factors, Disease Models, Animal, Endothelium, Vascular, Renin-Angiotensin System, Oxidative Stress, Dose-Response Relationship, Drug, Kidney Failure, Chronic, Genotype...
Detailed layer	30	Diabetes Mellitus, Type 2, Severity of Illness Index, Blood Pressure Monitoring, Ambulatory, Glomerular Filtration Rate, Diabetes Complications, Heart Failure, Drug Therapy, Combination, Double-Blind Method, Sympathetic Nervous System, Calcium Channel Blockers...

After analyzing the nodes in each layer, we can find that the semantic range of nodes from inner to outer gradually becomes concrete. The innermost nodes contain broader terms, such as Humans, Aged, Risk Factors, Multivariate Analysis, and Treatment Outcomes. These terms can be used in specific fields and seen as the basis of domain research, so we called it as the basic layer; The outermost nodes include Diabetes Mellitus, Type 2, Severity of Illness Index, Metabolic Syndrome X, Sympathetic Nervous System, Calcium Channel Blockers, and other specific terms. These terms can be characterized in specific areas, so we called it as the detailed layer. Other nodes between the above two layers contain Surveys and Questionnaires, Socioeconomic Factors, Disease Models, Animal, Vascular, Genotype and so on. These terms are neither broad nor specific, it can be seen as the knowledge concepts transitioned from the basic layer to the detailed layer, so it can be called as the middle layer. A representative list of 10 nodes in each layer was listed in Table 2.

4.3   The Position Analysis of Nodes in Various Layers in Chronic Disease Knowledge Network

The degree centrality and betweenness centrality of nodes in each layer were calculated, and their positions were determined in a two-dimensional plane, as shown in Fig. 6.

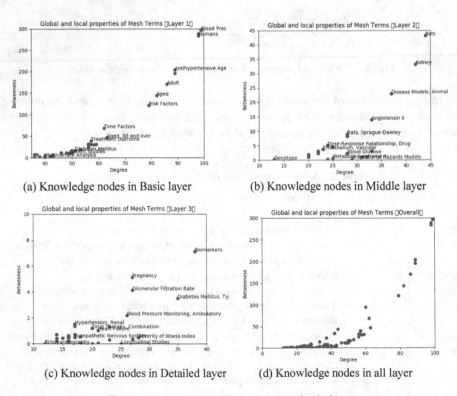

(a) Knowledge nodes in Basic layer   (b) Knowledge nodes in Middle layer

(c) Knowledge nodes in Detailed layer   (d) Knowledge nodes in all layer

Fig. 6. The positions of knowledge nodes in layers

In the basic layer (Fig. 6(a)), the degree centrality and betweenness centrality of nodes (such as Blood pressure, Humans, Antihypentensive age, and Risk factors) are relatively high, this indicates that these nodes are important both in locally and globally. Then the degree centrality of "Time factors" and "Treatment Outcomes" are high, while the betweenness centrality is relatively low, this indicates that the nodes are more important in the local area rather than in global area. In addition, the degree centrality and betweenness centrality of nodes (such as Multivariate Analysis, Diabetes Mellitus and et al.) are relatively low, which indicates that these nodes are relatively insignificant in the basic layer, and are closed to the next layer (middle layer).

In the middle layer (Fig. 6(b)), the degree centrality and betweenness centrality of nodes (such as Rats, kidney, Disease Models, Animals and et al.) are relatively high, this indicates that these nodes are both important in locally and globally. Then the degree centrality of nodes (such as Proportional Hazards Models and Blood Glucose) are relatively high, but their betweenness centrality are relatively low, this indicates that these nodes are more important in locally than in globally. The node of Genotype has a low degree centrality and betweenness centrality, this indicates that the node is not important in the middle layer.

In the detailed layer (Fig. 6(c)), the degree centrality and betweenness centrality of nodes (such as Biomarkers, Pregnancy, Glomerular Filtration Rate and et al.) are relatively high, this indicates that these nodes are both important in locally and globally. The degree centrality of the node Diabetes Mellitus, Type 2 is relatively high, while the betweenness centrality are relatively low, this indicates that these nodes are more important in locally than in globally. And the node of Echocardiography and RNA Messenger have a low degree centrality and betweenness centrality, this indicates that the nodes are not important in the detailed layer. The positions of all knowledge nodes are shown in Fig. 6(d).

4.4 Internal Correlation Analysis of Various Layers and Modules of Chronic Disease Knowledge Network

The subject terms' co-occurring matrix was imported into Gephi, and each knowledge node was merged as a community through the traditional community detection algorithm proposed by Blondel [11], until no new community emerged. Then we can obtain three relativity stable modules. In order to compare the correlations and differences among the three layers (obtained by the Tomographic Content Analysis method) and the three modules (obtained by the traditional social network analysis method), we constructed the degree centrality vector and betweenness centrality vector for each layer and each module, and calculated their cosine similarities to obtain the degree centrality similarity and betweenness centrality similarity, as shown in Table 3.

Then the similarity among layers and modules are represented in two-dimensional plane coordinates, as shown in Fig. 7. The red dots (L-1, L-2), (L-2, L-3), and (L-1, L-3) represent the similarity among layers. The three dots are all in the HL quadrant, indicating that the local similarity among layers are relatively high, while the global similarity is relatively low. For example, the coordinate (L-2, L-3) represents the similarity between middle layer and detailed layer. According to its position, we can find that the local similarity among the two layers are relatively high, while the global similarity is relatively low. The blue stars (M-1, M-2), (M-2, M-3) and (M-1, M-3) represent the similarity among modules. The three dots are basically in the HH quadrant, indicating that the local similarity among modules are relatively high. The yellow triangle represents the similarity among each layer and each module. The three nodes ((L-2, M-2), (L-2, M-3), (L-3, M-3)) are in the HL quadrant, indicating that the local similarity among the second layer with the second module and the third module, and the third layer with third module are relatively high, while the globally similarity are relatively low. And the three nodes ((L-1, M-1), (L-1, M-2), (L-1, M-3)) are all in the HH quadrant, indicating that the local similarity and global similarity among the first layer with the first module, the second module and the third layer are both high.

Table 3. Similarities among different layers and modules

	Degree similarity	Betweenness similarity		Degree similarity	Betweenness similarity
Layer1 vs Layer2	0.969	0.354	Layer1 vs Module1	0.866	0.768
Layer1 vs Layer3	0.961	0.265	Layer2 vs Module2	0.967	0.208
Layer2 vs Layer3	0.933	0.078	Layer3 vs Module3	0.928	0.232
Module1 vs Module2	0.898	0.95	Layer1 vs Module2	0.989	0.876
Module1 vs Module3	0.897	0.819	Layer1 vs Module3	0.946	0.761
Module2 vs Module3	0.947	0.898	Layer2 vs Module3	0.877	0.115

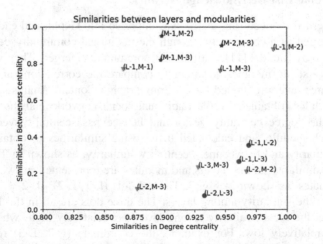

Fig. 7. Similarities among layers and modules (Color figure online)

Comparing the similarities among layers and modules, we can find that the local similarities of hierarchical classification results of the chronic disease based on the K-core value and clustering coefficient is relatively high, while the global similarities are relatively low, this indicates that layers in the network are important but their importance are different. However, the local similarity and global similarity of the modules obtained through the traditional community detection algorithm are both very high, this indicates that the differences among various modules are small, and it is difficult to distinguish the roles of each module.

5 Conclusion

This paper proposed a descriptive tomographic content analysis method to dissect the cross-section of chronic disease knowledge network from a hierarchical perspective. 26717 articles related to hypertension in the PubMed database were taken as an example to construct a subject terms co-occurring network. Then the network can be divided into three layers according to the K-core values and clustering coefficients. In order to compare the correlations and differences among various network layers, the degree centrality vector and betweenness centrality vector were constructed for each layer, then we can calculate their cosine similarities. Finally, the network stratification results were compared with the community modules obtained by traditional social network analysis method from a quantitative perspective.

It is found that: (1) The chronic disease knowledge network can be divided into three layers by K-core value and clustering coefficient. The basic layer mainly includes some relatively broad terms, which can be used as the research basic and research directions of chronic disease. The detailed layer mainly includes some specific terms, which can be used to characterize the specific research in the field of chronic diseases and reveal the microscopic forms of the network. The middle layer is between the two layers, and can be used to reveal the network intersection and evolution path. (2) The difference among layers obtained by Tomographic content analysis method are obvious, and each layer has different importance in the network. While the similarities among various modules obtained through the traditional SNA community detection algorithm are very high, it is difficult to distinguish their differences and roles. (3) The tomographic content analysis method can analyze the association and differences among layers from a quantitative perspective, we can obtain a more in-depth and detailed knowledge structures of the network than the traditional SNA method.

The tomographic content analysis method presents can analysis the micro-structure and correlation of knowledge network from the perspective of differentiation and quantification, and can facilitate exploring the knowledge structure and distribution of chronic disease. This method can also be applied to various knowledge networks, such as citation networks, co-authored networks, institutional cooperation networks and so on. However, this article is only a preliminary exploration. How can the most basic micro-unit (triads, small groups, etc.) of each layer of the network can be analyzed and extracted? More quantitative indicators automatically divide the hierarchical structure of network and other issues need to be further deepened.

Acknowledgment. This paper is an outcome of the international cooperation and exchange program "Research on Intelligent Home Care Platform Based on Chronic Disease Knowledge Management" (No. 71661167007) and the major international (regional) joint research project "Research on Knowledge Organization and Service Innovation in the Big Data Environments" (No. 71420107026) supported by National Nature Science Foundation of China.

References

1. NCG: Chronic disease management: the pioneer of online medical care. http://ncd.org.cn/Article/index/id/5641. Accessed 22 Oct 2017
2. Zhang, J.Z., Han, T., Wang, X.M.: Overview of complex network research and its application in library and information science. J. China Soc. Sci. Tech. Inf. **31**(9), 907–914 (2012)
3. Liu, X., Ma, F.C., Chen, X.J., et al.: Structure and evolution of knowledge network – concept and research review. China Inf. Sci. **29**(6), 801–809 (2011)
4. Yi, S., Choi, J.: The organization of scientific knowledge: the structural characteristics of keyword networks. Scientometrics **90**(3), 1015–1026 (2012)
5. Carmi, S., Havlin, S., Kirkpatrick, S., et al.: A model of internet topology using k-shell decomposition. Proc. Natl. Acad. Sci. U.S.A. **104**(27), 11150–11154 (2007)
6. Hu, C.P., Chen, G.: An exploration of hierarchical domain knowledge network and its micro-morphology based on co-word analysis with reliable relations. J. China Soc. Sci. Tech. Inf. **33**(2), 130–139 (2014)
7. Clauset, A., Moore, C., Newman, M.E.: Hierarchical structure and the prediction of missing links in networks. Nature **453**(7191), 98–101 (2008)
8. Sales-Pardo, M., Guimerà, R., Moreira, A.A., et al.: Extracting the hierarchical organization of complex systems. Proc. Natl. Acad. Sci. U.S.A. **104**(39), 15224–15229 (2007)
9. Teng, G.Q., Bai, S.C., Han, S.X., et al.: Analysis on the principle of knowledge network at level based on scale-free and fractal theory. Libr. Inf. Serv. **61**(14), 132–140 (2017)
10. Lee, K., Kim, S.Y., Kim, E.H., et al.: Comparative evaluation of bibliometric content networks by tomographic content analysis: an application to Parkinson's disease. J. Assoc. Inf. Sci. Technol. **68**(5), 1295–1307 (2016)
11. Blondel, V.D., Jean-Loup, G., Renaud, L., et al.: Fast unfolding of communities in large networks. J. Stat. Mech.: Theory Exp. **208**(10), 155–168 (2008)
12. Zhang, G.Q., Zhang, G.Q., Yang, Q.F., et al.: Evolution of the internet and its cores. New J. Phys. **10**(12), 123027 (2009)
13. Alvarez-Hamelin, J.I., Dall'Asta, L., Barrat, A., et al.: K-core decomposition of Internet graphs: hierarchies, self-similarity and measurement biases. Netw. Heterog. Media **3**(2), 371–393 (2005)
14. Liu, J.: Overall Network Analysis Handbook: Practical Guide of UCINET Software. Truth & Wisdom Press, Shanghai (2009)
15. Aristotelis, K., Laura, B., Henning, H., et al.: Organizational principles of the Reactome human BioPAX model using graph theory methods. J. Complex Netw. **4**(4), 604–615 (2016)
16. Cui, L.: Bibliographic Items Co-occurrence Matrix Builder, BICOMB 2.0. http://cid-3adcb3b569c0a509.skydnve.live.com/browse.aspx/BICOMB. Accessed 30 Sept 2017
17. Yang, Y., Wu, M., Cui, L.: Integration of three visualization methods based on co-word analysis. Scientometrics **90**(2), 659–673 (2012)

Health Informetrics

Visualizing the Intellectual Structure of Electronic Health Research: A Bibliometric Analysis

Tongtong Li[1], Dongxiao Gu[1(✉)], Xiaoyu Wang[2], and Changyong Liang[1]

[1] The School of Management, Hefei University of Technology, 193 Tunxi Road, Hefei 230009, Anhui, China
gudongxiao@hfut.edu.cn
[2] The 1st Affiliated Hospital, Anhui University of Traditional Chinese Medicine, 117 Meishan Road, Hefei 230031, Anhui, China

Abstract. The aim of this study is to detect the evolutionary track of the electronic health from its birth to the present, and then analyze its foundational knowledge and research hotspots. We conducted a bibliometric analysis on the 3085 literatures data collected from the Web of Science core data collection in 1992–2017. We used several bibliometric tools such as CiteSpace and Netdraw to complete time-and-space analysis and keywords co-occurrence network analysis. This research can provide important academic reference for international electronic health and medical informatics researchers.

Keywords: Electronic health · Medical informatics · Information technology Bibliometrics

1 Introduction

Based on information technologies and the fields of biomedical engineering and healthcare, e-health aims at providing collaborative healthcare services, integrating regional health resources, sharing and delivering medical information [1]. In the past 20 years, due to the significant breakthroughs in medical information construction around the world, electronic health represented by HIS, PACIS, and telemedicine has prospered. The widespread use of HIS, PACIS, etc. in hospitals has produced health big data represented by *EHR* (Electronic Health Records) and *EMR* (Electronic Medical Records) [2], which provide an important basis for disease diagnosis, health care and disease decision-making.

In recent years, the research and application of emerging information technologies such as artificial intelligence, cloud computing, Internet of things and wearable devices in the field of healthcare has expanded the content of electronic health. Mobile platforms use artificial intelligence, deep learning, advanced statistics and other technologies to dig up health changes in complex health big data, analyze the relationship between health changes and behavior, monitor outliers, and propose health promotion programmes. In this context, mobile health and smart health emerge as the important

© Springer Nature Switzerland AG 2018
H. Chen et al. (Eds.): ICSH 2018, LNCS 10983, pp. 315–324, 2018.
https://doi.org/10.1007/978-3-030-03649-2_31

part of constructing smart city. Electronic health has ushered in an unprecedented historical development opportunity, attracting more and more researchers around the world to carry out related research. For example, Heidi et al. conducted an 8-week tele-behavioral therapy program on 466 diabetic patients. The results showed that telehealth intervention elevated patients' depression, anxiety, and improved the frequency of blood glucose self-test [3]. Kathryn et al. studied existing mobile applications targeted toward reproductive endocrinology and infertility service providers [4]. Wang et al. systematically analyzed 16 studies about long-term health interventions for chronic diseases use smartphone. These studies found that the smartphone intervention was a completely effective tool to assist in managing some chronic diseases [5]. Yang et al. used bibliometrics to analyze the telemedicine articles published in the SCI–Expanded database from 1993 to 2012 [6].

Above studies have studied some hot issues in e-health from different perspectives, however it is difficult to meet the expectations of researchers in this field. In order to show the evolution process and identify the research hot spots of global knowledge in e-health, we conducted a series of bibliometric analyses on the retrieved 3085 litera-tures in 1992–2017 from the Web of Science database. The future research trends of e-health are discussed using visual analysis combined with systematic analysis. It will provide knowledge support for domestic and foreign research scholars to carry out research in related fields.

2 Methodology

2.1 Data Source

This article used SCI-E, SSCI, A&HCI, CPCI-S, CPCI-SSH, ESCI, CCR-E, and IC in Web of Science as data sources. We used advanced search methods, search #1 AND #2 AND #3, where #1 is TS = (health* OR "health management" OR "health service*" OR "medic*" OR #) (# represents 6 related keywords in the field of health), #2 is TS = ("Internet of things" OR "cloud computing" OR "information technology*" OR "information system*" OR ##) (## represents 7 related keywords about emerging technologies) and #3 is TS = ("electronic health" OR "e-health" OR "digital health-care" OR "telemedic*" OR ###) (### represents 6 keywords that emerged after new information technologies applied to the healthcare field). The literature type was selected as "Article", search period was 1992–2017, and the retrieval time was January 18, 2018. A total of 3085 literature data were collected.

2.2 Method and Data Analysis Tools

Bibliometrics is an interdisciplinary that utilizes mathematics, statistics, and bibliog-raphy to analyze academic literature quantitatively [7]. Scientific literature is one of the manifestations of scientific research achievements, which can reveal related research in a comprehensive and concrete way. For data statistics and visualization analysis, we comprehensively used CiteSpace, SATI3.2, UCINET and NETDRAW.

CiteSpace is a visualization software based on JAVA language and developed by Chen Chaomei, a Chinese scholar at Drexel University in the United States. CiteSpace is mainly based on co-citation analysis and path finding network algorithm (PFNET) to calculate specific domain literature to explore the critical evolution path and knowledge turning point of subject [8].

SATI was jointly developed by Liu Qiyuan and Ye Ying of Zhejiang University. It has four major functions: title format conversion, information extraction, word frequency statistics, and knowledge matrix construction [9]. After obtain the high-frequency keyword co-occurrence matrix, we used UCINET and NetDraw to draw the keyword co-occurrence network. Then the relationship among individual keywords can be visualized, which is convenient for analysis.

3   E-Health Knowledge Map of Time-and-Space Analysis

3.1   Time Distribution Map of the Published Literature Number

In order to examine the research outcomes in the health and medical fields under emerging information technology, this paper used CiteSpace to count literature amount from 1992 to 2017 and obtains the literature's quantity change yearly, as shown in Fig. 1.

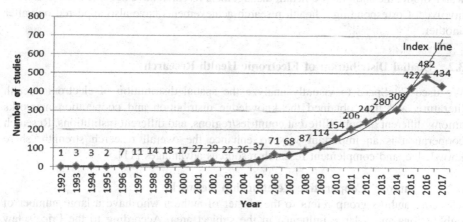

Fig. 1. Annual number of published articles.

The first article about e-health first began in 1992. The article titled "Current Status of Image Save and Carry (IS-AND-C) Standardization" was published in the journal named COMPUTER METHODS AND PROGRAMS IN BIOMEDICINE. It was also the first paper referring to electronic health and medical records. It was mainly about the image preservation and carrying plans for the transmission and exchange of medical information from different medical devices or medical institutions [10]. Since 2001, the number of scientific literature in the field of electronic health has increased significantly, and the number of relevant research scholars has also increased to 71.

The European commission's proposal for the "Electronic European Action Plan 2002" draft, which emphasized the importance of online medical, has effectively promoted scholars' research on telemedicine and electronic medical records at that time. With the introduction of cloud computing in 2006, the development of big data processing technologies and the improvement of residents' living quality, people have new pursuits for their own health management, and relevant scientific literature also shows an increasing trend year by year. For 2017, which has just ended, some documents may still be reviewed and not included in the Web of Science database. Thus the literature amount of 2017 is relatively less. According to the index trend line, the literature number after 2017 will still maintain a high growth rate. It can be seen that since the beginning of this century, internationally electronic health research has been developing vigorously.

In general, the annual input amount trend of authors in the field of electronic health is consistent with the change trend of the scientific literature number, which is roughly an exponential increase. The number of relevant authors in 2006 was 216. By the year 2016, the number of authors has grown to 2166, and the number of authors has turned 10 times in ten years. With the widely application of emerging technologies in telemedicine and mobile health as well as economic development and improvement of living standards in the past decade, the government is paying more attention to the national healthcare. Residents' demands for health have also shifted from being "disease-seeking" to full-life-cycle health. It can be seen that under the attention of all walks of life, the authors of e-health management research have become more and more involved. Corresponding e-health research achievements have also appeared one after another.

3.2   Spatial Distribution of Electronic Health Research

We used CiteSpace to visually analyze the spatial distribution of electronic health literature, and then obtained the knowledge distribution and cooperation networks among different authors, different countries/regions, and different institutions. Research cooperation is an important way to enhance the overall research strength, share knowledge, and complement research resources advantages [11].

3.2.1   Authors' Cooperative Relationship Network

The core authors group refers to the cluster of authors who have a large number of publications and a large influence in the subject area. According to the Price's law which uses to measure the literature authors distribution in specific subject area, $M = 0.749(NMax)/2$, where NMax refers to the papers number of the author who has the most publications, and the scholars with published papers number above M are the core authors in this field [12]. Based on the literature statistical analysis tool Hiscite, it shows that the author with the most publications is Sittig DF (with 50 articles) i.e. $NMax = 50$. According to Price law, $M = 18.7$, indicating that the authors with over 19 articles are the core authors in electronic health field, a total of 7 scholars. Table 1 reports the core authors and their cited information in the field of electronic health. The distribution of core authors is relatively concentrated, and they are mainly divided into two cooperation networks with Sittig DF as the core and Menachemi N as the core.

Most links of the authors' cooperation relationship are in warm colors, indicating that the core authors are closely collaborating.

Table 1. Core authors with high production of published papers

Author	Recs	TLCS	TGCS
Sittig DF	50	141	616
Bates DW	42	218	1123
Kaushal R	34	139	511
Singh H	33	97	445
Wright A	29	108	528
Jha AK	23	457	1779
Menachemi N	23	116	323

3.2.2   National/Regional Distribution and Cooperation Network

The distribution of knowledge possession and cooperation network for e-health research in different countries/regions is shown in Fig. 2. The size of the circles indicates the literature amount, and the different colors of circles and lines represent different years of publication. There are a total of 90 countries/regions in the map, and there are a total of 285 cooperative links between countries/regions. In general, in the field of electronic health, cooperation between countries/regions is very close.

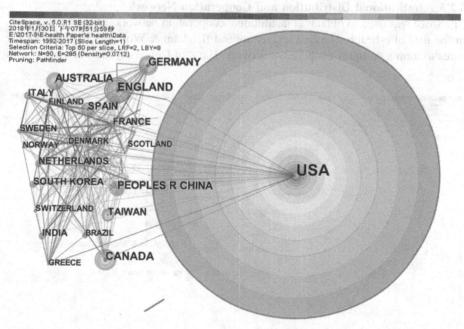

Fig. 2. National/regional distribution and cooperation network (Color figure online)

In terms of the number of published scientific and technical literature, the United States ranked first with 1,680 documents, and accounted for 54.4% of the total number of electronic health documents worldwide, far exceeding that of other countries/regions. China (including Taiwan) ranked second with 198 articles, but China started e-health research relatively late—began to produce literature in 1999. Taiwan began e-health research in 2007, but Taiwan has published 90 articles in a short period of ten years, surpassing Italy and France, which began research at the end of last century. China should follow the trend of the times, pay attention to health management, and emphasize cross-strait academic exchanges and cooperation in the future. Subsequent countries are Canada, Germany, and Australia, with 140, 134, and 132 articles respectively. The centrality describes the importance degree of the nodes, which is reflected in the purple circle of the nodes' outer edge on the cooperation network map. The highest centrality is the United States, which is 0.57, followed by the United Kingdom's 0.21 and France's 0.18. It can be seen that both the U.S. and U.K. have an advantage in terms of volume and importance. When it comes to the time of various countries began investing in e-health research, the earliest was still the United States, followed by Germany, which launched e-health research in 1994. Most countries began investing in this field in 1999. In the top ten countries/regions, from cooperation network it can be seen that the cooperation among European countries is the closest. At the same time these European countries all have an intimate cooperative relationship with the United States. Among them, the United States and Germany have the most cooperation. In contrast, cooperation between Asian countries is relatively small.

3.2.3   Institutional Distribution and Cooperation Network

CiteSpace was used to obtain an institutional cooperation network, as shown in Fig. 3. In the field of e-health, Harvard University and Brigham & Women's Hospital are the cores to form a complex cooperative network. Harvard University took first place with

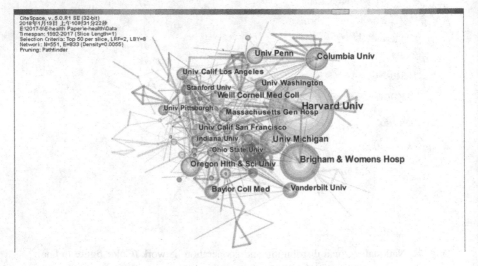

Fig. 3. Major institutional cooperation network

167 articles. The second-ranked Brigham & Women's Hospital is a well-known teaching branch of Harvard Medical School and has the most advanced resources for clinical care, medical research, doctor training and education. Most organizations that published more than 30 scientific articles are the world's top universities or affiliates in the United States. Since 2000, these authoritative academic institutions mainly from the U.S. cooperated very closely. This explains why U.S. has such a high output of e-health literature.

4 The Electronic Health Research Focus Analysis

One of the most important content of bibliometric analysis is the keywords analysis, which extracts the research hotspots in the field to summarize development trends and predict the future development direction. The research hotspot refers to the problems that are discussing and solving by a large number of related documents in a time period. By analyzing the keywords, it is easy to determine research hotspots in a certain field. The co-word analysis method holds that if two terms appear in a single document simultaneously, there is a certain co-occurrence relationship between these two. These two-two appearing keywords are constructed as a co-word network.

This paper uses the three-step method of co-word analysis: extraction keywords, constructing co-word matrix, and data analysis [13]. In order to construct a keyword co-occurrence network more rationally, the statistical analysis tool SATI 3.2 was used to perform statistics on documents. After the pre-processing such as synonym merging and irrelevant punctuation, we finally obtained a 65 * 65 co-occurrence matrix. Based on the co-word matrix, we used Ucinet 6.0 and Netdraw to generate a keyword co-occurrence network, as shown in Fig. 4.

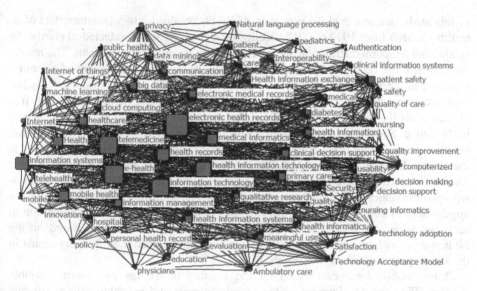

Fig. 4. Keywords co-occurrence network

Among all keywords, high-frequency keywords can best reflect research hotspots and research trends in specific areas [14]. Electronic health records, telemedicine, and e-health have become hot applications in electronic health research; Data mining, health information technology, and cloud computing have become hot technology topics in this area. Meanwhile, scholars have also paid close attention to hot issues such as privacy, security, and quality improvement.

Electronic Health Records (EHR) is the largest key node. Studies have shown that at least 80.5% of hospitals adopted a basic electronic health records system by 2015, an increase of 5.3% points compared to 2014; however, only 37.5% of hospitals used 8 or more EHR data for performance measurement, and 41.7% of hospitals used 8 or more EHR data for patient participation. The performance measurement and patient partic-ipation function of electronic health records are key factors in improving hospital performance. Although the "Economic and Clinical Health Information Technology Act" promotes the widespread adoption of EHR in hospitals, the application of advanced EHR functions has lagged behind. This situation is particularly present in some important hospitals [15]. In the current actual situation, there are still some limitations in the use of electronic health records. For example, because the lack of standards and regulations for electronic health records, different hospitals, mobile health companies issue various electronic health records or medical examination reports. Even the criteria for judging whether the index is normal are not the same, which is undoubtedly a significant impediment to integrate EHRs from different institutions and extract useful information from physical health changes. If there is no unified industry standard for electronic health records, it is difficult to achieve data interconnection and interoperability thoroughly.

5   Conclusion

In this study, we searched the core data of WOS, obtained 3,085 literature data of e-health research from 1992 to 2017. Bibliometric analysis was conducted to clarify the spatial and temporal distribution and research hotspots of electronic health. The results show that: First, during the period from 1992 to 2005, the annual output of scientific literature in the field of e-health was small; after 2005, the number of documents has been increasing year by year, and it has generally grown in an exponential manner. It is expected that the electronic health-related literature will continue to grow exponentially in the future. Secondly, the countries/regions that have issued documents in electronic health have relatively close cooperation and the cooperation between EU countries is the closest. In terms of the number of documents issued, the United States ranked first. Thirdly, the academic research studies in e-health have a strong co-citation relation-ship. Fourth, electronic health records, telemedicine, e-health, etc. have become hot applications in e-health research. Meanwhile, scholars have also paid close attention to such hot issues as privacy, security, and health quality improvement. Based on the bibliometric analysis and a systematic review, we summarized the following trends in the development of e-health research.

First, mobile healthcare based on the Internet of Things and smart wearable devices. With the development of the mobile Internet and wearable devices, mobile health management services are flourishing. Mobile health services quickly penetrate people's daily lives because of their convenience, economy, and personalization. Mobile health has a positive impact on the treatment of chronic diseases and daily care [16].

Second, smart health combined medical and health care. Smart health is an era product based on the concepts of e-Health and Smart City. For smart health, "smart" is just a form of expression, the core is still "health." Under the big data environment, only to build a smart community, a smart health care platform for the aged, and data interconnection can solve the problem of increasing global aging population and improving the quality of elderly care services [17].

Third, the deep integration of electronic health information in cloud environment and the dynamic knowledge service for the entire life cycle. Most traditional medical information integration systems mainly deal with basic patient information, diagnosis and treatment information in hospitals, and rarely involve external health information resources. The enlightenment from the development of big data and cloud computing platforms is that health information resources are very complicated, and medical health management is also facing the challenge of integrating information resources. It is very important to study the information fusion and service collaboration of the supply side of the health care service, and the mutual benefit mechanism of various service units in the pension industry.

Acknowledgements. This research were partially supported by the National Natural Science Foundation of China (NSFC) under grant Nos. 71331002, 71301040, 71771075, 71771077, 71573071, and 71601061.

References

1. Hesse, B.W., Shneiderman, B.: eHealth research from the user's perspective. Am. J. Prev. Med. **32**(5), S97–S103 (2007). https://doi.org/10.1016/j.amepre.2007.01.019
2. Fatehi, F., Wootton, R.: Telemedicine, telehealth or e-health? A bibliometric analysis of the trends in the use of these terms. J. Telemed. Telecare **18**(8), 460–464 (2012). https://doi.org/10.1258/jtt.2012.gth108
3. Mochari-Greenberger, H., Vue, L., Luka, A., Peters, A., Pande, R.L.: A tele-behavioral health intervention to reduce depression, anxiety, and stress and improve diabetes self-management. Telemed. e-Health **22**(8), 624–630 (2016). https://doi.org/10.1089/tmj.2015.0231
4. Shaia, K.L., Farag, S., Chyjek, K., Knopman, J., Chen, K.T.: An evaluation of mobile applications for reproductive endocrinology and infertility providers. Telemed. e-Health **23**(3), 254–258 (2017). https://doi.org/10.1089/tmj.2016.0079
5. Wang, J., et al.: Smartphone interventions for long-term health management of chronic diseases: an integrative review. Telemed. e-Health **20**(6), 570–583 (2014). https://doi.org/10.1089/tmj.2013.0243
6. Yang, Y.T., et al.: Trends in the growth of literature of telemedicine: a bibliometric analysis. Comput. Methods Programs Biomed. **122**(3), 471–479 (2015). https://doi.org/10.1016/j.cmpb.2015.09.008

7. Hood, W., Wilson, C.: The literature of bibliometrics, scientometrics, and informetrics. Scientometrics **52**(2), 291–314 (2001). https://doi.org/10.1023/a:1017919924342
8. Synnestvedt, M.B., Chen, C., Holmes, J.H.: CiteSpace II: visualization and knowledge discovery in bibliographic databases. In: AMIA Annual Symposium Proceedings, vol. 2005, p. 724. American Medical Informatics Association (2005)
9. Ying, L.Q.Y.: A study on mining bibliographic records by designed software SATI: case study on library and information science. J. Inf. Resour. Manag. **1**, 35–67 (2012)
10. Ando, Y., Hashimoto, S., Ohyama, N., Inamura, K.: Current status of Image Save and Carry (IS & C) standardization. Comput. Methods Programs Biomed. **37**(4), 319–325 (1992). https://doi.org/10.1016/j.joi.2015.08.002
11. Ebadi, A., Schiffauerova, A.: How to become an important player in scientific collaboration networks? J. Inf. **9**(4), 809–825 (2015). https://doi.org/10.1016/j.joi.2015.08.002
12. Ma, F., Hu, C., Chen, L.: Fundamentals of Information Management, pp. 83–90. Wuhan University Press, Wuhan (2002)
13. Wu, C.C., Leu, H.J.: Examining the trends of technological development in hydrogen energy using patent co-word map analysis. Int. J. Hydrog. Energy **39**(33), 19262–19269 (2014). https://doi.org/10.1016/j.ijhydene.2014.05.006
14. Huenteler, J., Ossenbrink, J., Schmidt, T.S., Hoffmann, V.H.: How a product's design hierarchy shapes the evolution of technological knowledge—evidence from patent-citation networks in wind power. Res. Policy **45**(6), 1195–1217 (2016). https://doi.org/10.1016/j.respol.2016.03.014
15. Adler-Milstein, J., Holmgren, A.J., Kralovec, P., Worzala, C., Searcy, T., Patel, V.: Electronic health record adoption in US hospitals: the emergence of a digital "advanced use" divide. J. Am. Med. Inform. Assoc. **24**(6), 1142–1148 (2017). https://doi.org/10.1093/jamia/ocx080
16. Beratarrechea, A., Lee, A.G., Willner, J.M., Jahangir, E., Ciapponi, A., Rubinstein, A.: The impact of mobile health interventions on chronic disease outcomes in developing countries: a systematic review. Telemed. e-Health **20**(1), 75–82 (2014). https://doi.org/10.1089/tmj.2012.0328
17. Sweileh, W.M., Al-Jabi, S.W., AbuTaha, A.S., Sa'ed, H.Z., Anayah, F.M., Sawalha, A.F.: Bibliometric analysis of worldwide scientific literature in mobile-health: 2006–2016. BMC Med. Inform. Decis. Mak. **17**(1), 72 (2017). https://doi.org/10.1186/s12911-017-0476-7

How Corporations Utilize Academic Social Networking Website?: A Case Study of Health & Biomedicine Corporations

Shengwei Yi[1], Qian Liu[1], and Weiwei Yan[1,2]

[1] School of Information Management, Wuhan University,
Wuhan 430072, China
yanww@whu.edu.cn
[2] Center for E-commerce Research and Development, Wuhan University,
Wuhan 430072, China

Abstract. Health & Biomedicine corporations are representatives that begin to flexibly utilize academic social networking websites to carry out research work and academic communications. As a typical academic social networking website of relatively high popularity and authority, ResearchGate (RG) was chosen as the study case. Data of RG users from 38 Health & Biomedicine corporations were crawled, including their RG metrics and research network formed, to support RG metrics analysis and social network analysis. The findings show that research level of Health & Biomedicine corporation RG users are closely correlated with their utilization of RG, with some social networking characteristics emerging at the same time. Specifically, universities are core subjects in organizing and coordinating research work in the field of Health & Biomedicine. Corporations and research institutions of different countries behave differently during their development of research work on RG, as North America shows its dominance in both focusing on research and authority recognized by others, while Europe lacks the former, and Asia is just the opposite of Europe.

Keywords: Health & biomedicine corporations · Academic social networking Research level · ResearchGate

1 Introduction

Academic social networking websites, a branch of social networking sites boasting popularity and massive usage, are virtual platforms specifically targeting scholars where researchers can create a research profile and communicate with other members [1, 2]. Over time, academic social networks are increasingly used by researchers of both theoretical and practical importance [3], especially thanks to the possibilities of sharing articles they offer [4].

As a typical academic social networking website first established in 2008, ResearchGate (RG) has verified more than 14+ million scientist or research professional members [5]. It allows uploading academic articles, abstracts, and links to published articles; tracks demand for published articles, and engages in professional interaction [6]. It is being increasingly used as a vehicle for publicizing research results

© Springer Nature Switzerland AG 2018
H. Chen et al. (Eds.): ICSH 2018, LNCS 10983, pp. 325–331, 2018.
https://doi.org/10.1007/978-3-030-03649-2_32

and facilitating collaboration [7], especially among researchers [4]. Although the mission of RG is to connect the world of science and make research open to all [5], most academics who have an RG account did not use it very heavily [8].

As core subjects of innovation, corporations have paid much attention to scientific research and academic communication during its operation and development. However, present utilization analyses of academic community mainly focus on universities and research institutions, which mainly fall into two arenas - promises and perils [9]. There is a lack of revealing on corporation users' characteristics and their participation in academic communities.

This paper aims at the evaluation of the effectiveness and the usage of RG among the corporation users through the crawling of their members' data. As a case study, all corporation users are specifically Health & Biomedicine ones. Besides, social networking analysis is conducted to demonstrate the research network during their utilization. With support from above, a preliminary overview of Health & Biomedicine corporations' utilization of academic communities can be given. Accordingly, we can have a deeper view on the correlation between research level of Health & Biomedicine corporations and their utilization of academic communities.

2 Methods

This study chose the top 100 research-oriented corporations according to the ranking of Nature 2016 [10]. Among them, 42 Health & Biomedicine corporations related (divided by their core business areas) were selected as the samples of study, for their largest proportion. Excluding the ones having no access to their RG homepages, a sample of 38 Health & Biomedicine corporations was finally confirmed.

As for each one of the 38 corporations, data of its members' url and their RG metrics (RG Score, Reads, Citations, Follower, Following) were successively crawled from its members' homepages. Besides, top 2 collaborating, top 3 Read_by_country and top 3 Read_by_institution on the corporation users' homepages were also collected. The data crawling date was from 30th Oct to 3rd Nov, 2017. In order to produce a more accurate result, data of the zombie users whose RG scores were lower than 0.01 were excluded. The total number of RG users is 33474, among which 62.54%, namely 20933 are real users.

3 Result

3.1 RG Metrics Analysis

To explore how the Health & Biomedicine corporations participate in research work and make use of RG, analysis is carried out through the view of 7 RG metrics including RG score, Reads (per research-item), Citations (per research-item), Follower, Following, Real Members and Total Members.

RG score is a metric provided by the platform of ResearchGate. It plays the role of the metric that reflects corporation users' utilization of RG and affected primarily by the members' engagement and activity in the site [11]. As shown in Table 1, the value of RG score varies in a relatively certain range according to its smaller SD among others, especially in contrast to Follower and Following.

Table 1. Overall RG metrics of Health & Biomedicine corporation users

	RG score	Reads	Citations	Follower	Following
Mean	18.82	42.46	35.80	12,021.00	11,039.76
Median	18.56	39.33	32.93	8,599.00	8,353.00
SD	2.91	14.34	14.14	11,268.21	9,965.87

Reads and Citations appear to have something in common due to their approximate values of Mean, Median and SD, similar to the relationship between Follower and Following. Nevertheless, Follower and Following tend to have lower values as the ranking descends, while Reads and Citations show a fluctuation instead.

The Krustal-Wallis test in SPSS 22.0 is utilized to conduct significant difference analysis of the RG metrics among the 38 corporations. Classified by the RG ranking, the 38 corporations have significant differences in all of the seven RG metrics under 95% confidence level ($p = 0.000 < 0.05$).

3.2 Social Network Analysis

From the perspective of scientific research cooperation network formed by the data of top 2 collaborating of the 38 corporations, the collaborators are divided into four groups, which are Company, University/College/School (abbreviated as University), Research Institution, and Others. Due to the relatively significant difference between the top 2 collaborating of each corporation, the development of scientific research cooperation and the corporation users' cooperation characteristics are presented on the level of institutional type.

We utilize Gephi 0.9.1 to visualize the cooperation network. Yifan Hu layout is chosen to reduce computation complexity due to its multilevel characteristic, and node degree is used to render the color and size of a node. As shown in Fig. 1, University ranks first among the four types of collaborating institutions. The degree of university is 41, much larger than Research Institution's 18 that ranks second. It means that University participates most highly in scientific research with Health & Biomedicine corporations. As for the 38 Health & Biomedicine corporations themselves, both profit-oriented (such as research institution) and research-oriented ones (such as company) are more likely to collaborate with research-dominating institutions, other than profit-driven ones.

From the visualization based on the metric of Read_by_institution (the following institutions are labeled by their institutional types), as shown in Fig. 2, University is second to none owing to its continuous sensitiveness and attention on corporations' research trends and achievements.

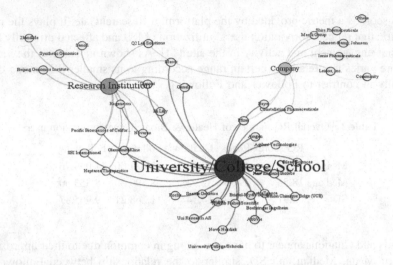

Fig. 1. The collaborating social network formed during research activities on RG, using Yifan Hu layout in Gephi. (Color figure online)

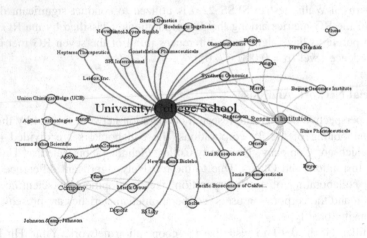

Fig. 2. The follower-followee social network based Read_by_institutions, using Yifan Hu layout in Gephi.

A directed social networking graph is constructed to reveal the Reads relations among countries. The countries of the 38 corporations and the top 3 countries of each who read their publications on RG most often are labeled. Both Fig. 3a and b following take Yifan Hu layout as pattern of manifestation, where direction represents the relationship of read.

As shown in the Fig. 3a, the four countries listing highest are successively United States, United Kingdom, Germany and Switzerland, which means their publications are ones most followed by others. Figure 3b indicates that United States, China, United Kingdom and India are the top 4 countries that keep a watchful eye on others' research achievements.

(a) **(b)**

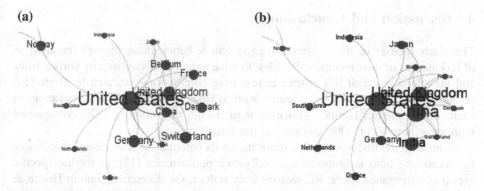

Fig. 3. (a) The follower-followee social network based on Read_by_countries (nodes are rendered by their in-degrees). (b) The follower-followee social network based on Read_by_countries (nodes are rendered by their out-degrees).

As a one-mode figure, further calculations of SNA metrics are conducted. The most important node "United States" which ranks first in both Fig. 3a and b, has the highest betweenness centrality and closeness centrality of 91.333 and 0.056 among all. Its own density is 0.343, much higher than the overall's 0.279. Another special node "United Kingdom" is 5.833 and 0.038 in betweenness and closeness, relatively low compared to that of the United States's, despite its significant social network status in being top 3 in both figures.

To simplify the communication relationship among countries, further continental division is implemented as the Table 2. Among all, Asia pays closest attention to North America (28.95%), which is also the highest percent (47.83%) within Group 1. North America contributes a lot to its own popularity with the total percentage of 20.18% and 33.33% within group. Followers of European publications mainly consists of North America and Asia.

Table 2. International research interactions on RG based on Read_by_countries

Group	Relationship of reads	Freq.	% (Within group)	% (Total)
1	North America → North America	23	33.33%	20.18%
	Asia → North America	33	47.83%	28.95%
	Europe → North America	13	18.84%	11.40%
2	North America → Europe	15	35.71%	13.16%
	Asia → Europe	16	38.10%	14.04%
	Europe → Europe	11	26.19%	9.65%
3	North America → Asia	1	66.67%	1.75%
	Asia → Asia	2	33.33%	0.88%
Total		114		100%

4 Discussion and Conclusions

This study focuses on the corporations of Health & Biomedicine through the analysis of RG metrics of their members. Besides, to what extent RG is utilized by corporations and the effectiveness of RG metrics in revealing corporations' research level are also considered. It is concluded that research level of Health & Biomedicine corporations in terms of RG metrics is much shown on their overall utilization of RG, accompanied with some networking characteristics at the same time.

Similar to the findings that RG score shows its potential to be an effective indicator for measuring both institutional and individual performance [12], as for the specific group of corporation users, RG metrics truly reflects the differences among Health & Biomedicine corporation users. What's more, utilization of RG proves to has its reflection on RG metrics, as Health & Biomedicine corporation users, who have higher real user ratio than top-level university users, also exceed them on every one of the RG metrics [13]. Present RG corporation users has already been on a higher research level than top-level university users. In other words, Health & Biomedicine corporations are representative ones who begin to flexibly apply RG to improving academic influence of their members and organizations. However, the regularity that users of lower rankings tend to have lower RG scores is not proved in this study [14], a value fluctuation is observed instead. It is probably because the scale of the original samples in this study is not large enough to contain several research levels that vary much in research conditions.

As for their utilization network, university plays a rather important role in organizing and coordinating research work in the field of Health & Biomedicine. They do not always act as initiators of such research collaborating relationships, but they engage in research activities as core subjects which facilitate the effective operation of RG and push the research work forward as well to some extent. And there are minor differences from above when the indicator of Read is used to describe the network among institutions. Read has its orientation that represents the type of the research subjects whose publications are followed by others, namely the mutual concern behaviors of the research-production-oriented corporations. But overall, it can be concluded that university prefers fundamental research, which is ultimately applied to industry by means of developing research cooperation with corporations.

In terms of international communication, America is an outstanding example for both its involvement in research activities and attention on research trends. It keeps high and continuous concentration on research productions on RG from home and broad, and at the same time is widely recognized as popular and authoritative in scientific research by others. In contrast, the two Asian countries, China and India, are dominant in their sensitive following of Europe and North America, while lacks acceptance by each other and their followings. According to the findings that RG users in Asia makes relatively little use of RG in spite of its active engagement [15], it's probably because that there are quite low-quality articles on the homepages of such corporation users despite their huge numbers, maybe given the fact that there's no quality control on RG. Corporation users in Europe are just the opposite of those in Asia, as they can learn to focus more on their peers during the following research process.

There are still limitations in this study such as the overall small variations in the research level among the chosen samples. However, comparisons with different industry sectors may help further reveal the true level of Health & Biomedicine corporations' utilization of academic social networking website represented by RG. Future study can further focus on the evaluation of the effectiveness and research interactions among corporations of various industries or those of different research levels, to have a deeper view of interdisciplinary user behavior difference on RG.

Acknowledgement. This work was supported by the Chinese National Funds of Social Science (No. 15CTQ025).

References

1. Abdulhayoglu, M.A., Thijs, B.: Use of ResearchGate and Google CSE for author name disambiguation. Scientometrics **111**(3), 1–21 (2017)
2. Sheikh, A.: Awareness and use of academic social networking websites by the faculty of CIIT. Qual. Quant. Methods Libr. **5**, 177–188 (2017)
3. Doleck, T., Lajoie, S.: Social networking and academic performance: a review. Educ. Inf. Technol. **23**, 1–31 (2017)
4. Boudry, C., Bouchard, A.: Role of academic social networks in disseminating the scientific production of researchers in biology/medicine: the example of ResearchGate. Med. Sci. **33** (6–7), 647–652 (2017)
5. ResearchGate. About. https://www.researchgate.net/about. Accessed 18 Oct 2017
6. Meishar-Tal, H., Pieterse, E.: Why do academics use academic social networking sites? Int. Rev. Res. Open Distrib. Learn. **18**(1), 1–22 (2017)
7. Hammook, Z., Misic, J., Misic, V.B.: Crawling ResearchGate.net to measure student/supervisor collaboration. In: 2015 IEEE Global Communications Conference (GLOBECOM), San Diego, CA, pp. 1–6 (2015)
8. Muscanell, N., Utz, S.: Social networking for scientists: an analysis on how and why academics use ResearchGate. Online Inf. Rev. **41**(5), 744–759 (2017)
9. Williams, A.E., Woodacre, M.A.: The possibilities and perils of academic social networking sites. Online Inf. Rev. **40**(2), 282–294 (2016)
10. Nature. 2017 tables: Institutions - corporate. https://www.natureindex.com/annual-tables/2017/institution/corporate/all. Accessed 19 Oct 2017
11. Copiello, S., Bonifaci, P.: A few remarks on ResearchGate score and academic reputation. Scientometrics **114**(2), 1–6 (2018)
12. Yu, M.C., Wu, Y.C.J., Alhalabi, W., Kao, H.Y., Wu, W.H.: ResearchGate: an effective altmetric indicator for active researchers? Comput. Hum. Behav. **55**, 1001–1006 (2016)
13. Yan, W., Zhang, Y.: Research universities on the ResearchGate social networking site: an examination of institutional differences, research activity level, and social networks formed. J. Informetr. **12**(1), 385–400 (2018)
14. Ali, M.Y., Wolski, M., Richardson, J.: Strategies for using ResearchGate to improve institutional research outcomes. Libr. Rev. **66**(8–9), 726–739 (2017)
15. Thelwall, M., Kousha, K.: ResearchGate: disseminating, communicating, and measuring scholarship? J. Assoc. Inf. Sci. Technol. **66**(5), 876–889 (2014)

Meta-analysis of the Immunomodulatory Effect of *Ganoderma Lucidum* Spores Using an Automatic Pipeline

Rui Liu[1], Yumeng Zhang[1], Ziwen Chen[1], Liqiang Wang[2],
Shuaibing He[2], Guifeng Hua[1], and Chang Liu[2(✉)]

[1] Central China Normal University, 152 Luoyu Road, 430079 Wuhan, China
[2] Institute of Medicinal Plant Development,
Chinese Academy of Medical Science,
151 Malianwa North Road, 100193 Beijing, China
cliu6688@yahoo.com

Abstract. Although many studies have been conducted on the chemistry and pharmacological activities of *Ganoderma lucidum* spores (GLS), there is a lack of systematic review on the health promoting functions especially immunomodulatory effects of GLS. In the current study, we constructed a data model and utilized R modules and PERL language to implement a pipeline that is capable of carrying out multiple meta-analyses automatically. Using GLS as the study subject, we carried out meta-analyses on 53 outcome measures using the automatic meta-analysis pipeline. Among them, 19 outcome measures were found to be significantly affected after GLS treatment (with p value < 0.05). 8 of them have I^2 less than 50%, indicating low level of study heterogeneity. Through the analysis of GLS, the automatic meta-analysis pipeline has been shown to be suitable for high-throughput meta-analysis and visualization. Also, the information derived from this study could assist policy-makers and functional food consumers to determine whether GLS could be a recommended choice for immunomodulatory effect.

Keywords: *Ganoderma lucidum* spore · Meta-analysis
Immunomodulatory effect

1 Introduction

A functional food is a food given an additional function, often one related to health-promotion or disease prevention. Functional food represents a significant type of products around the world. These types of products are particularly with an annual sale to more than 1 trillion Chinese Yuan in china. Traditional Chinese medicine is a major source of functional food production in China. Traditional Chinese Medicine can regulate the balance of the body and have fewer adverse reactions if its application is reasonable. Ganoderma lucidum has been a popular Traditional Chinese Medicine to treat various human diseases, such as hepatitis, hypertension, hypercholesterolemia and cancer [1–3]. Modern research also verified that Ganoderma lucidum spores (GLS) has multiple functions, such as blocking histamine release and inhibiting an overstimulated immune

© Springer Nature Switzerland AG 2018
H. Chen et al. (Eds.): ICSH 2018, LNCS 10983, pp. 332–341, 2018.
https://doi.org/10.1007/978-3-030-03649-2_33

system, and has an effect on regulating cellular and humoral immunity [4–6]. GLS has many bioactive components including bioactive compounds like polysaccharides, triterpenoids, alkaloids, amino acids, enzymes and proteins [7, 8]. The diversity of bio-active ingredients in GLS is associated with the universality of its multiple effects. Most systematic reviews and meta-analysis have looked at GLS for improving cancer-related fatigue [9, 10]. However, few meta-analyses were conducted on the health promoting function of GLS. This study is important because it looks at a broader range of outcome measures. It summaries the best available current quantitative evidence of the effec-tiveness of GLS. The information derived from this study could assist policy-makers for functional food administration as well as functional food consumers to determine whether GLS could be a recommended choice for immunomodulatory effect. The objective of the study was to evaluate whether GLS has any immunomodulatory effect, and a pipeline for automatic meta-analysis was developed and applied.

2   Method

2.1   Criteria for Considering Studies

Types of Studies. As described above, we intended to evaluate the health promoting functions, not the therapeutic effects of GLS. As a result, we did not included the studies using human as subject and following the standard randomized controlled trial design. We searched the literature for the following criteria: one of the 27 health promoting functions defined by China Food and Drug Administration (CFDA), subject include mouse, treatments include *Ganoderma lucidum* spores (GLS), Lingzhi spore powder, Reishi Spore Powder, Reishi Mushroom Powder, Ganoderma spore powder.

Types of Treatment. We surveyed the immunomodulatory literature and selected those papers using GLS as the treatment. There are a total of 2171 treatment doses, with a median of 470 mg/kg.bw. The maximum dose is 4000 mg/kg.bw.

Types of Outcome Measures. From these studies, 53 outcome measures were extracted including the increase of body weight, the number of antibody producing cells and the spleen index.

2.2   Search Methods

We searched the following electronic databases for primary studies: the China National Knowledge Infrastructure (CNKI, 1979 to December 2017) and the Pubmed (1950 to January 2018). Two strategies were applied when searching health promoting function literature. Firstly, we searched CNKI using the query of SU%' Lingzhi spore powder' AND SU%' function'; then, we used each of the 27 health promoting functions that are already approved by China Food and Drug Administration (CFDA) as a specification of function, such as SU%' Lingzhi spore powder' AND SU%' immunomodulation'. We searched Pubmed using the query of (((((Ganoderma lucidum spores) OR Lingzhi spore powder) OR Reishi Spore Powder) OR Reishi Mushroom Powder) OR Gano-derma spore powder) AND Function.

The full text of articles were retrieved and translated into English where required. We searched the bibliographies of pertinent articles, reviews and texts for additional citations. Two review authors independently assessed the eligibility of the trials, using a trial selection form. A third review author resolved discrepancies.

2.3   Data Model Construction

Data extraction was conducted by a dozen students and researchers. To minimize the time needed to discuss how to extract the data correctly. We first constructed a data

(a)

```
mysql> desc exp_data;
+-----------------------+------------------------------------------+------+-----+---------+----------------+
| Field                 | Type                                     | Null | Key | Default | Extra          |
+-----------------------+------------------------------------------+------+-----+---------+----------------+
| id_record             | int(10) unsigned                         | NO   | PRI | NULL    | auto_increment |
| id_material           | int(11)                                  | YES  |     | NULL    |                |
| id_source             | int(11)                                  | YES  |     | NULL    |                |
| test_category         | enum('function','toxicity')              | YES  |     | NULL    |                |
| test_type             | varchar(256)                             | YES  |     | NULL    |                |
| exp_name              | varchar(256)                             | YES  |     | NULL    |                |
| exp_group             | enum('normal','model','exp')             | YES  |     | NULL    |                |
| replicate_id          | int(11)                                  | YES  |     | NULL    |                |
| treatment_subject_name| varchar(45)                              | YES  |     | NULL    |                |
| treatment_subject_sex | enum('male','female','not_specified')    | YES  |     | NULL    |                |
| treatment_name        | varchar(45)                              | YES  |     | NULL    |                |
| treatment_dose        | float                                    | YES  |     | NULL    |                |
| treatment_unit        | varchar(45)                              | YES  |     | NULL    |                |
| treatment_time        | float                                    | YES  |     | NULL    |                |
| treatment_time_unit   | varchar(45)                              | YES  |     | NULL    |                |
| indicator_name        | varchar(45)                              | YES  |     | NULL    |                |
| indicator_value_unit  | varchar(45)                              | YES  |     | NULL    |                |
| indicator_value_mean  | float                                    | YES  |     | NULL    |                |
| indicator_value_std   | float                                    | YES  |     | NULL    |                |
| sample_size           | int(11)                                  | YES  |     | NULL    |                |
| desc                  | varchar(1024)                            | YES  |     | NULL    |                |
| create_time           | datetime                                 | YES  |     | NULL    |                |
| update_time           | datetime                                 | YES  |     | NULL    |                |
+-----------------------+------------------------------------------+------+-----+---------+----------------+
23 rows in set
```

(b)

```
mysql> desc material;
+-------------+--------------+------+-----+---------+----------------+
| Field       | Type         | Null | Key | Default | Extra          |
+-------------+--------------+------+-----+---------+----------------+
| id_material | int(11)      | NO   | PRI | NULL    | auto_increment |
| name        | varchar(45)  | YES  |     | NULL    |                |
| source      | varchar(45)  | YES  |     | NULL    |                |
| note        | varchar(256) | YES  |     | NULL    |                |
| create_time | datetime     | YES  |     | NULL    |                |
+-------------+--------------+------+-----+---------+----------------+
```

(c)

```
mysql> desc source;
+---------------+---------------+------+-----+---------+-------+
| Field         | Type          | Null | Key | Default | Extra |
+---------------+---------------+------+-----+---------+-------+
| id            | int(64)       | NO   | PRI | 0       |       |
| source_type   | varchar(45)   | YES  |     | NULL    |       |
| id_noteexpress| varchar(45)   | YES  |     | NULL    |       |
| citation      | varchar(1024) | YES  |     | NULL    |       |
| create_time   | datetime      | YES  |     | NULL    |       |
| update_time   | datetime      | YES  |     | NULL    |       |
+---------------+---------------+------+-----+---------+-------+
```

Fig. 1. Schema for the database supporting the automatic meta-analysis (a) exp_data; (b) material; (c) source.

model; all participants were then used the model as the references to extract data from the relevant data sources. As shown in Fig. 1(a). 23 columns were included in the data model indicating material name, information source, treatment materials, treatment unit, treatment subject name, treatment subject sex, experimental design (mostly for the dose-dependent treatment as well as time-series data), outcome measures, mean, standard deviations and sample sizes. Particularly, we used dose and unit to capture all information related to dose-dependent treatment. And time and unit were used to describe the time-series data. Several other fields were provided to capture any information that did not fit into the above fields and also some fields that were used for book-keeping, such the last time the information was collected and the last time the information were updated.

This model has been used to extract information from a total number of 5863 literatures and have been shown to be robust enough to incorporate all types of information needed.

2.4   Database Construction

Based on the above model, we constructed a relational database. The database schema contained three tables, which were exp_data, materials and sources. The table definitions were shown in Fig. 1(a), (b), (c). The database was running with mysql (5.6.38) on Operating System: CentOS Linux 7 (Core), CPE OS Name: cpe:/o:centos:centos:7, Kernel: Linux 3.10.0-693.11.1.el7.x86_64, Architecture: x86-64.

2.5   Implementation of Automatic Meta-analysis Pipeline

We performed the meta-analysis according to the recommendations of The Cochrane Collaboration. The pipeline was implemented using the Perl programming language (revision 5 version 24 subversion 0) with the meta library from the R package (version 3.2.0) [11, 12].

3   Results

3.1   Results of the Search

From the first round of data retrieval, 107 articles were retrieved and the second round resulted in 149 articles. Among all the 256 articles, 7 cannot be downloaded; 135 were excluded because their titles, abstracts or both were clearly irrelevant during the initial screen for potential relevance; 29 articles addressing on compound health promoting function analysis and 27 records lack of experimental data were also excluded. After eliminating duplication, we finally identified 51 articles for meta-analysis. See PRISMA study flow diagram (Fig. 2) for details.

3.2   Effects of Treatments

The pipeline was used to analyze GLS. Taken together, we selected 51 studies for our meta-analysis, corresponding to 89 meta-analysis data sets addressing

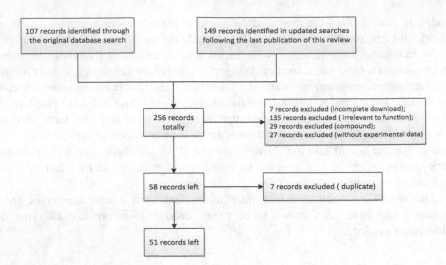

Fig. 2. PRISMA study flow diagram

immunomodulation, anti-fatigue, anti-oxidation and anti-radiation. 53 outcome measures of the immunomodulation function were reported from the data set which contained 419 records. Regarding the health promoting functions of GLS, a total of 89 outcome measures were carried out. Among them, 49 are related to the immunomodulatory functions. The data related to this function were extracted from the following references [13–38]. The Standard Mean Difference (SMD) of 19 outcome measures were found to be significantly from 0, among them, 8 have I^2 less than 50%, indicating low level of heterogeneity. The Standard Mean Differences (SMD) of the other 11 outcome measures were found not statistically significant from 0. Here we listed the characteristics of 4 articles (Table 1) regarding to 3 meta-analyses of immunomodulatory effect we reported in this paper.

Meta-analysis for Number of Antibody Producing Cells. There were 2 studies related to this outcome measure (Fig. 3). Heterogeneity analysis showed that the $I^2 < 50\%$, indicating that the level of heterogeneity is not significant, so fixed effects model was adopted for meta-analysis. The meta-analysis showed that the standard mean difference (SMD) is 1.1940, with the 95% confidence interval (CI) ranging from 0.5254 to 1.8627. The p value for the SMD $< 0.01(p = 0.0005)$. In summary, the analysis suggested that the treatment with GLS significantly increased the number of antibody producing cells.

Meta-analysis for Increase of Body Weight. There were 50 studies related to this outcome measure (Fig. 4). Heterogeneity analysis showed that the $I^2 < 50\%$, indicating that the level of heterogeneity is not significant, so fixed effects model was adopted for meta-analysis. The meta-analysis showed that the standard mean difference (SMD) is 0.1970, with the 95% confidence interval (CI) ranging from 0.0719 to 0.3222. The p value $< 0.01(p = 0.0020)$. In summary, the analysis suggested that the treatment with GLS significantly increased the body weight.

Table 1. Characteristic of included studies

Title	Author	Publication & year	Abstract	Outcome measure	Sample size
Study on spores of Ganoderma lucidum [13]	Wu Mingzhong	Master's degree thesis 2000	This study carried out delayed-type hypersensitivity, mice carbon clearance test and serolysin test, and proved that sporoderm-broken powder has immunomodulatory effect	Increase of body weight	10
A preliminary study on the effect of broken Ganoderma spore powder on immune function in mice [14]	Wu Mingzhong; Shen Aiguang	Edible fungi of China 2000	This study proved immunomodulatory effect of broken ganoderma lucidum spore powder in mice through the following experiments: delayed type hypersensitivity andserolysin test	Increase of body weight	10
Study on effect of broken Ganoderma lucidum spore powder on immune function in mice [15]	Zhang Rongbiao; Chen run; Chen Guanmin; Zheng Zhiwei	Preventive medicine tribune 2013	This study demonstrated the immunomodulatory effect of broken ganoderma lucidum spore powder in mice through the following experiments: the spleen lymphocyte transformation function induced by ConA, and the delayed type hypersensitivity response	Spleen index	10
Ganoderma lucidum spore powder capsule enhances immune function test in mice [16]	Zhang Qiang; Xie Genfa; Zhai Shuxiang; Qu Xianjun; Li Fengqin	Journal of pharmaceutical research 1998	This study carried out the macrophage phagocytic function test, Determination of the spleen index, Determination of serum agglutination and Determination of nonspecific acid esterase, and proved that Ganoderma lucidum spore powder capsules has immunomodulatory effect	Spleen index	19–20

Meta-analysis for Spleen Index. Spleen Index means the ratio of the Spleen Weight to the Body Weight. There were 4 studies related to this outcome measure (Fig. 5). Heterogeneity analysis showed that the $I^2 < 50\%$, indicating that the level of

Study	Experimental Mean	SD	Total	Control Mean	SD	Total	Weight	Std. Mean Difference IV, Fixed, 95% CI
20140079 subgroup	510.45	127.5600	11	360.50	101.3400	10	49.3%	1.24 [0.29; 2.19]
20150137 subgroup	510.00	165.9300	10	318.64	154.7300	11	50.7%	1.15 [0.21; 2.09]
Total (95% CI)			21			21	100.0%	1.19 [0.53; 1.86]

Heterogeneity: Tau² = 0; Chi² = 0.02, df = 1 (P = 0.89); I² = 0%

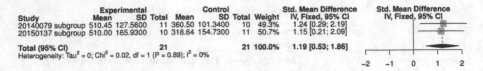

Fig. 3. Meta-analysis for number of antibody producing cells

Study	Experimental Mean	SD	Total	Control Mean	SD	Total	Weight	Std. Mean Difference IV, Fixed, 95% CI
20140079 subgroup	5430.00	390.0000	11	5550.00	480.0000	10	2.1%	-0.26 [-1.13; 0.60]
20140079 subgroup	5440.00	390.0000	11	5520.00	320.0000	10	2.1%	-0.21 [-1.07; 0.65]
20140079 subgroup	5570.00	340.0000	11	5490.00	420.0000	10	2.1%	0.20 [-0.66; 1.06]
20140079 subgroup	5530.00	320.0000	11	5360.00	260.0000	10	2.0%	0.56 [-0.32; 1.43]
20150269 subgroup	18000.00	1100.0000	10	17600.00	1500.0000	10	2.0%	0.29 [-0.59; 1.17]
20150269 subgroup	18000.00	1600.0000	10	17100.00	1400.0000	10	1.9%	0.57 [-0.33; 1.47]
20150269 subgroup	17300.00	1200.0000	10	17900.00	1700.0000	10	2.0%	-0.39 [-1.28; 0.50]
20150269 subgroup	18400.00	1500.0000	10	18400.00	2100.0000	10	2.0%	0.00 [-0.88; 0.88]
20150269 subgroup	17600.00	1500.0000	10	17300.00	1700.0000	10	2.0%	0.18 [-0.70; 1.06]
20150269 subgroup	17900.00	1500.0000	10	17800.00	1600.0000	10	2.0%	0.06 [-0.82; 0.94]
20040848 subgroup	14900.00	1800.0000	10	15300.00	2200.0000	10	2.0%	-0.19 [-1.07; 0.69]
20150137 subgroup	5430.00	1220.0000	10	5050.00	610.0000	11	2.1%	0.38 [-0.48; 1.25]
20150137 subgroup	5350.00	990.0000	11	5350.00	990.0000	11	2.1%	0.00 [-0.84; 0.84]
20150137 subgroup	5560.00	450.0000	11	5880.00	660.0000	11	2.1%	-0.55 [-1.40; 0.31]
20150137 subgroup	5220.00	610.0000	10	5240.00	630.0000	10	2.0%	-0.03 [-0.91; 0.85]
20150088 subgroup	14200.00	2000.0000	10	15000.00	2900.0000	10	2.0%	-0.31 [-1.19; 0.58]
20150088 subgroup	14200.00	1700.0000	10	14100.00	1600.0000	10	2.0%	0.06 [-0.82; 0.93]
20150088 subgroup	14700.00	1800.0000	10	14700.00	1800.0000	10	2.0%	0.00 [-0.88; 0.88]
20150088 subgroup	15100.00	1400.0000	10	14800.00	1700.0000	10	2.0%	0.18 [-0.69; 1.06]
20150719 subgroup	11800.00	1990.0000	10	10600.00	2880.0000	10	2.0%	0.46 [-0.43; 1.36]
20040559 subgroup	14000.00	500.0000	10	14000.00	1700.0000	10	2.0%	0.00 [-0.88; 0.88]
20040559 subgroup	14000.00	1000.0000	10	14000.00	1800.0000	10	2.0%	0.00 [-0.88; 0.88]
20040559 subgroup	14000.00	1200.0000	10	14000.00	1200.0000	10	2.0%	0.00 [-0.88; 0.88]
20040866 subgroup	15000.00	1000.0000	10	15000.00	1000.0000	10	2.0%	0.00 [-0.88; 0.88]
20040866 subgroup	15000.00	600.0000	10	15000.00	800.0000	10	2.0%	0.00 [-0.88; 0.88]
20040866 subgroup	16000.00	500.0000	10	15000.00	500.0000	10	1.3%	1.92 [0.82; 3.01]
20040866 subgroup	15000.00	700.0000	10	15000.00	800.0000	10	2.0%	0.00 [-0.88; 0.88]
20160280 subgroup	4840.00	1420.0000	10	5030.00	1460.0000	10	2.0%	-0.13 [-1.00; 0.75]
20160280 subgroup	5450.00	1580.0000	10	5450.00	2200.0000	10	2.0%	0.00 [-0.88; 0.88]
20160280 subgroup	6150.00	1680.0000	10	5440.00	1570.0000	10	2.0%	0.42 [-0.47; 1.31]
20160280 subgroup	5770.00	1550.0000	10	4780.00	1600.0000	10	1.9%	0.60 [-0.30; 1.50]
20160280 subgroup	5700.00	1680.0000	10	5150.00	1400.0000	10	2.0%	0.34 [-0.54; 1.23]
20140453 subgroup	5250.00	740.0000	12	5430.00	720.0000	12	2.4%	-0.24 [-1.04; 0.57]
20140453 subgroup	5550.00	670.0000	12	5590.00	770.0000	12	2.4%	-0.05 [-0.85; 0.75]
20140453 subgroup	5450.00	450.0000	12	5340.00	460.0000	12	2.4%	0.23 [-0.57; 1.04]
20140453 subgroup	5570.00	410.0000	12	5320.00	480.0000	12	2.3%	0.54 [-0.28; 1.36]
20160346 subgroup	11800.00	1870.0000	10	11300.00	2060.0000	10	2.0%	0.24 [-0.64; 1.12]
20160424 subgroup	13800.00	2000.0000	12	13200.00	3000.0000	12	2.4%	0.23 [-0.58; 1.03]
20160374 subgroup	4840.00	1420.0000	10	2150.00	400.0000	10	1.0%	2.47 [1.25; 3.69]
20160374 subgroup	4840.00	1420.0000	10	5030.00	1460.0000	10	2.0%	-0.13 [-1.00; 0.75]
20160374 subgroup	5700.00	1680.0000	10	2150.00	400.0000	10	0.9%	2.78 [1.48; 4.09]
20160374 subgroup	5700.00	1680.0000	10	5030.00	1460.0000	10	2.0%	0.41 [-0.48; 1.30]
20040791 subgroup	15000.00	900.0000	10	15000.00	700.0000	10	2.0%	0.00 [-0.88; 0.88]
20040791 subgroup	15000.00	700.0000	10	15000.00	500.0000	10	2.0%	0.00 [-0.88; 0.88]
20040791 subgroup	15000.00	700.0000	10	15000.00	700.0000	10	2.0%	0.00 [-0.88; 0.88]
20040791 subgroup	15000.00	500.0000	10	15000.00	700.0000	10	2.0%	0.00 [-0.88; 0.88]
20041380 subgroup	11830.00	1030.0000	12	11250.00	1140.0000	12	2.4%	0.52 [-0.30; 1.33]
11127 subgroup	6000.00	400.0000	10	4700.00	500.0000	10	0.9%	2.75 [1.46; 4.04]
11159 subgroup	5000.00	400.0000	10	4700.00	500.0000	10	1.9%	0.63 [-0.27; 1.54]
Total (95% CI)			518			515	100.0%	0.20 [0.07; 0.32]

Heterogeneity: Tau² = 0.0985; Chi² = 72.69, df = 49 (P = 0.02); I² = 33%

Fig. 4. Meta-analysis for the increase of body weight

Study	Experimental Mean	SD	Total	Control Mean	SD	Total	Weight	Std. Mean Difference IV, Fixed, 95% CI
20040559 subgroup	0.58	0.8500	10	0.56	0.1200	10	21.1%	0.03 [-0.85; 0.91]
20040866 subgroup	0.56	0.1200	10	0.50	0.0800	10	20.1%	0.56 [-0.33; 1.46]
15539 subgroup	0.32	0.0400	10	0.32	0.0200	10	21.1%	0.00 [-0.88; 0.88]
15484 subgroup	0.75	0.1390	20	0.64	0.1240	19	37.6%	0.82 [0.17; 1.48]
Total (95% CI)			50			49	100.0%	0.43 [0.03; 0.83]

Heterogeneity: Tau² = 0.0108; Chi² = 3.19, df = 3 (P = 0.36); I² = 6%

Fig. 5. Meta-analysis for spleen index

heterogeneity is not significant, so fixed effects model was adopted for meta-analysis. The meta-analysis showed that the standard mean difference (SMD) is 0.4302, with the 95% confidence interval (CI) ranging from 0.0273 to 0.8331. The p value for the SMD < 0.01(p = 0.0364). In summary, the analysis suggested that the treatment with GLS significantly increased the spleen index.

4   Conclusion

In this study, we have developed a complete pipeline that can be used to carry out meta-analysis on the health promoting effects of functional food products. Using GLS as an example, we demonstrated that the pipeline could be used to automatically analyze large numbers of outcome measures, and GLS's immunomodulatory effects on 19 outcome measures were also found.

5   Discussion

Although there were a large number of literatures related to the health promoting effects of Ganoderma lucidum spores (GLS), In addition, the outcome measures were not well defined. In this study, we setup a data model, constructed a database and implemented a pipeline that can be used to carry out a large number of meta-analysis automatically. Using GLS as an example, we obtained evidence that GLS have beneficial immunomodulatory effects based on results related to several outcome measures. Furthermore, the pipeline was approved to be robust.

Although the functional food has a large market share, the health promoting effects of functional food have not been analyzed using the meta-analysis approaches before. The difficulty lies in the facts that the outcome measures of health promoting effects are numerous. The study design was not always following standard design like the randomized control test (RCT) in human clinical trials. A data model is then needed to be able to capture the various designs. Furthermore, the number of outcome measures amounts to several hundred, making meta-analysis a daunting task for manual analysis. A pipeline is needed to (1) provide a standard for data extraction; (2) automatically reformat the data to the format that is acceptable for various analyses packages; (3) capable of carrying out a large number of meta-analysis simultaneously; (4) generate the result graph for visualization. All the goals have been achieved.

In the future, the data model needed to be further defined after integrating expert opinion. Algorithms and software tools designed for natural language processing are needed for automatic data processing from literature and internal documents. Various meta-analysis methods such as subgroup analyses, regression analyses needed to be tested for health promoting tests and be integrated into the pipelines.

Acknowledgement. This work was supported by grants from CAMS Innovation Fund for Medical Sciences (CIFMS) (2016-I2M-3-016 and 2017-I2M-1-013), From the Chinese Academy of Medical Science.

References

1. Liu, J., Shimizu, K., Konishi, F., Sato, M., Noda, K., et al.: Anti-androgenic activities of the triterpenoids fraction of Ganoderma lucidum. Food Chem. **100**, 1691–1696 (2007)
2. Yun, T.K.: Update from Asia: Asian studies on cancer chemoprevention. Ann. N. Y. Acad. Sci. **889**, 157–192 (1999)
3. Sliva, D., Loganathan, J., Jiang, J., Jedinak, A., Lamb, J.G., et al.: Mushroom ganoderma lucidum prevents colitis-associated carcinogenesis in mice. PLoS ONE **7**, e47873 (2012)
4. Jiang, Z.Y., Lin, C., Liu, X.C., et al.: Effects of ganoderma lucidum polysaccharide on humoral immune function in mice. J. Jinan Univ. (Health Sci.) **24**, 51–53 (2003)
5. Ho, Y.W., Yeung, J.S.L., Chiu, P.K.Y., et al.: Ganoderma lucidum polysaccharide peptide reduced the production of proinflammatory cytokines in activated rheumatoid synovial fibroblast. Mol. Cell. Biochem. **301**(1–2), 173–179 (2007)
6. Lin, Z.B.: Progress of studies on the anti-tumor activity and immunomodulating effect of Ganoderma. J. Peking Univ. (Health Sci.) **34**, 493–498 (2002)
7. Lin, Z.B., Wang, P.Y.: The pharmacological study of Ganoderma spores and their active components. J. Peking Univ. **38**, 541–547 (2006)
8. Gao, Y., Zhou, S., Chen, G., et al.: A phase I/II study of a Ganoderma lucidum (Ling Zhi, Reishi mushroom) extract in patients with chronic hepatitis B. Int. J. Med. Mushrooms **4**, 321–327 (2002)
9. Zhao, H., Zhang, Q., Zhao, L., et al.: Spore powder of Ganoderma lucidum improves cancer-related fatigue in breast cancer patients undergoing endocrine therapy: a pilot clinical trial. In: Evidence-Based Complementary and Alternative Medicine (2012)
10. Jin, X.Z., Beguerie, J.R., Sze, D.M.Y.: Ganoderma lucidum (Reishi mushroom) for cancer treatment. Cochrane Database Syst. Rev. **6**, CD007731 (2012)
11. Schwarzer, G.: meta: an R package for meta-analysis. R News **7**(3), 40–45 (2007)
12. Schwarzer, G., Carpenter, J.R., Rücker, G.: Meta-Analysis with R (Use-R!). Springer, Cham (2007)
13. Wu, M.Z.: Study on spores of Ganoderma lucidum—Technology of sporoderm-breaking and property. Nanjing Agricultural University (2000)
14. Wu, M.Z., Shen, A.G.: A preliminary study on the effect of broken Ganoderma spore powder on immune function in mice. Edible Fungi China **19**(2), 37–38 (2000)
15. Zhang, R.B., Chen, R., Chen, G.M., et al.: Study on effect of broken Ganoderma lucidum spore powder on immune function in mice. Pre. Med. Trib. **19**(12), 936–938 (2013)
16. Zhang, Q., Xie, G.F., Cui, S.X., et al.: Ganoderma lucidum spore powder capsule enhances immune function in mice. J. Pharm. Res. **17**(4), 24–25 (1998)
17. Yue, G.G., Fung, K.P., Leung, P.C., et al.: Comparative studies on the immunomodulatory and antitumor activities of the different parts of fruiting body of Ganoderma lucidum and Ganoderma spores. Phytother. Res. **22**(10), 1282–1291 (2010)
18. Bao, X., Liu, C., Fang, J., et al.: Structural and immunological studies of a major polysaccharide from spores of Ganoderma lucidum, (Fr.) Karst. Carbohydr. Res. **332**(1), 67–74 (2001)
19. Wu, M.Z., Shen, A.G., Xiong, X.H., et al.: Effect of Ganoderma lucidum spore powder on the immune function of mice before and after breaking. Edible Fungi **23**(6), 36–37 (2001)
20. Du, L.L., Zhao, M., Fu, Y.M., et al.: Study on the preparation and immune activity of broken Ganoderma lucidum spores. Edible Fungi **38**(6), 57–60 (2016)
21. Zhu, J.H., Li, T.M., Chen, Y., et al.: Effect of Ganoderma lucidum dry gum and Ganoderma spore powder on immune function in mice. Acta Edulis Fungi **11**(4), 24–27 (2004)

22. Chen, X.T., Wu, D., Gong, M., et al.: Effect of chewable tablets of Garoderma lucidum spore powder on immune function in mice. J. Jiangxi. Univ. Tra. Chin. Med. **28**(3), 73–75 (2016)

23. Cai, W.H., Wang, Y.X., Yang, J.Y.: The regulative effect of Ganoderma spore power on immune function of rats with severe acute pancreatitis. Inf. Trad. Chin. Med. **28**(6), 40–42 (2011)

24. Xing, E., Wu, S.Q.: Study on antitumor and immune function of two Ganoderma lucidum spores. Pharm. Today **18**(4), 57–59 (2008)

25. Yang, Y., Li, Z., Huang, J.M., et al.: Effect of Ganoderma lucidum spore on immunoregulation of immunosuppression mice. Chin. J. Health. Lab. Technol. **20**(6), 1286–1288 (2010)

26. Song, B.J., Zhu, X.J., Wei, L.N.: Effect of Ganoderma lucidum spores on immune modulation and inhibiting tumor in mice. J. Harbin. Med. Univ. **44**(5), 464–466 (2010)

27. Jiang, C.R., Zuo, L., Zhong, Z.Q.: Effect of Ganoderma lucidum spore on innate immunity of immunosuppression mice induced by Cyclosporin A. J. Guiyang Med. Coll. **34**(5), 546–549 (2009)

28. Wang, Y.H., Qu, Z.H., Zhao, Z.Y.: Effect of Ganoderma lucidum spores on immune function in patients with non small cell lung cancer during chemotherapy. China Prac Med. **9**(23), 20–21 (2014)

29. Ren, W., Zuo, L., Zhong, Z.Q.: The effect of the Ganoderma lucidum spore on the immunoregulation of the immunosuppression mice. Chin. J. Immunol. **23**(11), 979–984 (2007)

30. Li, Y.L., Qiao, S.S., Li, G.X.: Effect of glossy Ganoderma on antitumor and immune function in mice. Chin. J. Prev. Control Chronic Dis. **12**(4), 156–157 (2004)

31. Huang, S.X., Yu, S.Q., Liu, J.S., et al.: Effect of Ganoderma spore powder on immune function in mice. Hebei Med. J. **19**(1), 25 (1997)

32. Wu, C.M., Wang, L.J., Lin, J.M., et al.: Optimize the wall-breaking method of Ganoderma lucidum spore and research immunomodulatory and antitumor mechanism. Pharm. Today **27**(5), 307–311 (2017)

33. Liu, K.M., Li, Y.L.: Effect of broken Ganoderma lucidum spore powder on immune function in Kunming mice. J. Med. Pest Control **15**(2), 74–76 (1999)

34. Zhang, L.H., Wang, H.X., Wang, L.W., et al.: In vitro and in vivo immune effects of Ganoderma lucidum spore powder extract. Chin. J. Immunol. **10**(3), 169–172 (1994)

35. Xu, C.J., Zhang, R.H., Meng, J., et al.: Effect of nano spore powder of Ganoderma Lucidum on immune function of mice. Pharmacol. Clini. Chin. Mater. Med. **21**(5), 36–38 (2005)

36. Zhou, F.X.: Study on active components analysis and immune function of spore powder Ganoderma powder. Fujian University of Traditional Chinese Medicine (2014)

37. Fan, G.Y.: Effects of Ganoderma spores on liver function and cellular immune function after hepatocellular carcinoma. Sun Yat-sen University (2012)

38. Zhou, J.H., Zhang, Q.H.: Effects of Ganoderma lucidum spores on peripheral blood T lymphocyte subsets and VEGF in elderly patients with cervical cancer. Matern. Child Health Care. Chin. **29**(13), 2021–2022 (2014)

Section Identification to Improve Information Extraction from Chinese Medical Literature

Sijia Zhou[1,2(✉)] and Xin Li[1,2]

[1] Department of Information Systems, City University of Hong Kong,
Kowloon, Hong Kong
sjzhou3-c@my.cityu.edu.hk, Xin.Li@cityu.edu.hk
[2] Shenzhen Research Institute, City University of Hong Kong, Shenzhen, China

Abstract. The Chinese medical literature contains a large amount of knowledge. Reducing the effort needed by medical scholars to extract this knowledge requires a literature analysis to identify the key information in each paper. We argue that identifying the sections of a paper would help us filter noise from the paper and increase the accuracy of extracting the experimental findings. In this research in progress, we consider paper section identification as a sentence classification task and apply Conditional Random Fields (CRFs) to tackle the problem. In our model we combine both lexical and structural features to facilitate section identification. Experiments on a human-curated asthma dataset show that our approach achieves a 10%–20% performance improvement over Support Vector Machines (SVMs), and that use of both bag-of-words features and domain lexicons benefit the task.

Keywords: Section identification · Sentence classification · Chinese medicine

1 Introduction

As a valuable part of Chinese culture, traditional Chinese medicine is attracting increasing attention today. Cases, research, and other useful records of Chinese medicine have been documented in scientific publications. This medical literature has great value for medical research in accumulating evidence and developing hypotheses. However, to read such a vast amount of literature takes a great deal of time and effort. As a result, management of this medical literature can significantly assist medical research. In our previous study, we proposed a literature analysis system for Chinese medicine called MedC (http://medc.is.cityu.edu.hk/) [1], for which we collected the abstracts and metadata of about 1 million papers on Chinese medicine published since the 1950s. The system could reduce the effort of searching and digesting the literature by extracting and visualizing key information such as the syndrome, medicine, and treatment information documented in the literature.

When conducting meta-analyses and extracting the major findings from the medical literature, different sections of a paper have different levels of utility for the researcher. In general, more attention is paid to the experiment, including the sample (subjects), treatment, and treatment results. In this paper, we strengthen the information extraction process in medical literature analysis by improving the identification of the key parts of

© Springer Nature Switzerland AG 2018
H. Chen et al. (Eds.): ICSH 2018, LNCS 10983, pp. 342–350, 2018.
https://doi.org/10.1007/978-3-030-03649-2_34

a paper. Conducting section identification allows us to filter out irrelevant parts of the paper before information extraction. In this study, we explore different combinations of features using Conditional Random Fields (CRFs) to classify each sentence of a paper according to whether it relates to the subjects, method, or results. We compile a gold standard for Chinese medical papers on asthma treatment and compare the performance of CRFs with that of Support Vector Machines (SVMs). Chinese medical papers are more complex than Western papers, which receive less researches. The experiment shows that CRFs perform significantly better than SVMs, and that bag-of-words and domain lexicon features should be used in this task.

This paper is organized as follows: in Sect. 2, we review the literature on section classification. In Sect. 3, we discuss our problem setting. We introduce our features and model in Sect. 4 and describe the experimental process in Sect. 5. The results and discussion are found in Sects. 6, and 7 concludes the paper.

2 Literature Review

Section analysis is a research paper structure analysis task [2]. Most section analysis studies are conducted at the sentence level. Within a paper, sentences are a sequence of content that may have interdependencies in facilitating the expression of ideas. In addition to section identification, sentence classification is also used in sentiment labeling [3] topic labeling [4], etc.

Studies on section identification in research papers include Ito et al. [2], who use SVMs to label sentences according to their structural role, such as background, objectives, method, experimental results, and conclusions for Medline abstracts. Kim et al. [5] used CRFs to automatically annotate sentences in medical abstracts with a set of pre-defined medical categories. In addition to normal features, they also use semantic information to categorize the medical material. In addition, Lui [6] changed this process into a two-stage classification. First, he used logistic regression as the weak learner and naïve Bayes and an SVMs as the strong learner to increase classification performance. Most of these papers focus on medical material, which shows that this is important for research in the medical domain. But there are also exceptions. For instance, Angrosh et al. [7] tried to find the structural parts of research articles by focusing on citation features. Hachey and Grover [8] conducted sentence classification for section labels on legal judgments with many different models, such as naïve Bayes, SVMs, and maximum entropy models.

From an application domain perspective, section identification studies on the medical literature often focus on abstracts only, and guidelines for the section classification of full texts remain limited. In addition, most studies are based on English-language research papers, with very few on Chinese medical literature. Chinese text is different from that of English, and the language used in the literature on traditional Chinese medicine is unique, thus worthy of study.

From a technique perspective, more advanced techniques are being proposed in sentence classification. For example, Zhao et al. [3] applied the sentiment classification method based on CRFs by analyzing "context dependence" and "label redundancy." Kim [9] conducted a series of experiments with convolutional neural networks

(CNN) for sentence-level classification, including both polarity and topic classification. These techniques could be further explored in the section identification of Chinese medical literature.

3   Problem Setting

Figure 1 illustrates a typical Chinese medical paper. As we can see, after stating the purpose of the study, the Chinese medical literature often includes reports of medical experiments comparing the effects of applying a specific treatment to subjects versus another treatment. The end of the paper will include a discussion about the mechanism and theoretical reflection on the experiment. However, in evidence-based medical research, the most important part is the actual experiment and its findings. In this study, we aim to identify such sections within a medical paper. We adopt a sentence classification approach to classify the section label of each sentence. We focus on three types of section:

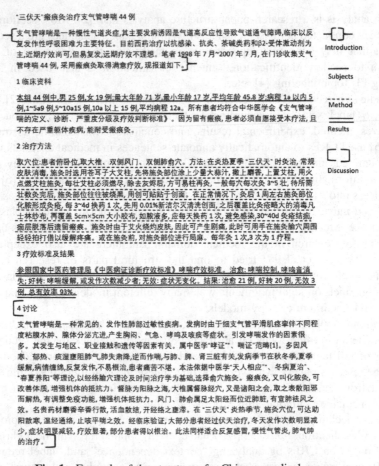

Fig. 1. Example of the structure of a Chinese medical paper

- Subjects: The group of people or objects that comprise the study sample.
- Method: The treatment and medicine that the study used to treat the disease.
- Results: The effect of the treatment, usually including the cure rate and improvement rate.

We plan to find the information belonging to these three labels to help clinicals or researchers extract information better. In addition, we define the following three hypothetical section types to facilitate the task.

- Introduction: The part before the first sentence of "Subjects" or "Method" or "Results".
- Discussion: The part after the last sentence of "Subjects" or "Method" or "Results".
- Other: Other sentences in the paper.

4   Method

In this study we convert the section-identification problem to a sentence-labeling problem in which the labels can be one of the six section labels. To facilitate this task, we first conduct sentence segmentation based on certain Chinese punctuation such as "。", "?" and "!". If a paragraph contains only a single line without punctuation, we consider it a single sentence. We need to build a classifier to classify each sentence using the features generated from the sentence and considering the interdependencies between sentences.

4.1   Feature Sets

In this research in progress, we choose three types of feature used in prior studies in an English context, and develop feature sets. These are bag-of-words, domain lexicons, and section headings.

The bag-of-words model is a widely used representation for classifying documents [5, 6, 10, 11]. As we are processing Chinese literature, it is necessary to conduct word segmentation to convert the documents into a set of words. We used Jieba to do the word segmentation based on a dictionary containing about 10 million Chinese words which we compiled using major lexicons available online. Following previous practice, we removed stop words and special characters from the representation of the common stop words list. Because there are often many different words in a document, the word-sentence matrices are too sparse, which limits the performance of machine learning models. Thus, we used latent Dirichlet allocation (LDA) to reduce the dimensionality and then use the LDA class probabilities as features. We tuned the number of LDA classes to maximize performance in experiments.

We also develop domain lexicons for the task, which are keywords selected by experts, and are often used in English literature analysis [5, 10]. In this paper, we chose high frequency words that appear in multiple documents and manually filter words that are more related to each section. Table 1 shows these selected keywords. We use the occurrence of these keywords in sentences as the feature value of the three features in the classification.

Table 1. Lexicons for different categories

Feature Name	Lexicon
S	男例，女例，男性，女性，性别，病程，本组，年龄
M	方法，疗程，检验，操作步骤，临床，取穴，注入，加服，小时，每次，每日，每周
R	治愈，痊愈，显效，显著，好转，明显好转，无效，不良反应，消失，缓解，治愈率，有效率

The last feature type we generate is section headings. Because the material we study does not have section heading labels, we define a rule to identify section headings. If a sentence has less than 6 words and lacks a complete sentence structure (punctuation at the end) we consider it a section heading. For each section heading, we apply bag-of-words and LDA operations to generate features. The section heading feature is associated with each complete sentence after the section heading before a new section heading appears.

4.2 Model

After generating the features, we use conditional random fields (CRFs) to do the sentence classification. CRFs are a type of discriminative undirected probabilistic graphical model often applied in pattern recognition and machine learning and used for structured prediction. In CRFs, each vertex represents a random variable whose distribution is to be inferred, with each edge representing the dependency between two random variables [12].

CRFs have an advantage in sentence classification for section labels because CRFs consider the sequencing of sentences. In the CRFs template of our model, we consider the two sentences before and after each sentence when classifying a focal sentence. The ability to consider the previous and following sentences is important for our task, as a paper has only a handful of sections and nearby sentences often have the same section label. The sections also appear in a specific order in a scientific paper.

5 Experiment

5.1 Dataset

For the evaluation we use a dataset provided by a Chinese medicine physician, who manually identified and downloaded Chinese medicine papers from CNKI, China's largest literature database, focused on the treatment of asthma by acupuncture and published from 1978 to 2008. We process the files, which are in pdf format, and convert them to text. To avoid the noise from OCR, we exclude files created from scanned documents that require OCR for conversion. To focus on section identification, we conduct noise filtering and remove footers, headers, and watermarks. To ensure that the content of all papers can be fully presented in text, we also remove some position papers or commentaries unrelated to empirical results. Our final dataset contains 386 Chinese medical papers. We employ an RA to code the papers and highlight the sentences about subjects, treatments, and results, which are later used to generate the 6 labels. Double checking of the RA's coding shows that it is of high quality, as the papers are written in modern Chinese and are generally easy to understand.

5.2 Baseline

To assess the performance of the CRFs method, we use the support vector machines (SVMs) as our baseline. An SVMs model seeks to separate data into categories so that the gap between them is as large as possible. It is a widely used method in previous sentence classification studies [2, 13, 14].

5.3 Evaluation Metrics

We use precision, recall, and the F_1-score to assess the performance of the different models. For each label, precision assesses if the ratio of predictions is correct. Recall assesses the ratio of sentences with an identifiable label. The F_1-score combines precision and recall as an overall assessment of the performance.

5.4 Experimental Procedure

The experiments on the combinations of features start with bag-of-words and then include domain lexicons, and finally section headings. We tune the number of LDA classes for bag-of-words features and section heading features to 40 and 6, respectively, in small experiments. The LDA processing works to an extent as feature selection and we do not have additional feature selection in the model. We put these features into SVMs and CRFs and conduct 10-fold cross-validation on the data set. With the 10-fold experiments, each paper has a precision, recall, and F_1-score for the classification of its sentences. We report the average precision, recall, and F_1-scores and conduct pair-wise t-tests to compare the performance of the model-feature combinations.

6 Results and Discussion

Because we aim to find useful information in key parts in Chinese medical literature, which means the sentence labeled Subjects, Method or Result, we just focus on the performance of these three labels. Our dataset has 15,346 sentences in total, containing 1049, 3184, and 1639 sentences labeled Subjects, Method, and Results, respectively, according to our annotation. For each paper, the average number of sentences is 40, with about 3, 8, and 4 sentences, respectively, for the different labels.

Tables 2, 3 and 4 show the performance of the different feature sets on SVMs and CRFs. In most experiments CRFs model outperforms SVMs model in prediction. For example, for the bag-of-words feature, the F_1 scores for CRFs are 0.825, 0.812, 0.760 for Subjects, Method, and Results, respectively, about 8%, 13%, and 21% better than the SVMs scores. For bag-of-words and domain lexicon features, CRFs outperform the SVMs by about 12%, 15%, and 19%. We conduct a pair-wise t-test to evaluate the improvement in our results. As shown in the tables, on the F_1 measure, CRFs are significantly better than the SVMs with a 99% confidence interval.

Tables 2, 3 and 4 together show performance differences when different feature sets are used. As the performance difference between CRFs and SVMs is large, our analysis focuses on CRFs. As we can see, when increasing the bag-of-words feature to include domain lexicons, the F_1-score for the label Subjects improves by about 2.4%, which is significant with a 95% confidence interval (p = 0.036). However, the performance for labels Method and Results are not significantly different (p equals 0.122 and 0.142, respectively).

When we further include the section headings, the performance of CRFs decreases for Subjects and Method but increases for Results, and the performance of Subjects for SVMs also decreases. Thus, in general, including section headings does not add much benefit with CRFs. We believe one reason for this phenomenon is that papers on Chinese medicine are often less clearly structured than Western medical papers. Because most Western medical papers follow a fixed format for each part, while Chinese medical papers don't have such format.

Table 2. Performance on bag-of-words

Model						
Label	Precision		Recall		F_1	
	SVMs	CRFs	SVMs	CRFs	SVMs	CRFs
Subjects	0.821	0.862**	0.676	0.793***	0.741	0.825***
Method	0.698	0.767***	0.668	0.867***	0.681	0.812***
Results	0.632	0.833***	0.488	0.706***	0.548	0.760***

Table 3. Performance on bag-of-words + domain lexicons

Model						
Label	Precision		Recall		F_1	
	SVMs	CRFs	SVMs	CRFs	SVMs	CRFs
Subjects	0.842	0.864	0.646	0.836***	0.730	0.849***
Method	0.697	0.795**	0.662	0.874***	0.679	0.829***
Results	0.666	0.816***	0.490	0.697***	0.559	0.749***

Table 4. Performance on bag-of-words + domain lexicons + section headings

Model						
Label	Precision		Recall		F_1	
	SVMs	CRFs	SVMs	CRFs	SVMs	CRFs
Subjects	0.837	0.810***	0.538	0.767***	0.654	0.785***
Method	0.618	0.773***	0.817	0.850*	0.700	0.808***
Results	0.757	0.794***	0.683	0.715*	0.715	0.752***

(p-value for comparison between SVMs and CRFs: *** < 0.01; ** < 0.05; * < 0.1)

7 Conclusion and Future Directions

In this research in progress, we conduct sentence classification to identify sections of Chinese medical papers to help extract the most useful and relevant information for knowledge management. We design a preliminary model using CRFs and propose several lexical and structural features for the task based on the English document analysis literature. Experiments show that the CRFs model can achieve about 80% in precision, recall, and F_1-measures, significantly outperforming SVMs on the task. In general, this research in progress shows the feasibility of using machine learning to address the section identification problem in Chinese medical papers.

As research in progress, we plan to improve our work in several ways. First, for feature development, we can improve the domain lexicons by seeking the opinions of practitioners. We aim to build a comprehensive lexicon that can be used in analyzing the literature on Chinese medicine. We will also consider other useful information in the documents and develop more features to tackle them. Second, for model development, there is room to design more complicated models, such as by using deep learning. Finally, from an evaluation perspective, it is necessary to understand how section identification and the follow-up noise filtering process influences the effectiveness of the knowledge management. We plan to recruit domain experts to assess the information extracted from filtered vs. unfiltered papers and get their views on how to better evaluate the impact of this design feature on the system's utility. In general, we see great potential in applying section identification and other text mining methods for knowledge management in the Chinese medical literature.

Acknowledgements. The research is partially supported by Digital Innovation Lab at City University of Hong Kong, GuangDong Science and Technology Project 2014A020221090, and the City University of Hong Kong Shenzhen Research Institute.

References

1. Li, X., Tong, Y., Wang, W.: MedC: a literature analysis system for chinese medicine research. In: Zheng, X., Zeng, D.D., Chen, H., Leischow, S.J. (eds.) ICSH 2015. LNCS, vol. 9545, pp. 311–320. Springer, Cham (2016). https://doi.org/10.1007/978-3-319-29175-8_29
2. Ito, T., Shimbo, M., Yamasaki, T., Matsumoto, Y.: Semi-supervised sentence classification for MEDLINE documents. Methods **138**, 141–146 (2004)
3. Zhao, J., Liu, K., Wang, G.: Adding redundant features for CRFs-based sentence sentiment classification. In: Proceedings of the Conference on Empirical Methods in Natural Language Processing, pp. 117–126. Association for Computational Linguistics (2008)
4. Naughton, M., Stokes, N., Carthy, J.: Sentence-level event classification in unstructured texts. Inf. Retr. **13**, 132–156 (2010). https://doi.org/10.1007/s10791-009-9113-0
5. Kim, S.N., Martinez, D., Cavedon, L.: Automatic classification of sentences for evidence based medicine. In: Proceedings of the ACM Fourth International Workshop on Data and Text Mining in Biomedical Informatics, pp. 13–22 (2010)
6. Lui, M.: Feature stacking for sentence classification in evidence-based medicine. In: Proceedings of the Australasian Language Technology Association Workshop 2012, pp. 134–138 (2012)

7. Angrosh, M.A., Cranefield, S., Stanger, N.: Context identification of sentences in related work sections using a conditional random field: towards intelligent digital libraries. In: Proceedings of the 10th Annual Joint Conference on Digital Libraries, pp. 293–302. ACM (2010)
8. Hachey, B., Grover, C.: Sequence modelling for sentence classification in a legal summarisation system. In: Proceedings of the 2005 ACM Symposium on Applied Computing, pp. 292–296 (2005)
9. Kim, Y.: Convolutional neural networks for sentence classification (2014)
10. Chung, G.Y.: Sentence retrieval for abstracts of randomized controlled trials. BMC Med. Inform. Decis. Mak. **9**, 1–13 (2009). https://doi.org/10.1186/1472-6947-9-10
11. Demner-Fushman, D., Lin, J.: Answering clinical questions with knowledge-based and statistical techniques. Comput. Linguist. **33**, 63–103 (2007)
12. Sutton, C., McCallum, A.: An Introduction to Conditional Random Fields for Relational Learning. In: Introduction to statistical relational learning. MIT Press (2006)
13. McKnight, L., Srinivasan, P.: Categorization of sentence types in medical abstracts. In: AMIA Annual Symposium Proceedings, pp. 440–444. American Medical Informatics Association (2003)
14. Yamamoto, Y., Takagi, T.: A sentence classification system for multi biomedical literature summarization. In: Proceedings of the 21st International Conference on Data Engineering, pp. 1163–1168 (2005)

Evolution of Research on Smart Health: A Bibliometrics Analysis

Xiao Huang[1], Ke Dong[2], and Jiang Wu[1(✉)]

[1] School of Information Management,
Center for E-commerce Development and Research,
Wuhan University, Wuhan 430072, China
jiangw@whu.edu.cn
[2] School of Information Management, Wuhan University, Wuhan 430072,
China

Abstract. Smart health is a new form of business created by the combination of the Internet and the medical industry and the research of smart health has gradually attracted much attention from the academic community. In this study, the scientific literatures of smart health included in Web of Science are analyzed to draw the knowledge map to find out the research trail in this field. The analysis results show that the number of literatures in the field continues to increase and that published journals have a certain degree of centrality. Reviews and commentary articles published earlier will receive more attention. The update of technology will significantly change the research trend, the content covered in this area will also be more extensive with the further development of smart health related technologies.

Keywords: Smart health · E-health · Online medical · Telemedical
Visualization

1 Introduction

Smart health [1], also known as e-health, is a new application of the internet in the medical industry. It includes various forms of online health services such as medical information inquiry, online disease consultation, teleconsultation and teletherapy. Smart health services have become very popular in American people's lives [2]. In recent years, the smart health applications are also rapidly developing in China. Smart health began to attract the attention of many researchers around the year 2000 in academia. Early research focused on the search behavior and evaluation of online health information in order to discriminate differences in online and offline medical information search behaviors [3, 4]. With the rapid development of social media and the emergence of community platforms of health care, the research hotspots in this field are gradually transformed into user behavior and content analysis in online communities [5]. At the same time, with the rapid spread of smart devices for healthcare, more research has been conducted on the technology research of smart devices for healthcare and its impact on ordinary people's lives [6].

With the development of information technology and the massive growth of data, visualization has become an important part of data processing, in which knowledge

© Springer Nature Switzerland AG 2018
H. Chen et al. (Eds.): ICSH 2018, LNCS 10983, pp. 351–358, 2018.
https://doi.org/10.1007/978-3-030-03649-2_35

mapping is an important application of this method. So far, the scientific knowledge mapping has been widely recognized because more and more researchers use knowledge mapping methods in their research. This study aims at complete visualization analysis of research literature in the field of smart health and concludes the development of the field by analyzing the publication time, journals and representative literatures. At the same time, this study outlines the research topics and research evolution maps and analyzes the research and development process and reveals research hotspots in the field of smart health.

2 Data and Method

The platform of WOS (Web of Science) is used as a data source and data objects are identified by keyword search. The search strategy is: TS = ("E-health" or "online medical" or "online health" or "smart health"). The time range is 1900–2015 and the result is 6305 records. Since there were few studies on smart health before the year 2000 and the cited volumes of these literatures were low, a lot of them were zero cited papers with an average of only 0.15 cited. It was not until 2000 that research on smart health began to take shape, so the data sampling was finally determined to be in the period 2000–2018. The final result was 6291 records and a total of 46,216 records were cited. The data collection time was March 1, 2018.

Each record includes the author, title, keywords, abstracts and references. This study analyzes the trends based on annual literatures and counts the top 10 journals and the top 10 cited papers in the field of smart health. The keyword frequency was counted and the word cloud of top 30 keywords in the field was drawn by visual tools. Based on the keywords of literatures, a map was developed showing the evolution of research from 2003 to 2018.

3 Results

3.1 Literatures Time Distribution

The number of literatures published in the smart health field from 2000 to 2018 is shown in Fig. 1. The research of smart health originated in the 1980s. The first paper about smart health was published in 1985. The literature entitled "ONLINE MEDICAL INFORMATION-SERVICES" was published in the journal named PRIMARY CARE, this research provides a comprehensive overview of online medical information services that can be accessed by personal computer users over telephone lines [7].

However, as mentioned above, there was not much research on smart health from 1985 to 1999 and there were only 63 articles in this period. Until 2000, research in this area gradually increased. After 2004, the volume of literatures grew at a faster rate, peaking in 2016 and the number reached 934. From the trend of literatures in this field in recent years, smart health has become a hot research field.

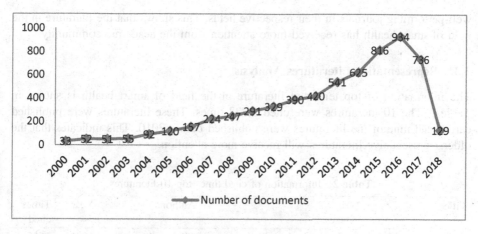

Fig. 1. Number of literatures from 2000 to 2018

3.2   Journal Distribution

Table 1 shows the information of the top 10 journals in the field of smart health. The number of literatures of top ten journals is 1119, which accounts for 17.79% of the total number in the field. This shows that there is a certain degree of concentration in published journals in the field of smart health.

Table 1. The top 10 journals in the number of literatures

Journal title	Number of literatures	Journal impact factor (2016)
Telemedicine and E-Health	427	2.031
Journal of Medical Internet Research	163	5.175
International Journal of Medical Informatics	87	3.21
Journal of Telemedicine and Telecare	77	2.008
Journal of Medical Systems	63	2.456
Bmc Medical Informatics and Decision Making	46	1.643
Health Communication	38	1.487
Journal of the American Medical Informatics Association	37	3.689
Computers in Human Behavior	36	3.455
Bmc Public Health	35	2.265
Total	1119	

From the titles of the journals, it can be seen that these journal topics all have a certain connection with smart health. The highest number in the Journal of Tele-medicine And E-Health, a total of 427 literatures, is much higher than the second-ranked journal. In addition, it can be seen from the impact factors that these journals are well-performing journals in their respective fields. This shows that the literature in the field of smart health has received more attention from the academic community.

3.3 Representative Literatures Analysis

The information of top ten cited literature in the field of smart health is shown in Table 2. The 10 literatures were cited 3,722 times. These literatures were published earlier and nine of the literatures were published before 2010. This indicates that the older representative literatures will receive more attention.

Table 2. Information of cited times top 10 literatures

Title	Author	Year	Times cited
Consumer health information seeking on the Internet: the state of the art	Cline and Haynes	2001	655
Trust and sources of health information - The impact of the Internet and its implications for health care providers: Findings from the first Health Information National Trends Survey	Hesse, Nelson, et al.	2015	637
What is e-health?	Eysenbach	2001	457
Characteristics of online and offline health information seekers and factors that discriminate between them	Cotten and Gupta	2004	340
A review of smart homes - Present state and future challenges	Chan and Esteve, et al.	2008	317
Influences, usage, and outcomes of Internet health information searching: Multivariate results from the Pew surveys	Rice	2006	306
Guest Editorial Introduction to the Special Section on M-Health: Beyond Seamless Mobility and Global Wireless Health-Care Connectivity	Istepanian, Jovanov and Zhang	2004	288
European citizens' use of E-health services: A study of seven countries	Andreassen, et al.	2007	257
Effectiveness of telemedicine: A systematic review of reviews	Ekeland, Bowes, Flottorp	2010	239
How Internet users find, evaluate, and use online health information: A cross-cultural review	Morahan-Martin	2004	226
Total			3722

Four of them are reviews. These four articles review literature on online health information search, smart home and wearable monitoring systems related to smart health, impact and costs of telemedicine services, how to retrieve, evaluate and use health information on the Internet [3, 8–10].

Two of them are commentaries. The third-ranked literature provides an overview of the concept and connotation of E-health. E-health is elucidated in terms of Efficiency,

Enhancing quality, Evidence based, Empowerment and so on [11]. The seventh-ranked literature briefly introduced the latest developments in the field of M-health, including telemedicine and wearable devices. This literature also elaborated some challenges and future implementation issues from the perspective of mobile health [12].

The rest of the literatures is empirical research. The second-ranked literature surveys 6,369 adults to study people's trust in health information sources and finds that the way patients discover health information changed and more patients will seek information online before communicating with their doctors [13]. The fourth-ranked literature explores the differences between online and non-online health information searchers and finds that most online and non-online health information searchers rely on professional medical personnel as sources of health information, but there is a significant difference from the age, income and education of these two groups of people [4]. The sixth-ranked literature explores the factors that influence people's search for online health information and finds that women who work part-time are more likely to search for health information on the Internet [14]. The eighth-ranked literature surveys the use of health-related online service and citizens' expectations for doctors to provide e-health services and find that compared with other health services, internet health services are more like supplements than alternatives to other services [15].

3.4   Research Focus and Research Trend Analysis

Figure 2 is a word cloud of keywords based on word frequency. As shown in the Fig. 2, the four most frequent keywords are E-Health, Internet, Care, and Telemedicine. This shows that telemedicine related to Internet technology in the field of smart health is a focus of academic attention. In addition to these four keywords, other high-frequency keywords include Web, Model, System, Telehealth, Quality, Trust, Security and other words, which shows that past researchers have paid more attention to issues such as the credibility of information in online health information search behavior in this field.

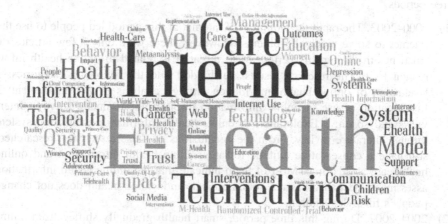

Fig. 2. Smart health keyword word cloud

Figure 3 is a map of the research evolution of smart health based on keywords using the analysis platform named cortext [16]. In this map, the start time was 2003 and the ending was June 2017. There were fewer literatures of smart health before 2003 and no one theme was the focus of this period, so the start time was 2003. At the same time, due to the inconsistency between publication time and online database time, the new literature does not represent future research trends, so the ending was selected in June 2017.

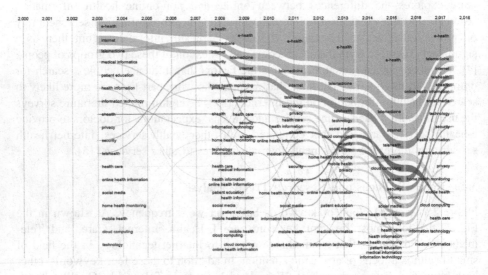

Fig. 3. Research evolution in smart health

Combining with Fig. 3 and related literatures and the development of technologies about smart health in reality, the research trends in the field can be divided into the three periods.

(1) 2000–2003. The rapid development of internet at this period led people to use the internet to solve medical problems. However, there were only a few articles on smart health during this period. Most research is related to online health information [17]. The research results are divided into the following categories: 1 Evaluation of online health information through analysis of website content; 2 Investigation of use of online information through questionnaire surveys, interviews and so on; 3 Exploration of online health information evaluation system through literature review. From the conclusions of these researches, researchers still have a conservative attitude towards online health information and online health care at this time. Most of them indicate that the online health information assessment mechanism is not sound enough and online health does not change people's lifestyles enough.

(2) 2004–2007. During this time period, smart health gradually shifted from online health information site to online discussion. The discussion on health topics is

mainly in the form of online support groups and later evolved into an online medical community [18]. This stage can be seen as a transition period in the field of smart health. Discussion of technology about smart health, learning and cooperation among online medical participants, the methods and tools related to this research are getting more attention [19].

(3) 2007–present. With the rapid growth of large online medical communities such as *Patientslikeme* and *DailyStrength*, the literatures have grown at a relatively rapid rate and researchers have focused more on online medical communities [20]. The typical research methods and results include the following types: 1 Exploring the features, credibility and role of online health information through content analysis, text mining and so on; 2 Exploring user participation, user needs and user acceptance of the online medical community through questionnaires and telephone interviews; 3 Research on the impact of online health information on user behavior through intervention experiments and randomized trials.

As can be seen from Fig. 3, although the number of papers in smart health continues to increase in the third phase of smart health research trend, the proportion of e-health keywords has declined after 2016. The reason is that the research of smart health involves more topics as the technology matures. Since 2007, the development of smart devices has brought more and more researchers concerned about the related research of the health home monitoring. Since 2010, research on mobile health has begun due to the popularity of mobile devices.

4 Summary

Based on the visual analysis of knowledge maps in the field of smart health, it can be found that smart health has gradually become the focus of researchers. In recent years, the literature published in the field has reached a peak. From the perspective of the journals, the literatures have a certain degree of centrality. The reviews and commentary articles published earlier will receive more attention. The research follows the actual application closely and the renewal of technology will make a significant change in research trends. With the further development of smart healthcare-related technologies, the content covered in this area of research will also be more extensive.

References

1. Farnan, J.M., et al.: Online medical professionalism: patient and public relationships: policy statement from the American college of physicians and the federation of state medical boards. Ann. Intern. Med. **158**(8), 620–627 (2013)
2. Fox, S.: The social life of health information [EB/OL] 2011 (2007). http://www.pewinternet.org/Reports/2011/Social-Life-of-Health-Info.aspx
3. Cline, R.J.W., Haynes, K.M.: Consumer health information seeking on the internet: the state of the art. Health Educ. Res. **16**(6), 671–692 (2001)
4. Cotten, S.R., Gupta, S.S.: Characteristics of online and offline health information seekers and factors that discriminate between them. Soc. Sci. Med. **59**(9), 1795–1806 (2004)

5. Munson, S.A., et al.: Sociotechnical challenges and progress in using social media for health. J. Med. Internet Res. **15**(10), e226 (2013)

6. Aungst, T.D., Belliveau, P.: Leveraging mobile smart devices to improve interprofessional communications in inpatient practice setting: a literature review. J. Interprofessional Care **29**(6), 570–578 (2015)

7. Bickers, R.G.: Online medical information services. Prim. Care **12**(3), 459–482 (1985)

8. Chan, M., Escriba, C., Campo, E.: A review of smart homes-present state and future challenges. Comput. Methods Programs Biomed. **91**(1), 55–81 (2008)

9. Ekeland, A.G., Bowes, A., Flottorp, S.: Effectiveness of telemedicine: a systematic review of reviews. Int. J. Med. Inform. **79**(11), 736–771 (2010)

10. Morahan-Martin, J.M.: How internet users find, evaluate, and use online health information: a cross-cultural review. Cyberpsychol. Behav. Impact Internet Multimed. Virtual R. Behav. Soc. **7**(5), 497 (2004)

11. Eysenbach, G.: What is e-health? J. Med. Internet Res. **3**(3), E20 (2001)

12. Istepanian, R.S.H., Jovanov, E., Zhang, Y.T.: Guest editorial introduction to the special section on m-health: beyond seamless mobility and global wireless health-care connectivity. IEEE Trans. Inf. Technol. Biomed. **8**, 405–414 (2004)

13. Hesse, B.W., et al.: Trust and sources of health information: the impact of the internet and its implications for health care providers: findings from the first health information national trends survey. Arch. Intern. Med. **165**(22), 2618–2624 (2015)

14. Rice, R.E.: Influences, usage, and outcomes of internet health information searching: multivariate results from the Pew surveys. Int. J. Med. Inform. **75**(1), 8–28 (2006)

15. Andreassen, H.K., et al.: European citizens' use of E-health services: a study of seven countries. BMC Public Health **7**(1), 53 (2007)

16. A digital platform powered by INRA with the support of IFRIS (2018). https://www.cortext.net/

17. Eysenbach, G., et al.: Empirical studies assessing the quality of health information for consumers on the world wide web: a systematic review. Jama **287**(20), 2691–2700 (2015)

18. Varlamis, I., Apostolakis, I.: Medical Informatics in the Web 2.0 Era. In: Tsihrintzis, G.A., Virvou, M., Howlett, R.J., Jain, L.C. (eds.) New Directions in Intelligent Interactive Multimedia. SCI, vol. 142, pp. 513–522. Springer, Heidelberg (2008). https://doi.org/10.1007/978-3-540-68127-4_53

19. Hughes, B., Joshi, I., Wareham, J.: Health 2.0 and Medicine 2.0: tensions and controversies in the field. J. Med. Internet Res. **10**(3), e23 (2008)

20. Sunderland, N., et al.: Moving health promotion communities online: a review of the literature. HIM J. **42**(2), 9 (2013)

Author Index

An, Bang 211
An, Lu 301

Ba, Zhichao 301

Cao, Gaohui 167
Chen, Haihua 154, 167
Chen, Jiangping 154, 167
Chen, Jing 3
Chen, Minghong 154
Chen, Shuqing 26
Chen, Ziwen 332
Chu, Chao-Hsien 249

Ding, Juncheng 154, 167
Dong, Jiancheng 292
Dong, Ke 351
Du, Kui 286
Du, Rong 119

Fan, Weiguo 240
Felka, Patrick 77
Freisleben, Bernd 77
Fu, Yucheng 53

Gan, Dan 211
Geng, Shupei 274
Geng, Xingyun 292
Gu, Bin 130
Gu, Dongxiao 263, 315
Guo, Chenhui 130
Guo, Xitong 26, 61, 90

Han, Xiaocui 90
He, Defu 292
He, Shuaibing 332
Hinz, Oliver 77
Hu, Xinping 292
Hua, Guifeng 332
Huang, Guanjie 249

Huang, Xiao 351
Huang, Yanli 286

Jiang, Kui 292
Ju, Xiaofeng 26, 90

Kakkar, Prerna 41
Khan, Salim 191

Lai, Kee-hung 61
Li, Chunxiao 130
Li, Jiexun 240
Li, Kang 263
Li, Liang 286
Li, Qi 142
Li, Shanshan 70
Li, Tongtong 315
Li, Xin 179, 185, 342
Li, Zhiyuan 301
Liang, Changyong 263, 315
Liu, Chang 332
Liu, Fei 90
Liu, Guanjun 204
Liu, Jing 231
Liu, Qian 325
Liu, Rong 53
Liu, Rui 332
Liu, Yang 53
Lu, Jiawei 53
Lu, Long 15
Lu, Quan 3
Luo, Xiaolu 286

Ma, Jingdong 231

Nagpal, Sushama 41
Nanda, Nalin 41
Ni, Xiaowei 292

Premkumar, Kalyani 107

Qu, Jingye   154
Qu, Zihan   179

Ran, Hua   274

Shah, Adnan Muhammad   191
Shah, Syed Jamal   191
Shang, Yujuan   292
Shen, Jiang   211
Sterz, Artur   77

Umaefulam, Valerie Onyinyechi   107

Wang, G. Alan   240
Wang, Jing   231
Wang, Lei   292
Wang, Liqiang   332
Wang, Xi   96
Wang, Xiaoyu   263, 315
Wang, Yu   240
Wu, Huiqun   292
Wu, Jiang   70, 204, 351
Wu, Xiaodan   249
Wu, Yi   61

Xia, Chenxi   231
Xiao, Di   274
Xie, Jiaheng   224

Xing, Chunxiao   179, 185
Xu, Man   211
Xu, Xiaoyu   142
Xu, Zeyuan   3

Yan, Weiwei   325
Yan, Xiangbin   191
Yi, Shengwei   325
Yin, Meng   142
Yuan, Xinlu   292

Zeng, Daniel   224
Zhang, Bin   224
Zhang, Guigang   179, 185
Zhang, Liangtao   3
Zhang, Wei   286
Zhang, Xiaofei   61
Zhang, Yong   185
Zhang, Yumeng   332
Zhao, Dong   231
Zhao, Tongyao   119
Zhao, Wang   15
Zhao, Yinghui   70
Zhou, Liqin   301
Zhou, Lusha   204
Zhou, Sijia   342
Zhu, Yushan   96
Zou, Ruyi   292

Printed in the United States
By Bookmasters